NCLEX-RN®
Prep
Twenty-sixth Edition

Practice Test **+** Proven Strategies

Also From Kaplan Nursing

Books

NCLEX-RN® Content Review Guide
The Basics: A Comprehensive Outline of Nursing School Content
NCLEX® Medication Review
Adult CCRN® Prep
Family Nurse Practitioner Certification Prep Plus
Dosage Calculation Workbook
Talk Like a Nurse

Online

www.kaptest.com/nclex

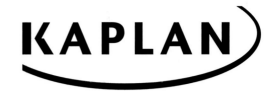

NCLEX-RN®
Prep

Twenty-sixth Edition

Practice Test + Proven Strategies

TABLE OF CONTENTS

ABOUT THE AUTHORS

Barbara Irwin, MSN, RN

Barbara Irwin is emeritus Executive Director of Nursing at Kaplan Test Prep. She supervised development of the Kaplan courses for preparation for the NCLEX-RN® examination for U.S. nursing students and international nurses, as well as integrated testing programs implemented by nursing schools. Irwin developed the Decision Tree, a framework of innovative test-taking strategies that help students achieve success on this high-stakes test. Her seminars about how to effectively study to achieve deep learning have guided thousands of student nurses. Her seminars to nursing faculty have shared important insights about the NCLEX-RN® and NCLEX-PN® examinations and how to overcome the challenge of non-self-efficacious nursing students. Irwin received a bachelor of science in nursing from the University of Oklahoma and a master of science degree in nursing and nursing education from Kaplan University. Her professional background includes experience as a nursing educator and director of a home health agency.

Judith A. Burckhardt, PhD, MSN, RN

Dr. Judith Burckhardt is former Dean of the Nursing and Health Programs for Kaplan Higher Education Campuses, Vice President of the Kaplan School of Nursing, and head of the Nursing division at Kaplan Test Preparation. Under Burckhardt's leadership, Kaplan introduced new methods of program provision, including online delivery. She is currently Dean of Nursing Programs at American Sentinel University. She also presents test preparation seminars to students, item-writing workshops to nursing faculty, and career development seminars to students, nurses, and health care professionals in the United States and abroad. Burckhardt received a bachelor of science in nursing from Loyola University in Chicago, a master's degree in education from Washington University in St. Louis, a master of science in nursing degree from Kaplan University, and a doctorate in educational administration from the University of Nebraska at Lincoln.

Kaplan thanks the following nursing professionals for their contributions to this book:

Barbara Arnoldussen, RN, MBA, CPHQ

Jean Blank, MSN, RN

Shawna M. Butler, RN, BSN, JD

Susan Compton, MSN, RN

Tamara Dolan, RN, MSN, OCN

Mary Fischer, MSN, CNM, RN

Terri Forehand, RN

Joseph Ryan Goble, MSN, RN, CEN, CPEN

Pamela Guillaume, MSN, RN

Janice Hoffman, PhD, RN, ANEF

Rene Jackson, MS, BSN, RN, LHRM, CPHRM

Amy Kennedy, MSN, RN

Constance Krueger, RN

Cheryl Martin, PhD, RNC-E, WHNP-E

Patricia Porta, MSN, RN

Rebecca Potter, PhD, MSIDT, MSN/ED, RN

Lindsey Unterseher, MSN, RN

For Any Test Changes or Late-Breaking Developments

kaptest.com/retail-book-corrections-and-updates

The material in this book is up-to-date at the time of publication. However, the National Council of State Boards of Nursing may have instituted changes in the test after this book was published. Be sure to carefully read the materials you receive when you register for the test. If there are any important late-breaking developments—or any changes or corrections to the Kaplan test preparation materials in this book—we will post that information online at **kaptest.com/retail-book-corrections-and-updates.**

HOW TO USE THIS BOOK

STEP 1: Read and Complete Part One

Part One, NCLEX-RN® Exam Overview and Test Taking Strategies, is a comprehensive, detailed strategy guide for each type of question on the NCLEX-RN® exam. This information will teach you how to analyze each question and use your nursing knowledge to select the correct answer choice.

STEP 2: Read and Complete Part Two

Part Two, NCLEX-RN® Exam Content Review and Practice, contains an essential review of all subject areas that appear on the exam, designed to help you master NCLEX-RN® exam questions. In the quiz at the end of each chapter, practice using the strategies you have learned and check your work against the detailed answer explanations provided.

STEP 3: Take the Practice Test

When you are nearing your exam date, take Kaplan's full-length practice test. It follows the NCLEX-RN® Exam Test Plan and simulates the format, content, question types, and difficulty of the actual test. This 150-question practice test will help you build your stamina for the real test and give you a good sense of your level of preparation. Detailed answer explanations follow the exam, and these can help you understand why you got off track on a particular question.

BONUS: Kaplan also offers a realistic NCLEX-RN practice test online, free. You may benefit from taking the online practice test first, because the exam software provides immediate feedback on your performance in the various content areas. You can then review your weaker areas before you tackle the test in the book. Sign up here: **kaptest. com/nclex/free/nclex-practice**

STEP 4: Register for the Exam

When you are prepared to take the NCLEX-RN® exam, contact your state/provincial/ territorial Board of Nursing to initiate the registration process. All the steps you'll need to follow are contained in Part Four, The Licensure Process.

Practice Makes Perfect

GO ONLINE

*www.kaptest.com/nclex/
practice/nclex-practice*

Looking for even more practice? Up your game with **Kaplan's NCLEX-RN® Qbank**.

- Over 2,200 test-like NCLEX questions
- Customizable: quiz yourself by category, incorrect questions, and more
- Comprehensive explanations for every answer option, correct and incorrect
- Topic refreshers and images that support learning
- Detailed performance feedback to measure your progress

Learn more at: **kaptest.com/nclex/practice/nclex-practice**

PART ONE

NCLEX-RN® EXAM OVERVIEW AND TEST TAKING STRATEGIES

[CHAPTER 1]

OVERVIEW OF THE NCLEX-RN® EXAM

The NCLEX-RN® exam is, among other things, an endurance test, like a marathon. If you don't prepare properly or approach it with confidence and rigor, you'll quickly lose your composure. Here is a sample, test-like question:

> A client had a permanent pacemaker implanted one year ago. The client returns to the outpatient clinic for suspected pacemaker battery failure. It is *most* important for the nurse to assess for which of these?
>
> 1. Abdominal pain, nausea, and vomiting.
> 2. Wheezing on exertion, cyanosis, and orthopnea.
> 3. Palpitations, shortness of breath, and dizziness.
> 4. Chest pain, headache, and diaphoresis.

As you can see, the style and content of the NCLEX-RN® exam is unique. It's not like any other exam you've ever taken, even in nursing school!

The content in this book was prepared by the experts on Kaplan's Nursing team, the world's largest provider of test prep courses for the NCLEX-RN® exam. By using Kaplan's proven methods and strategies, you will be able to take control of the exam, just as you have taken control of your nursing education and other preparations for your career in this incredibly challenging and rewarding field. The first step is to learn everything you can about the exam.

What Is the NCLEX-RN® Exam?

NCLEX-RN® stands for *National Council Licensure Examination for Registered Nurses.* The NCLEX-RN® examination is administered by the National Council of State Boards of Nursing (NCSBN), whose members include the boards of nursing in each of the 50 states in the United States, the District of Columbia, Canada, and four U.S. territories: American Samoa, Guam, the Northern Mariana Islands, and the Virgin Islands. These boards have a mandate to protect the public from unsafe and ineffective nursing care, and each board has been given responsibility to regulate the practice of nursing in its respective state. In fact, the NCLEX-RN® exam is often referred to as "the Boards" or "State Boards."

The NCLEX-RN® exam has only one purpose: to determine if it is safe for you to begin practice as an entry-level nurse.

Why Must You Take the NCLEX-RN® Exam?

The NCLEX-RN® exam is prepared by the NCSBN. Each state requires that you pass this exam to obtain a license to practice as a registered nurse. The designation *registered nurse* or *RN* indicates that you have proven to your state board of nursing or regulatory body that you can deliver safe and effective nursing care.

The NCLEX-RN® exam is a test of minimum competency and is based on the knowledge and behaviors that are needed for the entry-level practice of nursing. This exam tests not only your knowledge, but also your ability to make competent nursing judgments. Specifically, the National Council uses the NCLEX-RN® to verify that you have the cognitive skills and clinical judgment to do the following:

- Recognize concerning cues
- Analyze the significance or implications of the cues
- Identify the topic or the priority concern
- Generate solutions that enable you to plan your client's care
- Implement the care you have planned
- Evaluate whether the nursing interventions you took improved the client's condition

What Is Entry-Level Practice of Nursing?

In order to define *entry-level* practice of nursing, the National Council conducts a job analysis study every three years to determine what entry-level nurses do on the job. The kinds of questions they investigate include: In which clinical settings does the beginning nurse work? What types of care do beginning nurses provide to their clients? What are their primary duties and responsibilities? Based on the results of this study, the National Council adjusts the content and level of difficulty of the test to accurately reflect what is happening in the workplace.

What the NCLEX-RN® Exam Is *NOT*

The exam is not a test of achievement or intelligence. It is not designed for nurses who have years of experience. The questions do not involve high-tech clinical nursing or equipment. It is not predictive of your eventual success in the career of nursing. You will not be tested on all the content that you were taught in nursing school.

What Is a CAT?

CAT stands for *Computer Adaptive Test*. Each test is assembled interactively based on the accuracy of the candidate's response to the questions. This ensures that the questions you are answering are not "too hard" or "too easy" for your skill level. Your first question will be relatively easy; that is, below the level of minimum competency. If you answer that question correctly, the computer selects a slightly more difficult question. If you answer the first question incorrectly, the computer selects a slightly easier question (Figure 1.1). By continuing to do this as you answer questions, the computer is able to calculate your level of competence.

In a CAT, the questions are adapted to your ability level. The computer selects questions that represent all areas of nursing, as defined by the NCLEX-RN® detailed test plan and by the level of item difficulty. Each question is self-contained, so that all of the information you need to answer a question is presented on the computer screen.

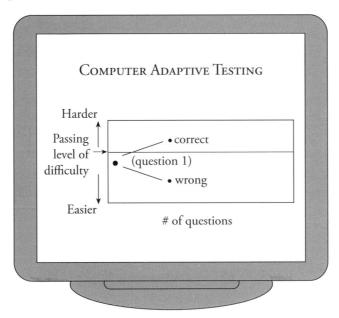

Figure 1.1

Taking the Exam

There is no time limit for each individual question. You have a maximum of five hours to complete the exam, but that includes the beginning tutorial, an optional 10-minute break after the first 2 hours of testing, and an optional break after an additional 90 minutes of testing. (Time that you spend in optional breaks, however, is counted as a part of your 5 hours of total testing time.) Everyone answers a minimum of 85 questions to a maximum of 150 questions. Regardless of the number of questions you answer, you are given 15 questions that are experimental. These questions, which are indistinguishable from the other questions on the test, are being tested for future use in NCLEX-RN® exams, and your answers do not count for or against you. Your test ends when one of the following occurs:

- You have demonstrated minimum competency and answered the minimum number of questions (85) (Figure 1.2)
- You have demonstrated a lack of minimum competency and answered the minimum number of questions (85) (Figure 1.3)
- You have answered the maximum number of questions (150)
- You have used the maximum time allowed (five hours)

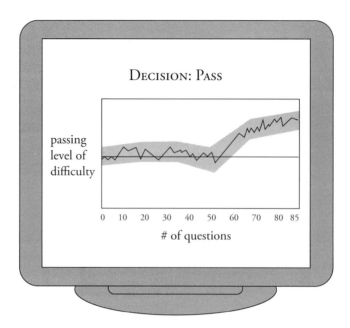

Figure 1.2

Remember, every question counts. There is no warm-up time, so it is important for you to be ready to answer questions correctly from the very beginning. Concentration is also key. You need to give your best to each question because you do not know which one will put you over the top.

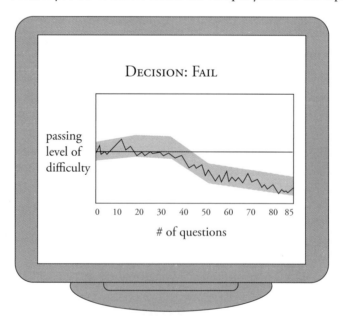

Figure 1.3

Structure of the NCLEX-RN® Exam

Whether you complete the exam in 85 questions (the minimum number) or 150 questions (the maximum), you will see a mix of standalone questions and case study question sets.

Standalone Questions

Standalone questions can be answered on their own, without considering any other question on the exam. These items may be text-based, or they may include a chart/exhibit in place of some of the text. The most common type of standalone question is also the most familiar type: text-based, four-option multiple choice question.

Some standalone questions will be case-based and start by introducing a client, the client's diagnosis or symptoms upon admission, and the client's medical record. Depending on the context, you may be required to analyze vital signs, physical assessment findings, and/or health care provider orders. Foundational nursing knowledge is a prerequisite for answering case-based questions, but sound clinical judgment is of equal importance.

In case-based questions, different categories of information may be visible under different "tabs" of the medical record, as shown in the following illustrations.

The nurse is caring for a 38-year-old client newly admitted to the medical-surgical floor with fatigue and dehydration.

Nurse's Notes | **Vital Signs**

The client has a history of diabetes mellitus and has been insulin dependent for over 20 years. The client has undergone hemodialysis for the last 4 years for end-stage kidney failure. The client's skin is warm and dry to touch with poor skin turgor, and the mucous membranes are dry. The client reports feeling nauseated for several days and has not been eating or drinking. The client also reports several episodes of diarrhea. Labs have been drawn, but results are not available yet.

Figure 1.4 First Tab of a Case-Based Question

The nurse is caring for a 38-year-old client newly admitted to the medical-surgical floor with fatigue and dehydration.

Nurse's Notes | **Vital Signs**

Vital Sign	Result
Blood Pressure	120/82 mmHg
Pulse	118
Respirations	12
Temperature	100.8° F (38.2° C)

Figure 1.5 Second Tab of a Case-Based Question

Case Study Question Sets

You will also see case-based questions in six-item sets. Like the standalone case-based questions, these case study question sets start by introducing a client case, passage, or vignette. In the six-item sets, however, you must apply information obtained in earlier questions to help answer later questions in the set.

Each "tab" of the medical record will show an aspect of the same client case, for example:

- Nurse's notes
- History and physical
- Laboratory or diagnostic results
- Flow sheets
- Admission notes or progress notes
- Intake and output
- Medications

Additional, "unfolding" tabs of the medical record may be added as you progress through the six questions in the set. Whenever a new tab of data is provided (such as laboratory results), the information in that tab will be available for the current question and for all subsequent questions in the set. Once you have navigated to a subsequent question in a six-item set, you cannot go back to previous questions in the set to alter your responses. However, you can "course correct" based on newly added information as you answer the remaining questions in the set.

The six questions within a set are counted as six different items. If question number 11 starts the set, the next question you see after the set ends will be question number 17.

Navigation

Case-based questions take the form of a split screen. In each case study question set, the case remains static on the left-hand side of the screen, while the right-hand side of the screen changes as you answer the individual questions. Within each set of six questions, you may also see a succession of different item types; for instance, the first question in a set might be a Highlight item, the second question a Matrix item, the third a Cloze item, and so on. (You will learn more about question types on the NCLEX-RN® exam in chapter 2.)

You can determine whether a case study is a standalone question or part of a question set by looking at the boldface text in the upper left-hand corner of the screen:

- **Case Study Screen 1 of 1** indicates a standalone question.
- **Case Study Screen 1 of 6** (or **Case Study Screen 2 of 6**, etc.) indicates a question in a six-item set.

Following is a series of examples illustrating how an unfolding case study will look. Only three sample screens are shown in this example. On the NCLEX-RN® exam, however, case study question sets will always have six items.

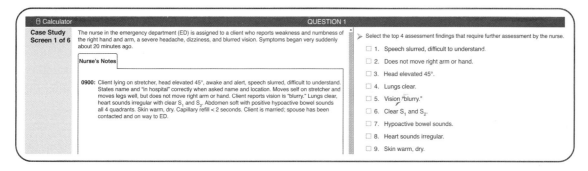

Figure 1.6 Screen 1 of 6 in an Unfolding Case Study

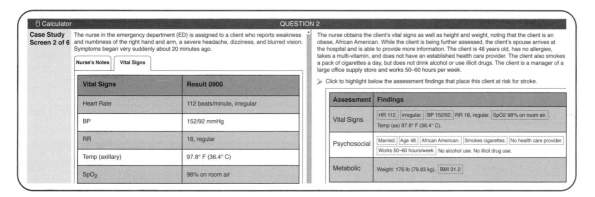

Figure 1.7 Screen 2 of 6 in an Unfolding Case Study

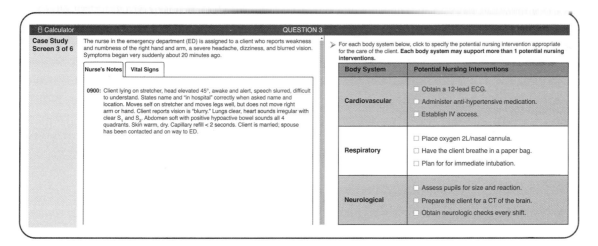

Figure 1.8 Screen 3 of 6 in an Unfolding Case Study

Structure of a Minimum Length Exam

The minimum length NCLEX-RN® exam is 85 questions. Within these first 85 questions, every test taker will receive three scored six-item question sets (18 scored questions) and 52 scored standalone items, for a total of 70 scored items. The other 15 questions are unscored, experimental items.

The scored case study question sets will be randomly selected and evenly distributed among the 70 scored questions, with the first set appearing in the first third, the second set in the middle third, and the third set in the final third (see Figure 1.9). All exam candidates will see case study question sets in the same region of the exam, but the sets will not appear in the same place for everyone. For example, you might receive the first set after the sixth item while another test taker receives the first set after the tenth item.

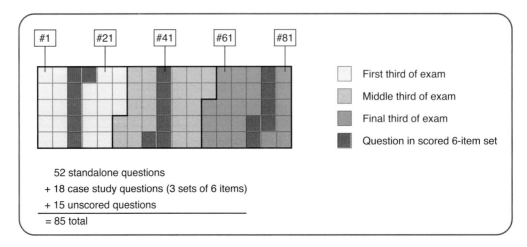

Figure 1.9 Example of a Minimum Length Exam

You may see as many as five case study question sets (30 items) on your NCLEX-RN® exam, but only three sets (18 items) will be scored. Any additional question sets you see will be part of the 15 unscored items randomly distributed in the first 85 questions. Looking at Figure 1.9, you can't tell which of the 85 items are unscored. The same is true when you are taking the exam. *You will not know* which items are scored for your NCLEX exam and which items are experimental.

Questions After the Minimum Length

If a stopping rule is not triggered after the minimum length of 85 questions, the exam will continue until either the computer reaches a pass/fail decision, you have answered 150 questions, or you have reached the maximum testing time of 5 hours. All remaining items will be scored. At this point, the computer will select only standalone questions.

- Case-based standalone items make up approximately 10% of the remaining questions.
- Non-case-based standalone items (such as "select all that apply" and four-option multiple choice questions) make up approximately 90% of the remaining questions.

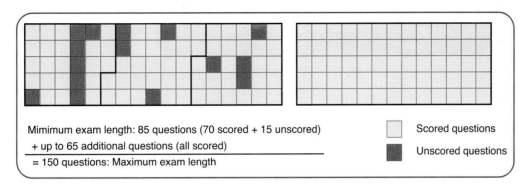

Figure 1.10 Example of a Maximum Length Exam

When you are taking the NCLEX-RN® exam, try not to be concerned with the length of your test. In fact, you should plan on testing for 5 hours and seeing 150 questions. You are still in the game as long as the computer continues to give you test questions, so focus on answering them to the best of your ability. If you are still getting questions, it means the computer has not made a decision on your ability level and you can still pass the NCLEX!

NCLEX-RN® Exam Scoring

In past versions of the NCLEX-RN®, no partial credit was given. If the correct answers to a question were answer choices (1), (2), and (4), for example, exam candidates had to select those three answers—and *only* those answers—as correct in order to receive credit for the question. Since 2023, however, NCSBN awards partial credit. Three different scoring methodologies are used:

- 0/1 Scoring Rule
- +/− Scoring Rule
- Rationale Scoring Rule

Let's look at how the NCLEX-RN® exam applies these scoring approaches.

0/1 Scoring Rule

The 0/1 Scoring Rule is the rule that you are probably most familiar with from nursing school. This is the classic approach used to score four-option Multiple Choice questions:

- Earn 1 point for correct response.
- Earn 0 points for incorrect response.

For an item that is worth more than 1 point, the sum of all correct responses is the total score. The illustration shows an example of how a multi-point Matrix Multiple Choice item would be scored using the 0/1 Scoring Rule.

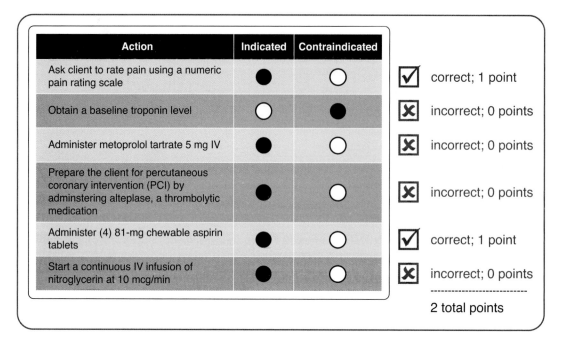

Figure 1.11 0/1 Scoring Rule Applied to a Matrix Item

$+/-$ **Scoring Rule**

The $+/-$ Scoring Rule awards a higher score when you identify and select information that is more pertinent. You probably remember "Select all that apply" (or SATA) questions from nursing school. You may have dreaded them too. The good news is that you can receive partial credit on the NCLEX exam for SATA questions! The $+/-$ Scoring Rule works like this:

- Earn 1 point for each correct selection.
- Forfeit 1 point for each incorrect selection.

While the $+/-$ Scoring Rule subtracts points for incorrect answers, there are no negative scores. The minimum score per item is zero.

The illustration shows an example of how a multi-point item would be scored using the $+/-$ Scoring Rule. In this example, the test-taker has selected all four correct answer options, and has also selected two incorrect options. This would result in a score of 2 out of a possible 4 points for this question.

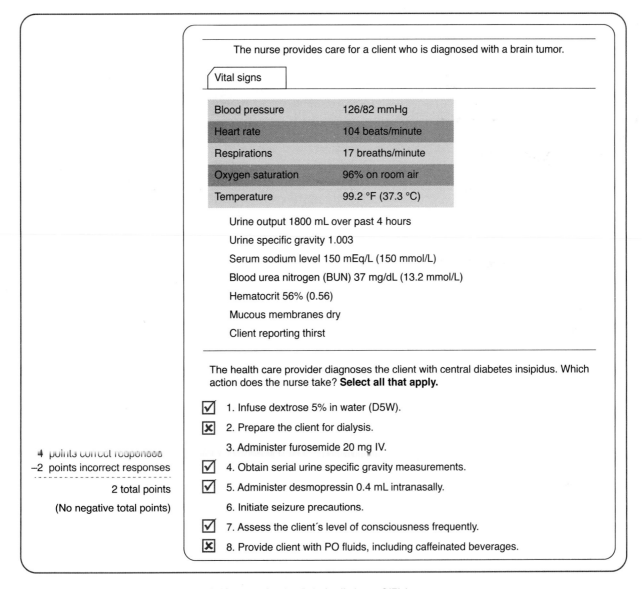

The nurse provides care for a client who is diagnosed with a brain tumor.

Vital signs	
Blood pressure	126/82 mmHg
Heart rate	104 beats/minute
Respirations	17 breaths/minute
Oxygen saturation	96% on room air
Temperature	99.2 °F (37.3 °C)

Urine output 1800 mL over past 4 hours

Urine specific gravity 1.003

Serum sodium level 150 mEq/L (150 mmol/L)

Blood urea nitrogen (BUN) 37 mg/dL (13.2 mmol/L)

Hematocrit 56% (0.56)

Mucous membranes dry

Client reporting thirst

The health care provider diagnoses the client with central diabetes insipidus. Which action does the nurse take? **Select all that apply.**

☑ 1. Infuse dextrose 5% in water (D5W).

☒ 2. Prepare the client for dialysis.

  3. Administer furosemide 20 mg IV.

☑ 4. Obtain serial urine specific gravity measurements.

☑ 5. Administer desmopressin 0.4 mL intranasally.

  6. Initiate seizure precautions.

☑ 7. Assess the client's level of consciousness frequently.

☒ 8. Provide client with PO fluids, including caffeinated beverages.

4 points correct responses
−2 points incorrect responses
----
2 total points
(No negative total points)

Figure 1.12 +/− Scoring Rule Applied to a SATA Item

Rationale Scoring Rule

Finally, the Rationale Scoring Rule awards points when both elements of a linked pair of concepts are correct. This scoring method tests concepts that require justification through a rationale—that is, situations in which a nurse must perform action X because of circumstance Y. Under the Rationale Scoring Rule:

- Earn 1 point when both X and Y are correct.
- Earn 0 points when any element of the answer selection is incorrect.

The Rationale Scoring Rule requires an understanding of paired information. The illustration shows an example of how a Cloze item would be scored using the Rationale Scoring Rule. Though the test taker has correctly selected "loss of visual fields or blindness" in this example, 0 points are earned because the other element of the paired information is incorrect.

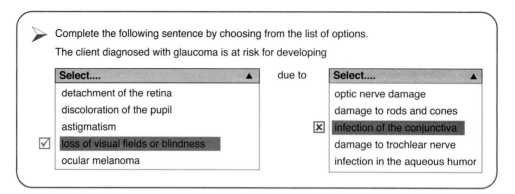

Figure 1.13 Rationale Scoring Rule Applied to a Cloze Item

Having a general familiarity with the scoring rules will help you avoid surprises. On the NCLEX exam, however, you should not try to calculate the number of points you may receive based on your responses. Similarly, you should not dwell on the difficulty level of the questions that the CAT has selected. Neither is a good use of your time. Instead, you should focus solely on making safe nursing judgments.

Content of the NCLEX-RN® Exam

The NCLEX-RN® exam is not divided into separate content areas. It tests integrated nursing content. Many nursing programs are based on the medical model. Students take separate medical, surgical, pediatric, psychiatric, and obstetric classes. On the NCLEX-RN® exam, all content is integrated.

Look at the following question.

> A client with type 1 diabetes returns to the recovery room one hour after an uneventful delivery of a 9 lb, 8 oz (4,309 g), newborn. The nurse would expect which change in the client's blood glucose level?
>
> 1. From 220 to 180 mg/dL (12.21 to 10 mmol/L).
> 2. From 110 to 80 mg/dL (6.1. to 4.4 mmol/L).
> 3. From 90 to 120 mg/dL (5 to 6.7 mmol/L).
> 4. From 100 to 140 mg/dL (5.6 to 7.8 mmol/L).

Is this an obstetrical question or a medical/surgical question? To select the correct answer, (2), you must consider the pathophysiology of type 1 diabetes along with the principles of labor and delivery. This is an example of an integrated question.

The NCLEX-RN® Exam Test Plan

The NCLEX-RN® exam is organized according to the framework "Client Needs." For the purposes of the NCLEX-RN® examination, a client is identified as the individual, family, or group, which includes significant others. There are four major categories of client needs; two of the major categories are further divided for a total of six subcategories. This information is distributed by NCSBN, the developer of the NCLEX-RN® exam.

Client Need #1: Safe and Effective Care Environment

The first subcategory for this client need is **Management of Care**, which accounts for **18** percent of the questions on the exam. Nursing actions that are covered in this subcategory include:

- Advance directives/self-determination/life planning
- Advocacy
- Assignment, delegation, and supervision
- Case management
- Client rights
- Collaboration with interdisciplinary team
- Concepts of management
- Confidentiality/information security
- Consultation
- Continuity of care
- Establishing priorities
- Ethical practice
- Information technology
- Informed consent
- Legal rights and responsibilities
- Organ donation
- Performance improvement (quality improvement)
- Referrals
- Supervision

Here is an example of a question from the Management of Care subcategory:

> Which assignment by the RN would be appropriate for an LPN/LVN?
>
> 1. A client with low back pain scheduled for a myelogram.
> 2. A client in traction for treatment of a fractured femur.
> 3. A client newly diagnosed with type 1 diabetes.
> 4. A client with emphysema scheduled for discharge.

The correct answer is (2). This client is in stable condition and can be cared for by an LPN/LVN with supervision of an RN.

Here is another example of a Management of Care question:

> After receiving a handoff of care report from the nurse on the prior shift, which client should the nurse see **first**?
>
> 1. A client refusing to take sucralfate before mealtime.
> 2. A client with left-sided weakness asking for assistance to the commode.
> 3. A client reporting chills who is scheduled for a cholecystectomy.
> 4. A client with a nasogastric tube who had a bowel resection yesterday.

The correct answer is (3). This is the least stable client.

You will learn more about the content covered by the Safe and Effective Care Environment: Management of Care subcategory in Chapter 4.

The second subcategory for this client need is **Safety and Infection Control**, which accounts for **13** percent of the questions on the exam. Nursing actions that are covered in this subcategory include:

- Accident/injury prevention
- Emergency response plan
- Ergonomic principles
- Error prevention
- Handling hazardous and infectious materials
- Home safety
- Reporting of incident/event/irregular occurrence/variance
- Safe use of equipment
- Security plan
- Standard precautions/transmission-based precautions/surgical asepsis
- Use of restraints/safety devices

Here is an example of a question from the Safety and Infection Control subcategory:

> The primary health care provider prescribes tobramycin sulfate 3 mg/kg IV every 8 hours for a 3-year-old client. The nurse enters the client's room to administer the medication and discovers that the client does not have an identification bracelet. Which action should the nurse take?
>
> 1. Ask the parents to state their child's name.
> 2. Ask the child to say the first and last name.
> 3. Have a coworker identify the child before giving the medication.
> 4. Hold the medication until an identification bracelet can be obtained.

The correct answer is (1). This action will allow the nurse to correctly identify the child and enable the nurse to give the medication on time.

You will learn more about the content covered by the Safe and Effective Care Environment: Safety and Infection Control subcategory in Chapter 5.

Client Need #2: Health Promotion and Maintenance

This client need accounts for **9** percent of the questions on the exam. Nursing actions that are covered in this category include:

- Aging process
- Ante/intra/postpartum and newborn care
- Developmental stages and transitions
- Heath promotion/disease prevention
- Health screening
- High-risk behaviors
- Lifestyle choices
- Self-care
- Techniques of physical assessment

It is important to understand that not everyone described in the questions will be sick or hospitalized. Some clients may be in a clinic or home-care setting. Some clients may not be sick at all. Wellness is an important concept on the NCLEX-RN® exam. It is necessary for a safe and effective nurse to know how to promote health and prevent disease.

This is an example of a question from the Health Promotion and Maintenance category:

> A client in active labor is admitted to the labor suite. An hour later, the client experiences spontaneous rupture of membranes. The nurse observes a glistening white umbilical cord protruding from the vagina. Which action should the nurse take **first**?
>
> 1. Return to the nurses' station and call the primary health care provider.
> 2. Administer oxygen by mask at 10 to 12 L/minute and assess vital signs.
> 3. Place a clean towel over the umbilical cord and wet it with sterile normal saline solution.
> 4. Apply manual pressure to the presenting part and have the client assume a knee-chest position.

The correct answer is (4). Umbilical cord prolapse is an emergency situation. The nurse must relieve pressure on the umbilical cord to prevent fetal anoxia.

You will learn more about the content covered by the Health Promotion and Maintenance category in Chapter 6.

Client Need #3: Psychosocial Integrity

This client need accounts for **9** percent of the questions on the exam. Nursing actions that are covered in this category include:

- Abuse/neglect
- Behavioral interventions
- Chemical and other dependencies
- Coping mechanisms
- Crisis intervention
- Cultural diversity/cultural influences on health
- End of life care
- Family dynamics
- Grief and loss
- Mental health concepts
- Religious and spiritual influences on health
- Sensory/perceptual alterations
- Stress management
- Support systems
- Therapeutic communication
- Therapeutic environment

This is an example of a question from the Psychosocial Integrity category:

> A client comes to the nurses' station and inquires about going to the cafeteria to get something to eat. The client becomes verbally abusive when told that personal privileges do not include going to the cafeteria. Which approach by the nurse would be **most** effective?
>
> 1. Tell the client to speak softly to avoid disturbing the other clients.
> 2. Ask what the client wants from the cafeteria and have it delivered to the client's room.
> 3. Calmly but firmly escort the client back to the client's room.
> 4. Assign the unlicensed assistive personnel (UAP) to accompany the client to the cafeteria.

The correct answer is (3). The nurse should not reinforce abusive behavior. Clients need consistent and clearly defined expectations and limits.

You will learn more about the content covered in the Psychosocial Integrity category in Chapter 7.

Client Need #4: Physiological Integrity

The first subcategory for this client need is **Basic Care and Comfort**, which accounts for **9** percent of the questions on the exam. Nursing actions that are covered in this subcategory include:

- Assistive devices
- Complementary therapies
- Elimination
- Mobility/immobility
- Nonpharmacological comfort interventions
- Nutrition and oral hydration
- Personal hygiene
- Rest and sleep

The following question is representative of the Basic Care and Comfort subcategory:

> The primary health care provider applies a cast to an infant client for the treatment of talipes equinovarus. Which instruction is **most** essential for the nurse to give to the client's parents regarding care?
>
> 1. Offer age-appropriate toys.
> 2. Visit clinic frequently for cast adjustments.
> 3. Give an analgesic as needed.
> 4. Check circulation in the casted extremity.

The correct answer is (4). Impaired circulation can result from cast application. All of these answer options might be included in parent teaching, but checking circulation in the casted extremity takes highest priority.

You will learn more about the content covered in the Physiological Integrity: Basic Care and Comfort category in Chapter 8.

The second subcategory for this client need is **Pharmacological and Parenteral Therapies**, which accounts for **16** percent of the questions on the exam. Nursing actions that are covered in this subcategory include:

- Adverse effects/contraindications/side effects/interactions
- Blood and blood products
- Central venous access devices
- Dosage calculation
- Expected actions/outcomes
- Medication administration
- Medication handling and maintenance
- Parenteral/intravenous therapies

- Pharmacological pain management
- Total parenteral nutrition

Try this question from the Pharmacological and Parenteral Therapies subcategory:

> The home health nurse prepares to insert an IV catheter for a client who is prescribed dextrose 5% in water (D_5W). Which venipuncture site should the nurse use to insert the IV catheter?
>
> 1. Ventral surface vein of the nondominant wrist.
> 2. Dorsal surface vein of the foot.
> 3. Dorsal surface vein of the nondominant forearm.
> 4. Ventral surface vein of the foot.

The correct answer is (3). A dorsal surface vein of the nondominant forearm provides the best venipuncture site for IV catheter insertion because it is easily accessible, is located away from an area of flexion, and promotes self-care.

You will learn more about the content covered in the Physiological Integrity: Pharmacological and Parenteral Therapies category in Chapter 9.

The third subcategory for this client need is **Reduction of Risk Potential**, which accounts for **12** percent of the questions on the exam. Nursing actions that are covered in this subcategory include:

- Changes/abnormalities in vital signs
- Diagnostic tests
- Laboratory values
- Potential for alterations in body systems
- Potential for complications of diagnostic tests/treatments/procedures
- Potential for complications from surgical procedures and health alterations
- System specific assessments
- Therapeutic procedures

This is an example of a question from the Reduction of Risk Potential subcategory:

> Parents bring a school-age client with a history of type 1 diabetes and several days of illness to the emergency department (ED). Which laboratory test result would the nurse expect if the client is experiencing diabetic ketoacidosis?
>
> 1. Serum glucose 140 mg/dL (7.8 mmol/L).
> 2. Serum creatinine 5.2 mg/dL (460 µmol/L).
> 3. Blood pH 7.28.
> 4. Hematocrit 38% (0.38).

The correct answer is (3). Normal blood pH range is 7.35 to 7.45. A blood pH of 7.28 indicates diabetic ketoacidosis.

You will learn more about the content covered in the Physiological Integrity: Reduction of Risk Potential category in Chapter 10.

The fourth subcategory for this client need is **Physiological Adaptation**, which accounts for **13** percent of the questions on the exam. Nursing actions that are covered in this subcategory include:

- Alterations in body systems
- Fluid and electrolyte imbalances
- Hemodynamics
- Illness management
- Medical emergencies
- Pathophysiology
- Unexpected response to therapies

The following question is an example of the Physiological Adaptation subcategory:

> The nurse delivers external cardiac compressions to a client during cardiopulmonary resuscitation (CPR). Which action by the nurse is **best**?
>
> 1. Maintain a position close to the client's side with the nurse's knees apart.
> 2. Position hands on the lower half of the sternum during compressions.
> 3. Lean on chest between compressions to prevent full chest wall recoil.
> 4. Check for return of the client's pulse after every 8 breaths by the nurse.

The correct answer is (2). The nurse's hands should be positioned on the lower half of the client's sternum during compressions with elbows locked, arms straight, and shoulders positioned directly over the hands. The nurse should avoid leaning on the chest between compressions to allow for full chest wall recoil.

You will learn more about the content covered in the Physiological Integrity: Physiological Adaptation category in Chapter 11.

The Nursing Process

Several processes are integrated throughout the NCLEX-RN® exam. The most important of these is *the nursing process*.

The nursing process involves the *assessment, analysis, planning, implementation,* and *evaluation* of nursing care. As a graduate nurse, you are very familiar with each step of the nursing process and how to write a care plan using this process. Knowledge of the nursing process is essential to the performance of safe and effective care. It is also essential to answering questions correctly on the NCLEX-RN® exam.

Now we are going to review the steps of the nursing process and show you how each step is incorporated into test questions. The nursing process is a way of thinking. Using it will help you select correct answers.

Assessment. Assessment is the first step in the nursing process. It involves establishing and verifying a database of information about the client, so you can identify actual and/or potential health problems. The nurse obtains subjective data (information given to you by the client that can't be observed or measured by others), and objective data (information that is observable and measurable by others). This data is collected by interviewing and observing the client and/or significant others, reviewing the health history, performing a physical examination, evaluating lab results, and interacting with members of the health care team.

Here is an example of an assessment test question:

> The nurse obtains a health history from a client admitted with acute glomerulonephritis. Which history finding is significant for the diagnosis of acute glomerulonephritis?
>
> 1. Personal history of sore throat 10 days prior.
> 2. Family history of chronic glomerulonephritis.
> 3. Personal history of renal calculus 2 years prior.
> 4. Personal history of renal trauma several years ago.

The correct answer is (1). Acute glomerulonephritis, an immunologic disorder that affects the kidneys, can be caused by group A Streptococcus. It usually occurs about 10 days after strep throat or scarlet fever and about 21 days after a group A Streptococcus skin infection.

Analysis. During the analysis phase of the nursing process, you examine the data that you obtained during the assessment phase. This allows you to analyze and draw conclusions about health problems. During analysis, you should compare the client's findings with what is normal. From the analysis, you establish nursing diagnoses. A nursing diagnosis is an actual or potential health problem that the nurse is licensed to manage.

Here is an analysis question:

> The nurse plans care for a client diagnosed with an acute myocardial infarction (MI). The client reports fatigue, and the nurse assesses clammy skin, prolonged capillary refill, and oliguria. Which nursing diagnosis is **most** appropriate for this client?
>
> 1. Impaired cardiac output.
> 2. Imbalanced energy field.
> 3. Activity intolerance.
> 4. Excess fluid volume.

The correct answer is (1). Based on the assessment findings of fatigue, clammy skin, prolonged capillary refill, and oliguria, decreased cardiac output is the most appropriate nursing diagnosis for the client diagnosed with an acute myocardial infarction.

Planning. During the planning phase of the nursing process, the nursing care plan is formulated. Steps in planning include:

- Assigning priorities to nursing diagnosis
- Specifying goals
- Identifying interventions
- Specifying expected outcomes
- Documenting the nursing care plan

Goals are anticipated responses and client behaviors that result from nursing care. Nursing goals are client-centered and measurable, and they have an established time frame. *Expected outcomes* are the interim steps needed to reach a goal and the resolution of a nursing diagnosis. There will be multiple expected outcomes for each goal. Expected outcomes guide the nurse in planning interventions.

This is an example of a planning question:

A client comes to the emergency department (ED) reporting nausea, vomiting, and severe right upper quadrant pain. The client's temperature measures 101.3° F (38.5° C), and an abdominal x-ray reveals an enlarged gallbladder. The client is scheduled for surgery. Which action should the nurse take **first**?

1. Assess the client's need for dietary teaching.
2. Evaluate the client's fluid and electrolyte status.
3. Examine the client's health history for allergies to antibiotics.
4. Determine whether the client has signed consent for surgery.

The correct answer is (2). Hypokalemia and hypomagnesemia commonly occur after repeated vomiting.

Implementation. Implementation is the term used to describe the actions that you take in the care of your clients. Implementation includes:

- Assisting in the performance of activities of daily living (ADLs)
- Counseling and educating the client and family
- Giving care to clients
- Supervising and evaluating the work of other members of the health care team

It is important for you to remember that nursing interventions may be:

- *Independent* actions that are within the scope of nursing practice and do not require supervision by others
- *Dependent* actions based on the written orders of a primary health care provider
- *Interdependent* actions shared with other members of the health care team

The NCLEX-RN® exam includes questions that involve all three types of nursing interventions.

Here is an example of an implementation question:

> A client is being treated in the burn unit for second- and third-degree burns over 45% of the body. The primary health care provider prescribes silver sulfadiazine cream application. Which method is **best** for the nurse to apply this medication?
>
> 1. Sterile dressings soaked in saline.
> 2. Sterile tongue depressor.
> 3. Sterile gloved hand.
> 4. Sterile cotton-tipped applicator.

The correct answer is (3). A sterile, gloved hand will cause the least trauma to tissues and will decrease the chances of breaking blisters.

Evaluation. Evaluation measures the client's response to nursing interventions and indicates the client's progress toward achieving the goals established in the care plan. You compare the observed results to expected outcomes.

This is an evaluation question:

> When caring for a client diagnosed with anorexia nervosa, which observation indicates to the nurse that the client's condition is improving?
>
> 1. The client eats all the food on the meal tray.
> 2. The client asks friends to bring special foods.
> 3. The client weighs self daily.
> 4. The client has gained weight.

The correct response is (4). The client's weight gain is the most objective outcome measure for evaluating improvement in the client's condition.

Integrated Processes

Several other important processes are integrated throughout the NCLEX-RN® exam. They are:

Caring. As you take the NCLEX-RN® exam, remember that the test is about caring for people, not working with high-tech equipment or analyzing lab results.

Communication and Documentation. For this exam, you are required to understand and utilize therapeutic communication skills with all professional contacts, including clients, their families, and other members of the health care team. Charting or documenting your care and the client's response is both a legal requirement and an essential method of communication in nursing. On this exam, you may be asked to identify appropriate documentation of a client behavior or nursing action.

Teaching/Learning Principles. Nursing frequently involves sharing information with clients so optimal functioning can be achieved. You may see questions that focus on teaching a client about diet and/or medications.

Culture and Spirituality. Nurses are entrusted to care for clients as whole persons—body, mind, and spirit. This requires caring for clients from cultures that are different from their own and whose spiritual beliefs may not be consistent with theirs. It is important for the nurse to be culturally and spiritually sensitive and to respond to the unique needs of each client. Interaction with the client must recognize and consider the client-reported, self-identified, unique, and individual preferences to client care.

Knowledge Is Power

The more knowledgeable you are about the NCLEX-RN® exam, the more effective your study will be. As you prepare for the exam, keep the content of the test in mind. Thinking like the test maker will enhance your chance of success on the exam.

Are you still thinking about that pacemaker battery from the beginning of the chapter? What do you think the correct answer is?

> A client had a permanent pacemaker implanted one year ago. The client returns to the outpatient clinic for suspected pacemaker battery failure. It is **most** important for the nurse to assess for which of these?
>
> 1. Abdominal pain, nausea, and vomiting.
> 2. Wheezing on exertion, cyanosis, and orthopnea.
> 3. Palpitations, shortness of breath, and dizziness.
> 4. Chest pain, headache, and diaphoresis.

The correct answer is (3). Palpitations, shortness of breath, dizziness, lightheadedness, syncope, irregular heart rate, and tachycardia or bradycardia may occur with pacemaker battery failure.

Gastrointestinal symptoms (1) are not found with pacemaker battery failure. The items listed in (2) are not symptoms of pacemaker battery failure. And although chest pain may occur with decreased cardiac output associated with pacemaker battery failure (4), chest pain is suggestive of angina. Headache and diaphoresis are not seen with pacemaker failure.

[CHAPTER 2]

GENERAL AND COMPUTER ADAPTIVE TEST STRATEGIES

As a nursing student, you are used to taking multiple choice tests. In fact, you've taken so many tests by the time you graduate from nursing school, you probably believe that there won't be any more surprises on any nursing test, including the NCLEX-RN® exam.

But if you've ever talked to graduate nurses about their experiences taking the NCLEX-RN® exam, they probably told you that the test wasn't like *any* nursing test they had ever taken. How can that be? How can the NCLEX-RN® exam seem like a nursing school test, but be so different? The reason is that the NCLEX-RN® exam is a standardized test that analyzes a different set of behaviors from those tested in nursing school.

Standardized Exams

Many of you have some experience with standardized exams. You may have been required to take the SAT or ACT to get into nursing school. Remember taking that exam? Was your experience positive or negative?

All standardized exams share the same characteristics:

- Tests are written by content specialists and test construction experts.
- The content of the exam is researched and planned.
- The questions are designed according to test construction methodology (all answer choices are about the same length, the verb tenses all agree, etc.).
- All the questions are tested before use on the actual exam.

The NCLEX-RN® exam is similar to other standardized exams in some ways, yet different in others:

- The NCLEX-RN® exam is written by nurse specialists who are experts in a content area of nursing.
- All content is selected to allow the beginning practitioner to prove minimum competency on all areas of the test plan.
- Minimum-competency questions are most frequently asked at the application level, not the recognition or recall level. All the responses to a question are similar in length and subject matter, and are grammatically correct.
- All test items have been extensively tested by NCSBN. The questions are valid; all correct responses are documented by two different sources.

What does this mean for you?

- NCSBN has defined what is minimum-competency, entry-level nursing.
- Questions and answers are written in such a way that you cannot, in most cases, predict or recognize the correct answer.
- NCSBN is knowledgeable about strategies regarding length of answers, grammar, and so on. It makes sure you can't use these strategies in order to select correct answers. English majors have no advantage!
- The answer choices have been extensively tested. The people who write the test questions make the incorrect answer choices look attractive to the unwary test taker.

What Behaviors Does the NCLEX-RN® Exam Test?

The NCLEX-RN® exam does *not* just test your nursing knowledge: It assumes that you have a body of knowledge and that you understand the material because you have graduated from nursing school. So what does the NCLEX-RN® exam test? Primarily, it tests your nursing judgment and discretion. It tests your ability to think critically and solve problems. The NCLEX-RN® exam recognizes that as a beginning practitioner, you will be managing LPN/LVNs and UAPs providing care to a group of clients. As the leader of the nursing team, you are expected to make safe and competent judgments about client care.

Critical Thinking

What does the term *critical thinking* mean? Critical thinking is problem solving that involves thinking creatively. It requires that the nurse do the following:

- Observe.
- Decide what is important.
- Look for patterns and relationships.
- Identify the problem.
- Transfer knowledge from one situation to another.
- Apply knowledge.
- Evaluate according to criteria established.

You successfully solve problems every day in the clinical area. You are probably comfortable with this concept when actually caring for clients. Although you've had lots of practice critically thinking in the clinical area, you may have had less practice critically thinking your way through test questions. Why is that?

During nursing school, you take exams developed by nursing instructors to test a specific body of content. Many of these questions are at the knowledge level. This involves recognition and recall of ideas or material that you read in your nursing textbooks and discussed in class. This is the most basic level of testing. Figure 2.1 illustrates the different levels of questions on nursing exams.

The following is an example of a knowledge-based question you might have seen in nursing school.

Which of the following is a complication that occurs during the first 24 hours after a percutaneous liver biopsy?

1. Nausea and vomiting.
2. Constipation.
3. Hemorrhage.
4. Pain at the biopsy site.

The question restated is, "What is a common complication of a liver biopsy?" You may or may not remember the answer. So, as you look at the answer choices, you hope to see an item that looks familiar. You do see something that looks familiar: "Hemorrhage." You select the correct answer based on recall or recognition. The NCLEX-RN® exam rarely asks questions at the recall/recognition level.

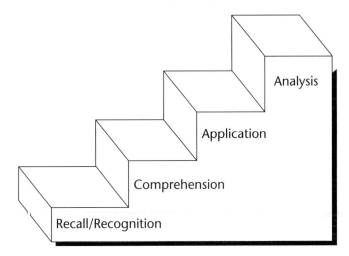

Figure 2.1 Levels of Questions in Nursing Tests

In nursing school, you are also given test questions written at the comprehension level. These questions require you to understand the meaning of the material. Let's look at this same question written at the comprehension level.

The nurse understands that hemorrhage is a complication of a liver biopsy due to which of the following reasons?

1. There are several large blood vessels near the liver.
2. The liver cells are bathed with a mixture of venous and arterial blood.
3. The test is performed on clients with elevated enzymes.
4. The procedure requires a large piece of tissue to be removed.

The question restated is, "Why does hemorrhage occur after a liver biopsy?" In order to answer this question, the nurse must understand that the liver is a highly vascular organ. The portal vein and the hepatic artery join in the liver to form the sinusoids that bathe the liver in a mixture of venous and arterial blood.

The NCLEX-RN® exam asks few minimum-competency questions at the comprehension level. It assumes you know and understand the facts you learned in nursing school.

Minimum-competency NCLEX-RN® exam questions are written at the application and/or analysis level. Remember, the NCLEX-RN® exam tests your ability to make safe judgments about client care. Your ability to solve problems is not tested with questions at the recall/recognition or comprehension level.

Let's look at this same question written at the application level.

Which symptom observed by the nurse during the first 24 hours after a percutaneous liver biopsy would indicate a complication from the procedure?

1. Anorexia, nausea, and vomiting.
2. Abdominal distention and discomfort.
3. P 112 beats/minute, BP 86/60 mmHg.
4. Redness and pain at the biopsy site.

Can you select an answer based on recall or recognition? No. Let's analyze the question and answer choices.

The question is: What is a complication of a liver biopsy? To begin to analyze this question, you must *know* that hemorrhage is the major complication. However, it's not listed as an answer. Can you find hemorrhage in one of the answer choices?

ANSWERS:

(1) "Anorexia, nausea, and vomiting." Does this indicate that the client is hemorrhaging? No, these are not symptoms of hemorrhage.

(2) "Abdominal distention and discomfort." Does this indicate that the client is hemorrhaging? Perhaps. Abdominal distention could indicate internal bleeding.

(3) "P 112 beats/minute, BP 86/60 mmHg." Does this indicate that the client is hemorrhaging? Yes. An increased pulse and a decreased blood pressure indicate shock. Shock is a result of hemorrhage.

(4) "Redness and pain at the biopsy site." Does this indicate the client is hemorrhaging? No. Pain and some redness at the biopsy site may occur as a normal result of the procedure.

Ask yourself, "Which is the best indicator of hemorrhage?" Abdominal distention or a change in vital signs? Abdominal distention can be caused by liver disease. The correct answer is (3).

This question tests you at the application level. You were not able to answer the question by recalling or recognizing the word *hemorrhage*. You had to take information you learned (hemorrhage is the major complication of a liver biopsy) and select the answer that best indicates hemorrhage. Application involves taking the facts that you know and using them to make a nursing judgment. You must be able to answer questions at the application level in order to prove your competence on the NCLEX-RN® exam.

Let's look at a question that is written at the analysis level.

> The nurse is caring for a client receiving haloperidol 2 mg PO twice per day. The nurse assists the client to choose which menu?
>
> 1. 6 oz (168 g) roast beef, baked potato, salad with dressing, dill pickle, baked apple pie, and milk.
> 2. 3 oz (84 g) baked chicken, green beans, steamed rice, 1 slice of bread, banana, and milk.
> 3. 6 oz (168 g) burger on a bun, french fries, apple, chocolate chip cookie, and milk to drink 30 minutes after mealtime.
> 4. 3 oz (84 g) baked fish, slice of bread, broccoli, ice cream, and pineapple juice to drink 60 minutes after mealtime.

Many students panic when they read this question because they can't immediately recall any diet restriction required by a client taking haloperidol. Because students can't recall the information, they assume that they didn't learn enough information. Analysis questions are often written so that a familiar piece of information is put in an unfamiliar setting. Let's think about this question.

What type of diet do you choose for a client receiving haloperidol? To begin analyzing this question, you must first recall that haloperidol is an antipsychotic medication used to treat psychotic disorders. There are no diet restrictions for clients taking haloperidol. Because there are no diet restrictions, you must problem-solve to determine what this question is *really* asking. Based on the answer choices, it is obviously a diet question. What kind of diet should you choose for this client? Because you have been given no other information, there is only one type of diet that can be considered: a regular balanced diet. This is an example of taking the familiar (a regular balanced diet) and putting it into the unfamiliar (a client receiving haloperidol). In this question, the critical thinking is deciding what this question is *really* asking.

QUESTION: "Which is the most balanced regular diet?"

ANSWERS:

(1) "6 oz (168 g) roast beef, baked potato, salad with dressing, dill pickle, baked apple pie, and milk." Is this a balanced diet? Yes, it certainly has possibilities.

(2) "3 oz (84 g) baked chicken, green beans, steamed rice, 1 slice of bread, banana, and milk." Is this a balanced diet? Yes, this is also a good answer because it contains foods from each of the food groups.

(3) "6 oz (168 g) burger on a bun, french fries, apple, chocolate chip cookie, and milk to drink 30 minutes after mealtime." Is this a balanced diet? No. This diet is high in fat and does not contain all of the food groups. Eliminate this answer.

(4) "3 oz (84 g) baked fish, slice of bread, broccoli, ice cream, and pineapple juice to drink 60 minutes after mealtime" Does this sound like a balanced diet? The choice of foods isn't bad, but why would the intake of fluids be delayed? This sounds like a menu to prevent dumping syndrome. Eliminate this answer.

Which is the better answer choice: (1) or (2)? Dill pickles are high in sodium, so the correct answer is (2).

Choosing the menu that best represents a balanced diet is not a difficult question to answer. The challenge lies in determining that a balanced diet is the topic of the question. Note that answer choices (1) and (2) are very similar. Because the NCLEX-RN® exam is testing your discretion, you will be making a decision between answer choices that are very close in meaning. Don't expect obvious answer choices.

These questions highlight the difference between the knowledge/comprehension-based questions that you may have seen in nursing school, and the application/analysis-based questions that you will see on the NCLEX-RN® exam.

Strategies That Don't Work on the NCLEX-RN® Exam

Whether you realize it or not, you developed a set of strategies in nursing school to answer teacher-generated test questions that are written at the knowledge/comprehension level. These strategies include the following:

- "Cramming" in hundreds of facts about disease processes and nursing care
- Recognizing and recalling facts rather than understanding the pathophysiology and the needs of a client with an illness
- Knowing who wrote the question and what is important to that instructor
- Predicting answers based on what you remember or who wrote the test question
- Selecting the response that is a different length compared to the other choices
- Selecting the answer choice that is grammatically correct
- When in doubt, choosing answer choice (3)

These strategies will not work on the NCLEX-RN® exam. Remember, the NCLEX-RN® exam is testing your ability to make safe, competent decisions.

Becoming a Better Test Taker

The first step to becoming a better test taker is to assess and identify the following:

- The kind of test taker you are
- The kind of learner you are

Successful NCLEX-RN® Exam Test Takers

- Have a good understanding of nursing content.
- Have the ability to tackle each test question with a lot of confidence because they assume that they can figure out the right answer.
- Don't give up if they are unsure of the answer. They are not afraid to think about the question, and the possible choices, in order to select the correct answer.

- Possess the know-how to correctly identify the question.
- Stay focused on the topic of the question.

Unsuccessful NCLEX-RN® Exam Test Takers

- Assume that they either know or don't know the answer to the question.
- Memorize facts to answer questions by recall or recognition.
- Read the question, read the answers, read the question again, and pick an answer.
- Choose answer choices based on a hunch or a feeling instead of thinking carefully.
- Answer questions based on personal experience rather than nursing theory.
- Give up too soon, because they aren't willing to think hard about questions and answers.
- Don't stay focused on the topic of the question.

If you are a successful test taker, congratulations! This book will reinforce your test taking skills. If you have many of the characteristics of an unsuccessful test taker, don't despair! You can change. If you follow the strategies in this book, you will become a successful test taker.

What Kind of Learner Are You?

It is important for you to identify whether you think predominantly in images or words. Why? This will assist you in developing a study plan that is specific for your learning style. Read the following statement:

> A nurse walks into a room and finds the client lying on the floor.

As you read those words, did you hear yourself reading the words? Or did you see a nurse walking into a room, and see the client lying on the floor? If you heard yourself reading the sentence, you think in words. If you formed a mental image (saw a picture), you think in images.

Students who think in images sometimes have a difficult time answering nursing test questions. These students say things like:

> *"I have to study harder than the other students."*

> *"I have to look up the same information over and over again."*

> *"Once I see the procedure (or client), I don't have any difficulty understanding or remembering the content."*

> *"I have trouble understanding procedures from reading the book. I have to see the procedure to understand it."*

> *"I have trouble answering test questions about clients or procedures I've never seen."*

Why is that? For some people, imagery is necessary to understand ideas and concepts. If this is true for you, you need to visualize information that you are learning. As you prepare for the NCLEX-RN® exam, try to form mental images of terminology, procedures, and diseases. For example, if you're reviewing information about traction but you have never seen traction, it would be ideal for you to see a client in traction. If that isn't possible, find a picture of traction and rig up a traction setup with whatever material you have available. As you read about traction, use the photo or model to visualize care of the client. If you can visualize the theory that you are trying to learn, it will make recall and under-standing of concepts much easier for you.

It is also important that you visualize test questions. As you read the question and possible answer choices, picture yourself going through each suggested action. This will increase your chances of select-ing correct answer choices.

Let's look at a test question that requires imagery.

An adolescent sustains a left femur fracture during a sledding accident. The health care provider reduces the fracture and applies a cast. The client is taught how to use crutches for ambulating without bearing weight on the left leg. The nurse expects the client to learn which crutch-walking gait?

1. Two-point gait.
2. Three-point gait.
3. Four-point gait.
4. Swing-through gait.

Don't panic if you can't remember crutch-walking gaits. Instead, visualize!

STEP 1. "See" a person (or yourself) walking normally. First the right leg and left arm are extended, and then the left leg and right arm are extended.

STEP 2. Put crutches in your hands. Now walk. Each foot and each crutch is a point.

STEP 3. "See" a person (or yourself) with a full cast on the left leg, with the foot never touching the ground.

STEP 4. Visualize the answers.

(1) Two-point gait. One leg and one crutch would be touching the ground at the same time. Sounds like normal walking. Eliminate this choice because the client is non-weight-bearing.

(2) Three-point gait. Both crutches and one foot are on the ground. This would be appropriate for a non-weight-bearing client.

(3) Four-point gait. This would require both legs and crutches to touch the ground. However, in this question the client is non-weight-bearing. Eliminate this option.

(4) Swing-through gait. This gait means advancing both crutches, then both legs, and requires weight-bearing. The gait is not as stable as the other gaits. Eliminate this option: the client in this question is non-weight-bearing.

The correct answer is (2). Even if you are unsure of crutch-walking gaits, imagining and thinking through the answer choices will enable you to select the correct answer.

NCLEX-RN® Exam Question Types

NCSBN has developed a variety of question types designed to assess your nursing knowledge and critical thinking ability. Some are most likely familiar to you already. Some are new to the NCLEX-RN® as of 2023. Broadly speaking, the exam is composed of multiple choice questions with four options and alternate format question types—that is, questions that take a form other than four-option, text-based multiple choice.

Take a moment to review this list of all the question types and subtypes that you may encounter on the exam.

(1) **Multiple Choice**

(2) **Multiple Response**

   • Multiple Response Select All That Apply (SATA)

   • Multiple Response Grouping

   • Multiple Response Select N

(3) **Highlight**

   • Highlight Table

   • Highlight Text

(4) **Hot Spot**

(5) **Fill-in-the-Blank**

(6) **Drag-and-Drop**

   • Drag-and-Drop Ordered Response

   • Cloze Drag-and-Drop

   • Drag-and-Drop Rationale

(7) **Dropdown**

   • Cloze Dropdown

   • Cloze Dropdown Rationale

   • Dropdown Table

(8) **Matrix**

   • Matrix Multiple Choice

   • Matrix Multiple Response

(9) **Bowtie**

(10) **Trend**

After reading this list, you may be thinking, "That's a lot of question types, and I've never even heard of some of them!" Don't panic. The following sections contain strategies that will help you correctly answer alternate format questions and four-option, text-based, multiple choice questions. We will identify each question type in the following sections and walk you through how to tackle them. Let's get started.

Multiple Choice Test Questions

Multiple choice questions with four answer options may take the form of a text-based question or may include an exhibit/chart or graphics in place of some of the text. Each of the four options will be preceded by an empty circle. To select an option as correct, you will click on that empty circle to fill it in. While you can click to a different circle to change your answer before confirming it as your selection, the computer will allow you to fill in *only one* of these circles, or "radio buttons," at any time.

No matter the form, you need to understand the components of a multiple choice NCLEX-RN® exam question to effectively apply the strategies discussed in this book. They are as follows:

- The *stem* of the question. The stem includes the situation that describes the client, the client's problems or health care needs, and other relevant information. It also includes a question or an incomplete statement. This is the question that you must answer.
- Three incorrect answer options, referred to here as *distracters*.
- The correct answer.

The three distracters will probably sound logical to you. They may even be based on information provided in the stem, but they don't really answer the question. Other incorrect answers may be actions that are common nursing practice but not ideal nursing practice.

The correct answer is the only choice that is recognized as correct by the NCLEX-RN® exam, so you need to learn to select it. Remember that most answer choices are written at the application level, so you will not be able to select answers based on recognition or recall. You must understand the *whys* of nursing care in order to select the correct response.

Read the following exam-style Multiple Choice question. In addition to selecting an answer, identify the components of this question.

The nurse is planning care for a 4-year-old client who has been sexually abused by the parent. Play therapy is scheduled. The nurse knows that the **primary** goal of play therapy for a 4-year-old client is which of these?

1. Provide the opportunity to express anger and hostility by playing with dolls.
2. Promote communication because the client may lack capacity to verbally express perceptions.
3. Assess whether the client functions at an age-appropriate developmental level.
4. Reveal the type of abuse experienced through direct observation of the client at play.

The Components

- The stem:
  - 4-year-old client
  - Sexually abused by the parent
  - Play therapy is scheduled
  - What is the primary goal of play therapy for a 4-year-old client?

- The answer choices:

    (1)   Provide the opportunity to express anger and hostility. Play therapy will allow children to express anger and hostility if that's what they want to communicate. Some students select this answer because they focus on the treatment of sexual abuse mentioned in the situation. This is a distracter.

    (2)   Promote communication. Play is the universal language of children. The purpose of play therapy is to give children the opportunity to communicate using their own "language." This is the correct answer.

    (3)   Assess the client's developmental level. The nurse might be able to assess whether a child is functioning at an age-appropriate developmental level, but this is not the primary purpose of play therapy. This is a distracter.

    (4)   Find out what type of abuse the client has experienced. The child might communicate the type of abuse experienced if that is what the child chooses to communicate. The nurse should focus on the purpose of play therapy, not the type of abuse. This is a distracter.

Let's try another question.

A client is being treated for heart failure with diuretic therapy. Which assessment finding **best** indicates to the nurse that the client's condition is improving?

1. The client's weight has remained stable since admission.
2. The client's systolic blood pressure has decreased.
3. There are fewer crackles heard when auscultating the client's lungs.
4. The client's urinary output is 1,500 mL per day.

The Components

- The stem:

    - Heart failure

    - Treatment is diuretic therapy

    - How do you know the client's condition is improving?

- The answer choices:

    (1)   Weight has remained stable. The client's weight should decrease with diuretic therapy. Weight addresses issues involved with diuretic therapy. However, it is not the best indication of improvement in a client with heart failure. This is a distracter.

    (2)   The systolic blood pressure has decreased. Decreased blood pressure may be the result of diuretic therapy, but it could also be due to other causes (change of position, calm rather than in an excited state, etc.). This is not the best indication of improvement in a client with heart failure. This is a distracter.

    (3)   There are fewer crackles. A client with heart failure has crackles due to pulmonary edema. Diuretics are given to promote excretion of sodium and water through the kidneys. Decreased crackles would indicate that the pulmonary edema is improving. This is the correct answer.

(4)   Urinary output of 1,500 mL in 24 hours. This is within normal limits. Although a normal output addresses diuretic therapy, it is not the best indication of improvement of heart failure. This is a distracter.

Alternate Format Test Questions

If a question is not a four-option multiple choice item, it is known as an *alternate format question*. As outlined earlier, the NCLEX-RN® exam uses several different alternate format question types. These may appear either as standalone questions or as questions in a six-item case study question set. Let's look at each alternate format question type and the strategies that will help you correctly answer these questions.

Multiple Response

Like multiple choice questions, Multiple Response alternate format questions present a list of options for you to evaluate. Unlike traditional multiple choice questions, where there is a single best answer choice, more than one option may be correct. In a Multiple Response item, you must identify and select *all of the correct answer options*.

The NCLEX-RN® exam includes three varieties of Multiple Response questions:

- Multiple Response Select All That Apply (SATA)
- Multiple Response Grouping
- Multiple Response Select N

Take a look at the following Multiple Response question.

> The nurse is caring for a client diagnosed with a right-sided stroke with dysphagia. Which action by the nurse reflects appropriate care for the client? **(Select all that apply.)**
>
> ☐   1. The nurse assesses the client's ability to swallow.
>
> ☐   2. The nurse positions the client with the head of bed elevated 25 degrees.
>
> ☐   3. The nurse offers the client scrambled eggs.
>
> ☐   4. The nurse instructs the client to place food on the left side of the mouth.
>
> ☐   5. The nurse turns off the client's television.

You will know that the question is a "Select all that apply" (SATA) alternate format question because it gives you the instruction **(Select all that apply)** after the question stem and before the answer choices. You will see that there are more than four possible answer choices; usually five or six are provided, and up to ten are possible. Instead of the radio buttons you see with multiple choice, four-option, text-based questions, there is a box in front of each answer choice.

To answer this type of question, determine which of the answer choices provided are correct. To receive full credit for a **Multiple Response SATA** question, you must select *all* of the answer choices that apply, not just the best response. Left-click on the box in front of each answer choice that you think is correct. A small check mark will appear in the box indicating that you have selected that answer. If you change your mind about a particular answer choice, simply click on the box again. The check mark will disappear and the answer choice will no longer be selected.

How should you approach this type of question? What *does not* work is to compare and contrast the individual answer choices. In a Multiple Response SATA question, any number of answer choices may be correct. Instead, consider each answer choice a True/False question. Reword this question to ask, "What is appropriate care for a client with a right-sided stroke who has dysphagia?" Dysphagia means the client is having difficulty swallowing; if the stroke involves the right hemisphere, the client's left side is affected.

Let's look at the answers. The strategy is to change each answer choice into a statement, and then determine if the statement is true or false.

(1)   "I should assess the client's ability to swallow." Is this true for a client with dysphagia? Yes. This is a correct response because the nurse needs to make sure that the client can swallow food before providing anything to eat. The results of the evaluation will also determine whether the nurse should offer the client clear liquids or thickened liquids. Some clients will require thickened liquids while others will not. Select this answer choice.

(2)   "I should position the client with the head of bed elevated 25 degrees." Is this the correct position for a client with dysphagia? No. The client should be sitting upright in a chair or with the head of bed elevated at least 30 degrees. Eliminate this answer choice.

(3)   "I should offer the client scrambled eggs." Is this an appropriate food for a client with dysphagia? Yes. Soft or semi-soft foods are more easily tolerated than a regular diet. Select this answer choice.

(4)   "I should instruct the client to place food on the left side of the mouth." Is this what should be done? If the client has a right-sided stroke that means the left side of the client's body is affected. The food should be placed on the unaffected side—the right side of the mouth for this client. Eliminate this answer.

(5)   "I should turn off the television." What are they getting at with this statement? Many clients are easily distracted after a stroke. If the client has dysphagia, you don't want the client to aspirate while being distracted by the television. It is best to turn off the TV during meals. Select this answer choice.

So, which answers should be checked as correct? For this question, choices (1), (3), and (5) are correct. Left-click on the box in front of each of these answer choices to select it. When you have selected all the responses you believe to be correct, click on the NEXT (N) button in the bottom left of the screen or press the Enter key on the keyboard to lock in your answer and go on to the next question. Remember, once you click on the NEXT (N) button or press the Enter key, you have entered your answer to the question and you cannot return to the question.

The nurse is caring for a client diagnosed with a right-sided stroke with dysphagia. Which action by the nurse reflects appropriate care for the client? **(Select all that apply.)**

☑ 1. The nurse assesses the client's ability to swallow.

☐ 2. The nurse positions the client with the head of bed elevated 25 degrees.

☑ 3. The nurse offers the client scrambled eggs.

☐ 4. The nurse instructs the client to place food on the left side of the mouth.

☑ 5. The nurse turns off the client's television.

A variation of the Multiple Response item type is **Multiple Response Grouping**. In this question type, you will again see a box in front of each answer option, and you will be prompted to select all of the correct answers. However, the options are arranged in groupings within a table. The figure gives an example of a Multiple Response Grouping question.

➤ For each body system below, click to specify the potential nursing intervention appropriate for the care of the client. **Each body system may support more than 1 potential nursing intervention.**

Body System	Potential Nursing Interventions
Cardiovascular	☐ Obtain a 12-lead ECG. ☐ Administer anti-hypertensive medication. ☐ Establish IV access.
Respiratory	☐ Place oxygen 2L/nasal cannula. ☐ Have the client breathe in a paper bag. ☐ Plan for immediate intubation.
Neurological	☐ Assess pupils for size and reaction. ☐ Prepare the client for a CT of the brain. ☐ Obtain neurologic checks every shift.

Figure 2.2 Example of Multiple Response Grouping Question

As in a Multiple Response SATA question, the strategy is to reword each answer option as a True/False question and consider it individually. In the first row of the figure, for example, you would reword the first option as "Is obtaining a 12-lead ECG an appropriate cardiovascular intervention for this client?", the second option as "Is administering anti-hypertensive medication an appropriate nursing intervention for this client?", and so on.

The last variation of the Multiple Response item type is **Multiple Response Select N**, in which the question tells you the correct number of responses to choose, for example:

- "Which 3 findings are most concerning?"
- "Which 3 findings require follow-up?"

Read the question stem carefully. If the question stem directs you to choose three answers, choose *exactly three answers*—and no fewer—before proceeding to the next question. Again, reword each answer option as a True/False question and consider it individually.

Which **3** findings are **most** concerning to the nurse?

1. Not walking.
2. Attends daycare 6 days per week as both parents work.
3. Eats with fingers.
4. Watches television most of day.
5. Drinks only from a bottle.
6. Has home babysitter.
7. Used bouncy walker until age 12 months.

Figure 2.3 Example of Multiple Response Select N Question

Highlight

This type of alternate format question asks you to identify relevant text within a passage. For example, a Highlight question may ask you to select concerning or priority findings that require follow-up by the nurse or health care provider or, alternatively, to select client findings that indicate an improvement in condition. Highlight questions may take either of two forms: a table or a paragraph.

The figure shows an example of a **Highlight Table** question.

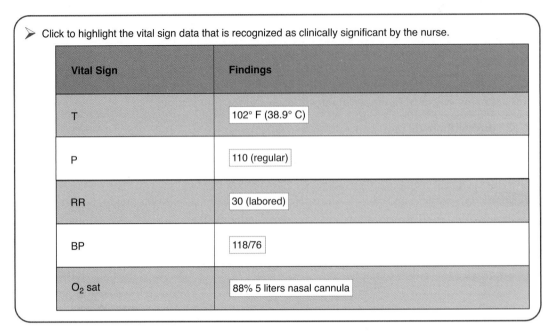

➤ Click to highlight the vital sign data that is recognized as clinically significant by the nurse.

Vital Sign	Findings
T	102° F (38.9° C)
P	110 (regular)
RR	30 (labored)
BP	118/76
O$_2$ sat	88% 5 liters nasal cannula

Figure 2.4 Example of Highlight Table Question

Highlighting is achieved by selecting "tokenized text"—that is, preselected phrases or words that can be highlighted in response to an exam question. The tokenized text may be a mix of "keys" (correct answers) and distracters (incorrect answers).

Highlighting tokenized text on the NCLEX-RN® exam is much like physically marking a book with a highlighter pen. Hover the cursor over tokenized text and click once to highlight the text. Hovering the cursor over the tokenized text and clicking again would remove the highlighting.

To answer a Highlight question, analyze each piece of tokenized text individually. As in a Multiple Response SATA question, the strategy is to change each answer choice into a statement, then determine if the statement is correct/incorrect, right/wrong, true/false, significant/insignificant, priority/nonpriority, indicated/contraindicated, expected/unexpected, and so on.

Here is how you would begin to answer the Highlight question in the example:

(1) T 102° F (38.9° C). Is this finding significant? Yes, it is outside the normal range. Hover the cursor over the tokenized text and left-click.

(2) P 110 (regular). Is this finding significant? Yes, it is outside the normal range. Hover the cursor over the tokenized text and left-click.

(3) RR 30 (labored). Is this finding significant? Yes, respiratory rate is high, and labored breathing is significant. Hover the cursor over the tokenized text and left-click.

Continue with this method of questioning for each remaining assessment finding. Then enter your answer by clicking on the NEXT (N) button or pressing the Enter key.

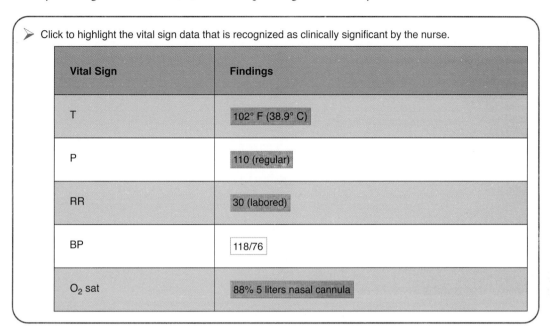

➤ Click to highlight the vital sign data that is recognized as clinically significant by the nurse.

Vital Sign	Findings
T	102° F (38.9° C)
P	110 (regular)
RR	30 (labored)
BP	118/76
O$_2$ sat	88% 5 liters nasal cannula

Figure 2.5 Example of Highlight Table Question, Marked

In a **Highlight Text** question, the tokenized text is located in a sentence or text-based paragraph.

- Hover the cursor over tokenized text and click once to mark an answer choice as correct.
- Hover the cursor over tokenized text and click again to remove the highlighting.

Approach it in the same way as in a table. The figure shows an example of a Highlight Text alternate format question.

> ➤ Click to highlight the information in the Nurse's Notes that concerns the nurse at this time.

Client was brought to the urgent care clinic by spouse due to abdominal pain. The client states, "I have been having pain on and off for several days, but today the pain was very severe." The client has a history of atrial fibrillation, myocardial infarction, hypertension, and hyperlipidemia. The client also reports a 40-pound (18 kg) weight loss over the last three months. Vital Signs: T 99.9° F (37.7° C), P 76, RR 20, BP 148/90, pulse oximetry reading 95% on room air. Upon assessment the client's breathing is unlabored, and lungs are clear bilaterally. Pain intermittent, located in the epigastric area and often radiates to the right shoulder, rated "7" on 1-10 pain scale. Abdomen slightly distended, and firm to palpation. Client is alert and oriented to person, place, and time. Currently taking digoxin, metoprolol, and atorvastatin.

Figure 2.6 Example of Highlight Text Question

Hot Spot

This type of alternate format question asks you to identify a location on a graphic or table and select it by clicking it with the mouse. This is not a test of your fine motor skills. **Hot Spot** questions are designed to evaluate your knowledge of nursing content, anatomy, and physiology and pathophysiology.

Let's take a look at a question that involves a hot spot.

The nurse is performing a physical assessment on an adult client. Identify the area where the nurse should place the stethoscope to auscultate heart sounds heard in the tricuspid area.

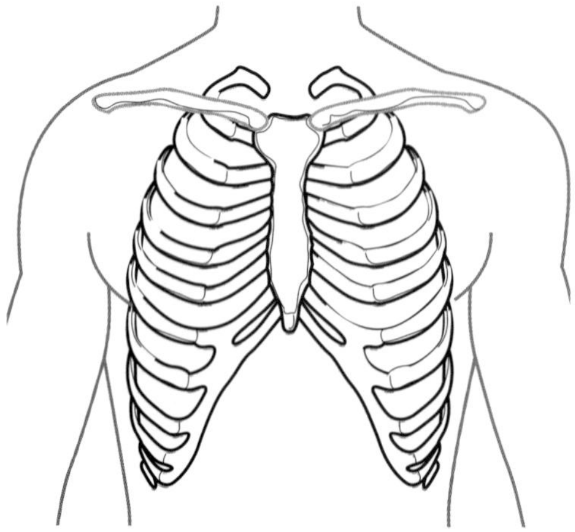

This question asks you to identify where you would listen to heart sounds in the tricuspid area. The strategy you should use is to locate anatomical landmarks. You need to know that the tricuspid area is located on the client's left side. It is found in the space between ribs, two ribs up from the bottom of the seven true ribs. The tricuspid area is located in the fourth and fifth intercostal spaces at the lower left of the sternal border.

Move the cursor to the location you think is correct. Then, left-click the mouse. Check to make sure that you have selected the location you wanted. Then enter your answer by clicking on the NEXT (N) button or pressing the Enter key. If you click on the right side of the chest, or four ribs up from the bottom, or at the midclavicular area instead of the sternal border, the location would be inaccurate for the tricuspid area and the question would be counted as incorrect. Just do your best and use anatomical landmarks to get your bearings and select the location.

Here's the answer to this Hot Spot question.

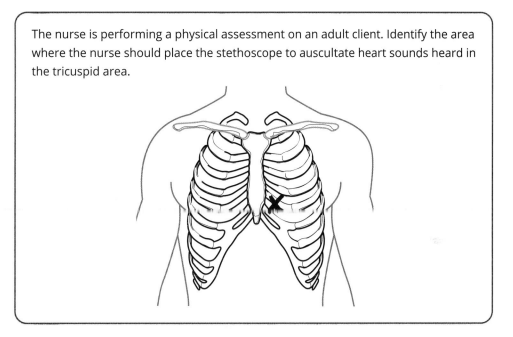

The nurse is performing a physical assessment on an adult client. Identify the area where the nurse should place the stethoscope to auscultate heart sounds heard in the tricuspid area.

It is important for you to know where to listen to specific heart sounds. In addition to the tricuspid area, you should be able to locate other anatomical landmarks to evaluate heart sounds:

- Angle of Louis—manubrial sternal junction at the second rib
- Aortic area—second intercostal space to the *right* of the sternum
- Pulmonic area—second intercostal space to the *left* of the sternum
- Erb's point—third intercostal space to the *left* of the sternum
- Mitral area—fifth intercostal space at the *left* midclavicular line

In the mitral area of an adult is the *apical impulse*, also known the point of maximal impulse (PMI), where the impulse of the left ventricle is felt most strongly; on an infant, the apical impulse is lateral to the left nipple.

Fill-in-the-Blank

This type of alternate format question asks you to fill in the blank with a number based on a calculation.

The following is an example of a **Fill-in-the-Blank** question.

> The nurse is caring for a client receiving hourly peritoneal dialysis exchanges. During a one-hour exchange, the nurse infuses 2,000 mL of dialysate and 1,900 mL of outflow returns. During the exchange, the client drinks 8 oz of apple juice, 2 cups of water, and voids 150 mL of urine. Calculate and record the client's intake in milliliters.
>
> _____ milliliters

To answer this question, calculate the client's intake from the information provided. **Note: Pay close attention to the unit of measure you need for your final answer.** In this situation, you are asked for the client's intake in milliliters, not cups or ounces.

You can use the drop-down calculator provided on the computer to do the math. The button that displays the calculator is on the bottom of the right side of the computer screen. Use your mouse to click on the numbers or functions you want. Remember, the slash (/) is used for division.

To answer this question you need to know that intake includes what the client drinks along with the amount of dialysate that is retained after the one-hour exchange of solution.

First, convert cups into ounces. One cup of fluid = 8 oz. Then convert ounces into milliliters. One ounce = 30 milliliters.

The client's intake is:

8 oz apple juice = 240 mL

2 cups = 16 oz water = 480 mL

100 mL = retained dialysate

Move the cursor inside the text box, and left-click on the mouse. Type in the correct intake using the number keys on the keyboard. The correct answer is 820. Do not put "mL" or any other unit of measure after the number. *Only the number* goes into the box. Rules for rounding are typically provided with the question.

> The nurse is caring for a client receiving hourly peritoneal dialysis exchanges. During a one-hour exchange, the nurse infuses 2,000 mL of dialysate and 1,900 mL of outflow returns. During the exchange, the client drinks 8 oz of apple juice, 2 cups of water, and voids 150 mL of urine. Calculate and record the client's intake in milliliters.
>
> 820_____ milliliters

Drag-and-Drop

Drag-and-Drop alternate format questions ask you to arrange answers in the correct order or to supply missing information to complete a passage of text. The NCSBN defines three Drag-and-Drop varieties.

- Drag-and-Drop Ordered Response
- Cloze Drag-and-Drop
- Drag-and-Drop Rationale

Drag-and-Drop Ordered Response questions direct you to place answers in a specific order.

Take a look at the following question.

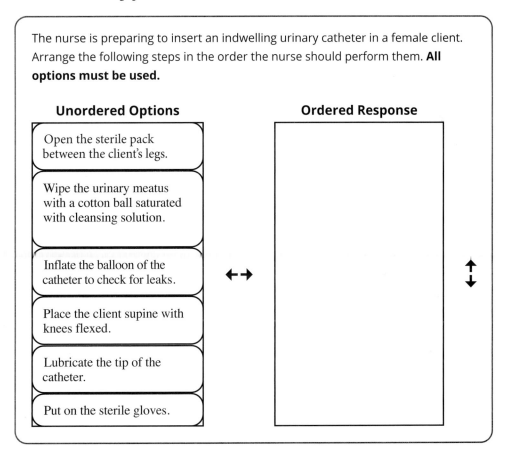

The nurse is preparing to insert an indwelling urinary catheter in a female client. Arrange the following steps in the order the nurse should perform them. **All options must be used.**

Unordered Options

Open the sterile pack between the client's legs.

Wipe the urinary meatus with a cotton ball saturated with cleansing solution.

Inflate the balloon of the catheter to check for leaks.

Place the client supine with knees flexed.

Lubricate the tip of the catheter.

Put on the sterile gloves.

Ordered Response

The strategy to use when answering this kind of question is to visualize: Picture yourself performing the procedure. First, prepare the client. Next, prepare the equipment in the correct order, using sterile technique. Open the sterile insertion kit. Then, put on the sterile gloves. Next, inflate the balloon of the catheter to check for leaks. (NOTE: This step may vary per facility policy and manufacturer guidelines. Silicone catheter balloons should not be pre-inflated.) Lubricate the tip of the catheter. After preparing the equipment, prepare the client for the insertion of the catheter. The last step from those provided is to cleanse the periurethral area using swabsticks or cotton balls saturated with cleansing solution.

To place the options in the correct order, click on an option and drag it to the box on the right. You can also move an answer from the left column to the right column by highlighting the option and clicking the arrow key that points to the column on the right. You may also rearrange the order of the options in the right column using the arrow keys pointing up and down.

Here's the answer to this question.

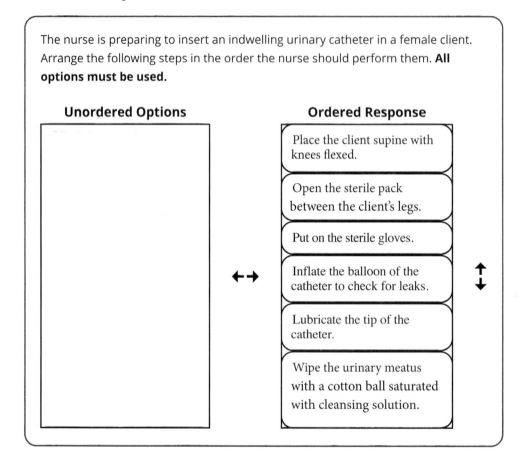

The nurse is preparing to insert an indwelling urinary catheter in a female client. Arrange the following steps in the order the nurse should perform them. **All options must be used.**

Unordered Options | **Ordered Response**

Place the client supine with knees flexed.

Open the sterile pack between the client's legs.

Put on the sterile gloves.

Inflate the balloon of the catheter to check for leaks.

Lubricate the tip of the catheter.

Wipe the urinary meatus with a cotton ball saturated with cleansing solution.

A variation is **Cloze Drag-and-Drop**, in which you choose a word or words from an answer well to complete a sentence. (The word *cloze* is derived from "closure.") With the cursor, drag "tokens" (answer choices) from the answer well to complete the sentence. If you mistakenly drag an incorrect token into the sentence, you can remove it by either returning it to the answer well or dragging the correct token from the answer well to replace the incorrect token.

The figure shows an example of a Cloze Drag-and-Drop alternate format question.

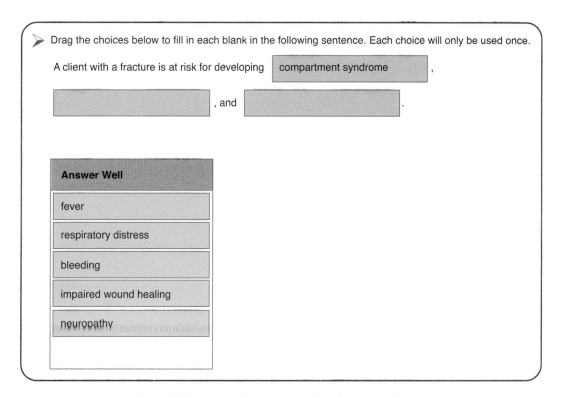

Figure 2.7 Example of Cloze Drag-and-Drop Question in Progress

Another variation is **Drag-and-Drop Rationale**. Again, you use the cursor to drag tokens from the answer well to complete a sentence. In this question type, however, the word or words you choose complete a *rationale-based* sentence. A Drag-and-Drop Rationale question requires you to recognize a cause-and-effect relationship.

Take a look at the following question.

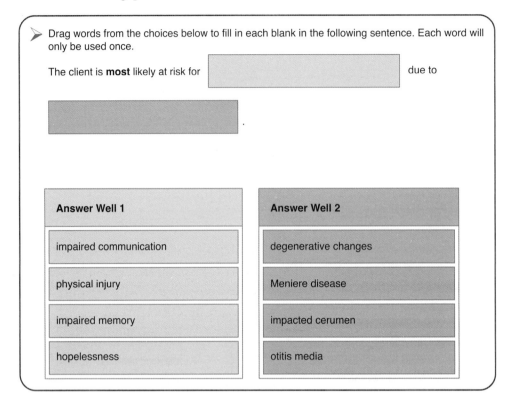

Figure 2.8 Example of Drag-and-Drop Rationale Question

You will know that an item is a rationale-based question because it includes the words "due to" or "as evidenced by."

To complete the sentence, drag a color-coded token from each answer well and drop it into the blank in the sentence with the corresponding color. Note that a token "dropped" into a noncorresponding blank will be rejected and automatically returned to its answer well.

Drag-and-Drop Rationale questions on the NCLEX-RN® exam come in two forms:

- A single dyad has one cause and one effect. (The sample question is an example of a single dyad.)
- A single triad has one cause and two effects.

How should you approach this question? The strategy you should use is to identify the client's priority problem based on cues in the case study. Starting with the first answer well, consider each answer choice: Is it related to the priority problem or potential condition you identified for this client? If the answer is yes, select the answer option. Identifying the priority problem or potential condition in the first answer well is essential to earning any credit on the item.

After choosing your answers from the answer wells, pause to consider each of your selections. Ask yourself:

- "Do the answers I chose make sense?"
- "Have I selected answers based on my foundational nursing knowledge?"
- "Have I selected answers based on the client's priority problem/condition?"

If you can answer "Yes," you have selected the best choices to answer the Drag-and-Drop Rationale item.

Dropdown

Dropdown alternate format questions ask you to select a word or phrase from a dropdown menu to complete a passage of text or table. There are three Dropdown varieties.

- Cloze Dropdown
- Cloze Dropdown Rationale
- Dropdown Table

The **Cloze Dropdown** question type asks you to complete a sentence by choosing a word or words from a dropdown list.

Take a look at the following question.

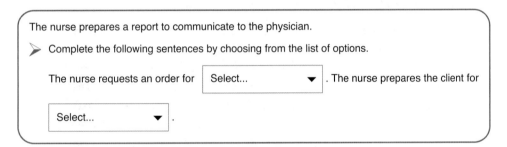

Figure 2.9 Example of Cloze Dropdown Question

To populate the answer choices, place the cursor on the first dropdown, labeled with the instruction "Select" beside an inverted triangle, and left-click. Typically, three to five answer choices are provided in each dropdown.

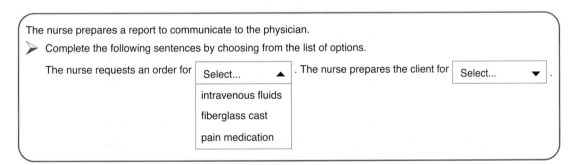

Figure 2.10 Example of Cloze Dropdown Options

The first step to answer a Cloze Dropdown question is to identify the client's priority problem based on cues in the case study. Next, consider each answer choice in the first dropdown menu.

- Does the answer choice help validate or address the priority problem or potential condition you identified for this client?
- Will the action in the answer choice help the client "right here, right now"?

If not, eliminate that answer choice. Repeat this process with each answer choice in each dropdown menu. After choosing your answers, pause to consider each of your selections. Ask yourself:

- "Do the answers I chose make sense?"
- "Have I selected answers based on my foundational nursing knowledge?"

If you can answer "Yes," you have selected the best choices to answer the Cloze Dropdown item.

A variation of the dropdown question type is **Cloze Dropdown Rationale**, in which you complete a rationale-based sentence. Like Drag-and-Drop Rationale, this question type requires you to recognize a cause-and-effect relationship. In Cloze Dropdown Rationale questions, however, you select answers to complete the sentence from dropdown menus rather than answer wells. As in any rationale-based question, the sentence will include the words "due to" or "as evidenced by."

Look at the following Cloze Dropdown Rationale question.

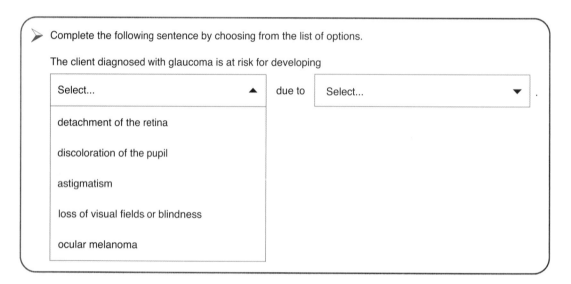

Figure 2.11 Example of Cloze Dropdown Rationale Question, First Dropdown

To answer a Cloze Dropdown Rationale question, identify the client's priority problem based on cues in the case study. Then, starting with the first dropdown, consider each answer choice: Is it related to the priority problem or potential condition you identified for this client? If not, eliminate that answer choice. Identifying the priority problem or potential condition in the first dropdown is essential to earning any credit on the item.

Repeat this process with each answer choice in each dropdown. After choosing your answers, pause to consider each of your selections. Ask yourself:

- "Do the answers I chose make sense?"
- "Have I selected answers based on my foundational nursing knowledge?"
- "Have I selected answers based on the client's priority problem/condition?"

If you can answer "Yes," you have selected the best choices to answer the Cloze Dropdown Rationale question.

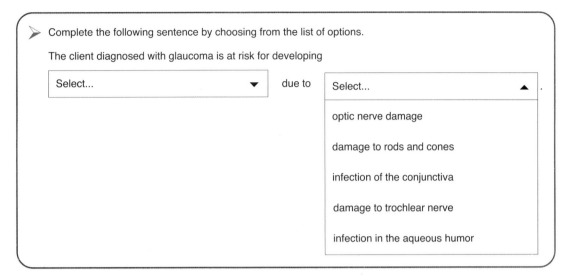

Figure 2.12 Example of Cloze Dropdown Rationale Question, Second Dropdown

Another dropdown variation is **Dropdown Table**, in which you select from a series of dropdowns incorporated into a chart. As in the other dropdown question types, you select only one answer choice per dropdown.

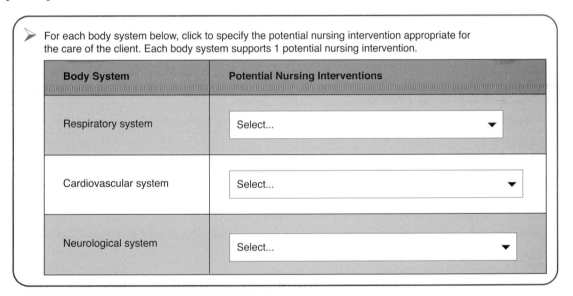

Figure 2.13 Example of Dropdown Table

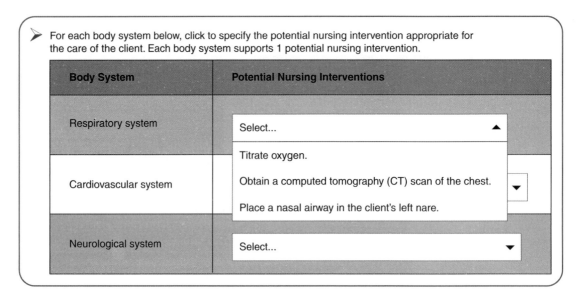

Figure 2.14 Example of Dropdown Table, First Dropdown

The strategy you should use in a Dropdown Table question is to reword each answer option as a True/False question and consider it individually. In the first row of the figure, for example, you would reword the first option as "Is titrating oxygen an appropriate respiratory intervention for this client?", the second option as "Is obtaining a CT scan of the chest an appropriate respiratory intervention for this client?", and so on.

After choosing your answers, pause to consider each of your selections. Ask yourself:

- "Do the answers I chose make sense?"
- "Have I selected answers based on my foundational nursing knowledge?"

If you can answer "Yes," you have selected the best choices to answer the Dropdown Table question.

Matrix

Matrix alternate format questions present answer options arranged in a table and prompt you to select an answer or answers from each row. There are two varieties, Matrix Multiple Choice and Matrix Multiple Response.

In the **Matrix Multiple Choice** question type, there is only one correct answer per row, which you will select from a set of radio buttons. The question will prompt you to evaluate each item of a series against the same set of answer options. For instance, you would decide for each item in a series:

- Is the intervention indicated or contraindicated?
- Is the intervention priority or nonpriority?
- Does the client response indicate that teaching is effective or ineffective?

Look at the following Matrix Multiple Choice question.

On day 3 of the client's hospitalization, the nurse assesses the client and documents care. The nurse provides additional discharge teaching.

➤ For each client statement, click to indicate if the client understands discharge teaching or requires **further** education.

Statement	Understands	Further education
"If my blood glucose is below 60 mg/dL (3.33 mmol/L), I should drink 4 ounces of fruit juice or cola."	●	●
"Fifteen minutes after I eat or drink something to correct hypoglycemia, I should recheck my blood glucose."	○	○
"If my blood glucose remains low after I eat or drink something, I should come to the emergency department (ED)."	●	●
"I should keep hard candies with me at all times."	○	○
"It is very important for me to eat as soon as I have injected my regular insulin dose."	●	●

Figure 2.15 Example of Matrix Multiple Choice Question

The strategy you should use to answer a Matrix Multiple Choice question is the same as for SATA questions. Change each answer choice into a statement, and then determine if the statement is correct. Let's look at the answers.

- "If my blood glucose is below 60 mg/dL (3.33 mmol/L), I should drink 4 ounces of fruit juice or cola." Does this statement indicate client understanding? Yes, this statement indicates understanding of the "15–15" rule. Select "Understands" for this row.

- "Fifteen minutes after I eat or drink something to correct hypoglycemia, I should recheck my blood glucose." Does this statement indicate client understanding? Yes, this statement indicates understanding of the "15–15" rule. Select "Understands" for this row.

- "If my blood glucose remains low after I eat or drink something, I should come to the emergency department (ED)." Does this statement indicate client understanding? No. As the immediate next step, the client should follow the "15–15" rule and ingest an additional 15 grams of carbohydrates. Select "Further education" for this row.

- "I should keep hard candies with me at all times." Does this statement indicate client understanding? Yes, this statement indicates understanding of the "15–15" rule. Select "Understands" for this row.

- "It is very important for me to eat as soon as I have injected my regular insulin dose." Does this statement indicate client understanding? Yes. Having injected regular insulin, the client needs to take in a bolus of food so that there is glucose in the bloodstream when the peak action of insulin occurs. Select "Understands" for this row.

Matrix Multiple Response questions may prompt you to correlate a set of client symptoms or nursing assessment findings with a medical problem. In this question type, there is *potentially more than one correct answer* per row. Instead of radio buttons, you will see a box for each answer option. Left-click in the box to select the option. Remember, you may select more than one option per row.

It is important to note that each column in a Matrix Multiple Response question must have at least one option selected. Otherwise, you will be unable to progress to the next question.

Here is a sample Matrix Multiple Response question.

> For each assessment finding below, click to specify whether the finding is consistent with the disease process of pneumonia, heart failure, or sepsis. Each finding may support more than one disease process. **Each column must have at least 1 response option selected.**

Assessment Finding	Pneumonia	Heart failure	Sepsis
Shortness of breath.	☐	☐	☐
BP 94/62 mmHg.	☐	☐	☐
1+ edema to lower extremities.	☐	☐	☐
Temperature 101.4° F (38.8° C).	☐	☐	☐
Coarse crackles to lung bases.	☐	☐	☐

Figure 2.16 Example of Matrix Multiple Response Question

Let's look at the answer options for the first two rows of the table. The strategy for this type of question is, once again, to change each answer choice into a statement, and then determine if the statement is true or false based on your foundational nursing knowledge.

- "Shortness of breath is expected with pneumonia." Yes, this is a true statement. Select this answer choice.
- "Shortness of breath is expected with heart failure." True. Select this answer choice.
- "Shortness of breath is expected with sepsis." True. Select this answer choice.
- "Hypotension is expected with pneumonia." No, this statement is false. Eliminate this answer.
- "Hypotension is expected with heart failure." Perhaps, if the client has a reduced ejection fraction. Refer to information in the case to determine whether the client has a reduced ejection fraction.
- "Hypotension is expected with sepsis." True. Select this answer choice.

Continue with this method for each remaining assessment finding.

Bowtie

This is a standalone, case-based alternate format question type in which you "drag and drop" answer choices into a bowtie-shaped diagram. The **Bowtie** question type requires you to make multiple clinical decisions that range from recognizing concerning cues to evaluating client outcomes.

Take a look at the following Bowtie question.

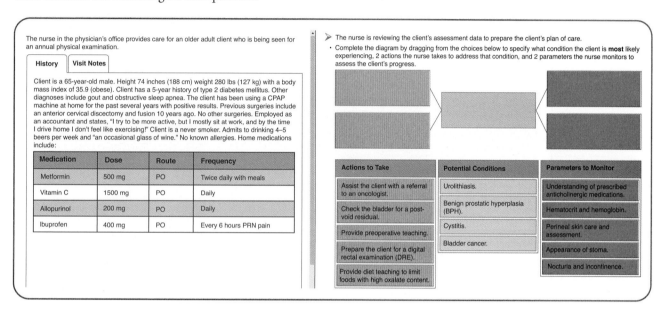

Figure 2.17 Example of Bowtie Question and Case Study

The answer choices in a Bowtie item are laid out in an uneven table with five options in the left column, four in the middle column, and five in the right column. In each Bowtie item, two options are correct in the left and right columns, and one answer is correct in the middle column.

The color-coded columns of these answer wells correspond with the targets above each column. For example, tokens from the "Actions to Take" column can only be dragged to a corresponding-colored "Actions to Take" target location directly above it. As with other drag-and-drop question types, a token dropped into a noncorresponding blank will be rejected and automatically returned to its answer well.

To remove a token that you have mistakenly dragged into the diagram, you can either return it to its answer well or drag the desired token to the target to replace the discarded token. Note that paired options, such as the two options chosen for "Actions to Take" and "Parameters to Monitor" in the example, are interchangeable and do not need to be in a specific order in the diagram.

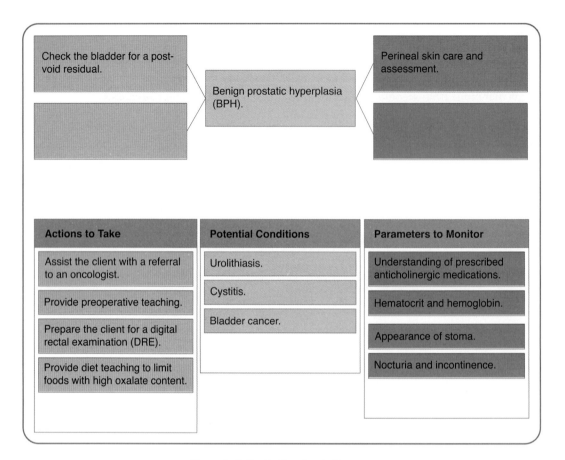

Figure 2.18 Bowtie Question in Progress

To answer a Bowtie question, start with the middle of the diagram.

- First, identify the Potential Condition you believe the client is experiencing, and place it in the middle target. You should derive the Potential Condition by recognizing cues in the case record and analyzing their significance based on your foundational nursing knowledge.

- Next, select the two Actions to Take based on the Potential Condition you have identified, and place them (in either order) in the left-hand targets of the diagram.

- Finally, select the two Parameters to Monitor based on the Potential Condition you have identified, and place them (in either order) in the right-hand targets of the diagram.

The Potential Condition that you select will help you determine which Actions to Take are appropriate and which Parameters to Monitor are necessary. Use the *if/then* principle as you consider these: "If the potential condition is most likely _____, then the actions the nurse will take are _____ and _____, and the parameters to monitor are _____ and _____."

Trend

This standalone, case-based alternate format question type also requires clinical decision-making skills and clinical judgment. The name of the question, **Trend**, is representative of what you will be asked to do: recognize and interpret a pattern of changes over a period of time. Some trends may be desired and therapeutic, such as a decline in blood glucose readings after starting an antidiabetic medication. Other trends may be harmful, such as steady increases in blood pressure readings after increasing sodium intake in the diet.

Different "tabs" in the medical record provide different categories of information gathered over a period of time, such as:

- Nurse's Notes
- Laboratory Results
- Diagnostic Results
- Vital Signs
- Intake and Output

The time evolution could occur over minutes, hours, days, and so on. For example, a Trend question might provide a "Nurse's Notes" tab documenting a client's vital signs throughout the shift, and then ask you to interpret the vital signs and make a clinical decision regarding care of the client. Trend items can feature any item response type except Bowtie, so you could see a Trend question in the form of Cloze, Matrix, Highlight, Multiple Response, or four-option multiple choice.

Following is an example of a Trend question.

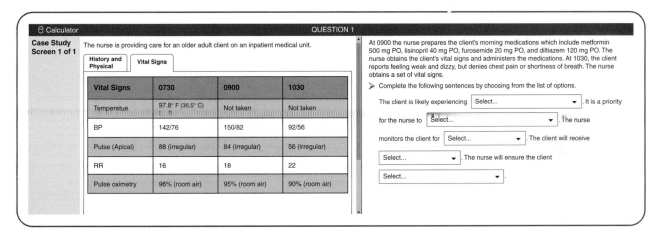

Figure 2.19 Example of Trend Question

Each time you receive a set of trended data, analyze it and consider whether the trend is therapeutic or nontherapeutic for the client's condition. Making that determination sets the stage for you to respond successfully to the trended data.

Critical Thinking Strategies

- The NCLEX-RN® exam is not a test about recognizing facts.
- You must be able to correctly identify what the question is asking.
- Do not focus on background information that is not needed to answer the question.
- The NCLEX-RN® exam focuses on thinking through a problem or situation.

Now that you are more knowledgeable about the components of a multiple choice test question and the structure of the various alternate format question types, let's talk about specific strategies that you can use to problem-solve your way to correct answers on the NCLEX-RN® exam.

Remember, the NCLEX-RN® exam is testing your ability to think critically. Critical thinking for the nurse involves the following:

- Observation (recognizing cues)
- Applying knowledge and deciding what is important (analyzing cues and prioritizing)
- Looking for patterns and relationships (trends)
- Identifying the problem (based on cue recognition)
- Transferring knowledge from one situation to another
- Discriminating between possible choices and/or courses of action
- Evaluating according to criteria established

Are you feeling overwhelmed as you read these words? Don't be! We are going teach you a step-by-step method to choose the appropriate path. The Kaplan Nursing team has developed a Decision Tree that shows you how to approach every NCLEX-RN® exam question. In this book, these strategies appear as 10 critical thinking paths.

There are some strategies that you must follow on *every* NCLEX-RN® exam test question. You must *always* figure out what the question is asking, and you must *always* eliminate answer choices.

Choosing the right answer often involves choosing the best of several answers that have correct information. This may entail your correct analysis and interpretation of what the question is really asking. So let's talk about how to figure out what the question is asking.

Reword the Question

The first step to correctly answering NCLEX-RN® exam questions is to find out what each question is *really* asking.

STEP 1. Read each question carefully from the first word to the last word. Do not skim over the words or read them too quickly.

STEP 2. Look for hints in the wording of the question stem. The adjectives *most, first, best, primary,* and *initial* indicate that you must establish priorities. The phrase *further teaching is necessary* indicates that the answer will contain incorrect information. The phrase *client understands the teaching* indicates that the answer will be correct information.

STEP 3. Reword the question stem in your own words so that it can be answered with a *yes* or a *no*, or with a specific bit of information. Begin your questions with *what, when,* or *why*. We will refer to this reworded version as THE REWORDED QUESTION in the examples that follow.

STEP 4. If you can't complete step 3, read the answer choices for clues.

Let's practice rewording a question.

> A preschool-age child is brought to the emergency department (ED) by the parents for treatment of a femur fracture. When asked how the injury occurred, the parents state that the child fell from the sofa. On examination, the nurse finds old and new lesions on the child's buttocks. Which statement **most** appropriately reflects how the nurse should document these findings?
>
> 1.
> 2.
> 3.
> 4.

We omitted the answer choices to make you focus on the question stem this time. The answer choices will be provided and discussed later in this chapter.

STEP 1. Read the question stem carefully.

STEP 2. Pay attention to the adjectives. *Most appropriately* tells you that you need to select the best answer.

STEP 3. Reword the question stem in your own words. In this case, it is, "What is the best documentation for this situation?"

STEP 4. Because you were able to reword the question, the fourth step is unnecessary. You didn't need to read the answer choices for clues.

We have all missed questions on a test because we didn't read accurately. The following question illustrates this point.

> A client is admitted to the hospital for treatment of active tuberculosis (TB). The nurse teaches the client about TB. Which statement by the client indicates to the nurse that further teaching is necessary?
>
> 1.
> 2.
> 3.
> 4.

Again, just the question stem is given to encourage you to focus on rewording the question. We will discuss the answer choices for this question later in this chapter.

STEP 1. Read the question stem carefully.

STEP 2. Look for hints. Pay particular attention to the statement "further teaching is necessary." You are looking for negative information.

STEP 3. Reword the question stem in your own words. In this case, it is, "What is incorrect information about TB?"

STEP 4. Because you were able to reword the question, the fourth step is unnecessary. You didn't need to read the answer choices for clues to determine what the question is asking.

Try rewording this test question.

A client admitted to the hospital in premature labor has been treated successfully. The client is to receive a regimen of betamethasone. Which statement by the client indicates to the nurse that the client understands the teaching about the medication?

1.

2.

3.

4.

Again, just the question stem is given to encourage you to focus on rewording the question. We will discuss the answer choices for this question later in this chapter.

STEP 1. Read the question stem carefully.

STEP 2. Look for hints. Pay attention to the words *client understands*. You are looking for true information.

STEP 3. Reword the question stem. This question is asking, "What is true about betamethasone?"

STEP 4. Because you were able to reword this question, the fourth step is unnecessary. You didn't need to obtain clues about what the question is asking from the answer choices.

Eliminate Incorrect Answer Choices

Now that you've mastered rewording the question, let's examine how to select the correct answer.

Remember the characteristics of unsuccessful test takers? One of their major problems is that they do not thoughtfully consider each answer choice. They react to questions using feelings and hunches. Unsuccessful test takers look for a specific answer choice. The following strategy will enable you to consider each answer choice in a thoughtful way.

STEP 1. Do not look at any of the answer choices except answer choice (1).

STEP 2. Read answer choice (1). Then repeat THE REWORDED QUESTION after reading the answer choice. Ask yourself, "Does this answer THE REWORDED QUESTION?" If you know the answer choice is wrong, eliminate it. If you aren't sure, leave the answer choice in for consideration.

STEP 3. Repeat the above process with each remaining answer choice.

STEP 4. Note which answer choices remain.

STEP 5. Reread the question to make sure you have correctly identified THE REWORDED QUESTION.

STEP 6. Ask yourself, "Which answer choice best answers the question?" That is your answer.

Let's practice the elimination strategy using the same questions.

> A preschool-age child is brought to the emergency department (ED) by the parents for treatment of a femur fracture. When asked how the injury occurred, the parents state that the child fell from the sofa. On examination, the nurse finds old and new lesions on the child's buttocks. Which statement **most** appropriately reflects how the nurse should document these findings?
>
> 1. "Six lesions in various stages of healing noted on buttocks."
> 2. "Multiple lesions noted on buttocks due to child abuse."
> 3. "Lesions noted on buttocks from unknown causes."
> 4. "Several lesions noted on buttocks caused by cigarettes."

THE REWORDED QUESTION: "What is good documenting?"

STEP 1. Do not look at any of the answer choices except for answer choice (1). Thoughtfully consider each answer choice individually.

STEP 2. Read answer choice (1). Does it answer the question, "What is good documenting for this situation?"

(1) "Six lesions noted on buttocks at various stages of healing." Is this good documenting? Maybe. Leave it in for consideration.

STEP 3. Repeat the process with each remaining answer choice.

(2) "Multiple lesions noted on buttocks due to child abuse." Is this good documenting? No, because the nurse is making a judgment about the cause of the lesions.

(3) "Lesions noted on buttocks from unknown causes." Is this good documenting? Maybe. Leave it in for consideration.

(4) "Several lesions noted on buttocks caused by cigarettes." Is this good documenting? No. The question does not include information about how the lesions occurred.

STEP 4. Answer choices (1) and (3) remain.

STEP 5. Reread the question to make sure you have correctly identified THE REWORDED QUESTION. This question asks you to identify good documenting.

STEP 6. Which is better documenting? "Six lesions noted on buttocks at various stages of healing," or "Lesions noted on buttocks from unknown causes"? Good charting is accurate, objective, concise, and complete. It must reflect the client's current status. The correct answer is (1).

Some students will select answer (3), thinking, "How can I be sure about the stages of healing?" But the purpose of this question is to test your ability to select good documenting.

Select the answer choice that shows you are a safe and effective nurse. Remember, questions on the NCLEX-RN® exam are not designed to trick you. Stay focused on the question.

Let's select the correct answer for the second question.

> A client is admitted to the hospital for treatment of active tuberculosis (TB). The nurse teaches the client about TB. Which statement by the client indicates to the nurse that further teaching is necessary?
>
> 1. "I will have to take medication for 6 months."
> 2. "I should cover my nose and mouth when coughing or sneezing."
> 3. "I will remain in isolation for at least 6 weeks."
> 4. "I will always have a positive skin test for TB."

THE REWORDED QUESTION: "What is incorrect information about TB?"

STEP 1. Do not look at any of the answer choices except answer choice (1).

STEP 2. Read answer choice (1). Does it answer THE REWORDED QUESTION, "What is incorrect (or wrong) information about TB?"

(1) "I will have to take medication for 6 months." Is this wrong information? No, it is a true statement. The client will need to take a medication, such as isonicotinyl hydrazine (INH), for 6 months or longer. Eliminate this choice.

STEP 3. Repeat the process with each remaining answer choice.

(2) "I should cover my nose and mouth when coughing or sneezing." Is this wrong information about TB? No, this is a true statement. TB is transmitted by droplet contamination. Eliminate it.

(3) "I will remain in isolation for at least 6 weeks." Is this wrong information about TB? Maybe. Leave it in for consideration.

(4) "I will always have a positive skin test for TB." Is this a wrong statement about TB? No, this is true. A positive skin test indicates that the client has developed antibodies to the tuberculosis bacillus. Eliminate this choice.

STEP 4. Only answer choice (3) remains.

STEP 5. Reread the question to make sure you have correctly identified THE REWORDED QUESTION. The question is, "What is incorrect information about TB?"

STEP 6. The correct answer is (3). You "know" this is the correct answer because you've eliminated the other three answer choices. The client does not need to be isolated for 6 weeks. The client's activities will be restricted for 2–3 weeks after medication therapy is initiated.

A couple of things to remember when using this strategy:

- Eliminate only what you know is wrong. However, once you eliminate an answer choice, do not retrieve it for consideration. You may be tempted to do this if you do not feel comfortable with the one answer choice that is left. Resist the impulse!

- Stay focused on THE REWORDED QUESTION. How many times have you missed a question that asked for negative information because you selected the answer choice that contained correct information?

Here's another question.

> A client admitted to the hospital in premature labor has been treated successfully. The client is to receive a regimen of betamethasone. Which statement by the client indicates to the nurse that the client understands the teaching about the medication?
>
> 1. "As long as I receive my medication, I won't deliver prematurely."
> 2. "It is important that I count the fetal movements for one hour, twice a day."
> 3. "I may have insomnia and a rapid heart beat while on this medication."
> 4. "Bed rest is necessary in order for the medication to work properly."

THE REWORDED QUESTION: "What is true about antenatal betamethasone?"

STEP 1. Do not look at any of the answer choices except answer choice (1).

STEP 2. Read answer choice (1). Does it answer the question, "What is true about betamethasone?"

(1) "As long as I receive my medication, I won't deliver prematurely." Is this true about betamethasone? No. Betamethasone will help fetal lung maturation in case the client delivers prematurely, but it doesn't prevent premature delivery. Eliminate it.

STEP 3. Repeat the process with each remaining answer choice.

(2) "It is important that I count the fetal movements for one hour, twice a day." Is this true about betamethasone? Maybe. Clients are told to be aware of fetal movement. Keep it as a possibility.

(3) "I may have insomnia and a rapid heart beat while on this medication." Is this true of betamethasone? Yes. Betamethasone is a corticosteriod. Side effects include insomnia, increased maternal heart rate, and hypertension. Leave this choice in for consideration.

(4) "Bed rest is necessary for the medication to work properly." Is this true about betamethasone? No. Betamethasone will work whether the client is on bed rest or not. Eliminate it.

STEP 4. Note that only answer choices (2) and (3) remain.

STEP 5. Reread the question to make sure you have correctly identified THE REWORDED QUESTION. The reworded question is, "What is true about betamethasone?"

STEP 6. Which choice best answers the question, (2) or (3)? If you are focused on the question, you will select (3). Some students focus on the background information (pregnancy). This question has nothing to do with pregnancy. If you chose (2), you fell for a distracter.

Remember: Focus on the question, and not the background information. If you can answer the question—"What is true about betamethasone?"—without considering the background information (pregnancy), do it. Many students answer a question incorrectly because they don't focus on THE REWORDED QUESTION. Don't fall for the distracters.

At this point you're probably thinking, "Will I have enough time to finish the test using these strategies?" or "How will I ever remember how to answer questions using these steps?" Yes, you will have time to finish the test. Unsuccessful test takers spend time agonizing over test questions. By using these strategies, you will be using your time productively. You will remember the steps because you are going to practice, practice, practice with test questions. You will not be able to absorb this strategy by osmosis; the process must be practiced repeatedly.

Don't Predict Answers

On the NCLEX-RN® exam, you are asked to select the best answer from the four choices that you are given. Many times, the "ideal" answer choice is not there. Don't sit and moan because the answer that you think should be there isn't provided. Remember:

- Identify THE REWORDED QUESTION.
- Select the best answer *from the choices given*.

Look at this question.

> The nurse is explaining the procedure for clean-catch urine specimen collection for culture and sensitivity testing to a male client. Which explanation by the nurse would be **most** accurate?
>
> 1. "The urinary meatus is cleansed with an iodine solution and then a urinary drainage catheter is inserted to obtain urine."
> 2. "You will be asked to empty your bladder one-half hour before the test; you will then be asked to void into a container."
> 3. "Before voiding, the urinary meatus is cleansed with an iodine solution and urine is voided into a sterile container; the container must not touch the penis."
> 4. "You must void a few drops of urine, then stop; then void the remaining urine into a clean container, which should be immediately covered."

STEP 1. Read the question stem.

STEP 2. Focus on the adjectives. "Most accurate" tells you that more than one answer may seem correct.

STEP 3. Reword the question stem. What is true about a clean-catch urine specimen for culture and sensitivity?

STEP 4. Read each answer choice and ask yourself, "Is this true about a clean-catch urine specimen for culture and sensitivity?"

(1) "The urinary meatus is cleansed with an iodine solution and then a urinary drainage catheter is inserted to obtain urine." This choice describes how to obtain a catheterized urine specimen. Urine isn't usually collected by catheterization due to the increased risk of infection. This answer does not answer the question about a clean-catch urine specimen. Eliminate.

(2) "You will be asked to empty your bladder one-half hour before the test; you will then be asked to void into a container." This describes a double-voided specimen. This action is usually done when testing urine for glucose and ketones. It is not relevant to a clean-catch urine specimen. Eliminate.

(3) "Before voiding, the urinary meatus is cleansed with an iodine solution and urine is voided into a sterile container; the container must not touch the penis." This is true of a clean-catch urine specimen for culture and sensitivity. The urinary meatus is cleansed, a sterile container is used, and the penis must not touch the container. Leave it in for consideration.

(4) "You must void a few drops of urine, then stop; then void the remaining urine into a clean container, which should be immediately covered." This does describe a clean-catch urine specimen. The client does void a few drops of urine, stops, and then continues voiding into the container. There is only one problem. For a culture and sensitivity, the container must be sterile. Eliminate.

The correct answer is (3). Many students will select answer choice (4) because they see the expected words: "Void a few drops, then stop; continue voiding." Be careful. This question is a good example of why scanning for expected words could get you into trouble. You may see expected words in an answer choice that is not correct.

Okay. You've practiced how to identify the topic of the question and how to eliminate answer choices. You know that predicting answers does not work on the NCLEX-RN® exam. You are well on your way to correctly answering NCLEX-RN® exam test questions. Unfortunately, this is just the starting point. Let's talk about specific paths and how you can correctly decide which paths to use on the NCLEX-RN® exam. Remember, the correct answer is at the end of the path!

Recognize Expected Outcomes

You spent much of your time in nursing school learning about what might go wrong with clients and their care. This makes sense; after all, nurses need to deal with problems and illnesses. Many test questions that your nursing school faculty wrote focused on what was wrong with clients and their care. In order to prove minimum competence, the beginning practitioner must demonstrate the ability to make appropriate nursing judgments. Competent nursing judgments include recognizing both expected and unexpected behaviors, so it is important for you to recognize expected outcomes on the NCLEX-RN® exam. Expected outcomes are the behaviors and changes you think are going to occur as a result of nursing care. These outcomes allow the nurse to evaluate whether goals have been met.

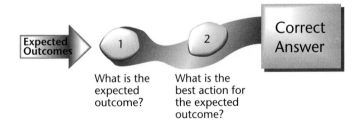

Look at the following question.

> The primary health care provider prescribes arterial blood gas (ABG) analysis for a client receiving oxygen at 6 L/minute. Results show pH 7.37, HCO_3 26 mmHg, pCO_2 42 mmHg, and pO_2 90 mmHg. Which should the nurse do **first**?
>
> 1. Increase the client's oxygen flow rate.
> 2. Elevate the head of the client's bed.
> 3. Document results in the medical record.
> 4. Instruct the client to cough and deep-breathe.

If this question were included on one of your medical/surgical tests, you would assume that a problem was being described. So you would choose an answer choice that involves "fixing" the problem. Let's look at this question.

THE REWORDED QUESTION: "What should you do for a client with these ABG results?"

STEP 1. Interpret the ABG results. Recognize normal. All the results are within normal limits.

STEP 2. Decide how you should use this information. Because all the results normal, let's reword the question again to include this information.

Now THE REWORDED QUESTION is: "What should you do for a client with normal ABG results?"

ANSWERS:

(1) "Increase the client's oxygen flow rate." This is unnecessary because the O_2 level is within normal limits. Eliminate.

(2) "Elevate the head of the client's bed." This is unnecessary because the ABG results are within normal limits. Eliminate.

(3) "Document the results in the medical record." This action should be done because the ABG results are normal.

(4) "Instruct the client to cough and deep-breathe." This is usually recommended in a situation in which there is some limitation of respiratory function, due to immobility or post-operative conditions, for example. The only information you are given in this question is the client's ABG results, which are within normal limits. Although this could be done, you are given no indication that it is necessary. Eliminate.

The correct answer is (3). The ABG results are within normal limits. Some students select answer choice (2) because they think there's something they missed, or it must be a trick question. The "trick" is deciding whether the information that you are given is normal or abnormal, and then answering the question accordingly.

Try this question.

> A client reporting chest pressure is brought to the emergency department (ED). Vital signs include blood pressure 150/90 mmHg, pulse 88 beats/minute, and respirations 20 breaths/minute. The nurse administers nitroglycerin 0.4 mg sublingually as prescribed. After five minutes, the client's vital signs include blood pressure 100/60 mmHg, pulse 96 beats/minute, and respirations 20 breaths/minute. Which action should the nurse take next?
>
> 1. Notify primary health care provider of hypotension and obtain a prescription for IV fluids.
> 2. Place the client in semi-Fowler position and administer oxygen at 4 L/minute.
> 3. Administer a second dose of nitroglycerin 0.4 mg sublingually, as prescribed.
> 4. Document the vital signs and continue to closely monitor the client.

THE REWORDED QUESTION: "What should you do for this client?" To answer this question you need to know what these vital signs indicate.

STEP 1. Recognize normal. Nitroglycerin is a potent vasodilator with anti-anginal, anti-ischemic, and antihypertensive actions. It increases blood flow through the coronary arteries. Side effects include orthostatic hypotension, tachycardia, dizziness, and palpitations. Decreased blood pressure, increased pulse rate, and stable respiratory rate after administration of a potent vasodilator are normal and expected.

STEP 2. Decide how you should use this information. The question should be reworded as, "What should you do for a client who has responded as expected to a dose of nitroglycerin?"

ANSWERS:

(1) "Notify primary health care provider of hypotension and obtain an prescription for IV fluids." The blood pressure has decreased due to vasodilatation. Decreased blood pressure is expected. Eliminate.

(2) "Place the client in semi-Fowler position and administer oxygen at 4 L/minute." Respiratory rate is stable and there is no indication of respiratory distress. Eliminate.

(3) "Administer a second dose of nitroglycerin 0.4 mg sublingually, as prescribed." The nurse should assess the client for chest pain first and administer a second dose of the medication only if the client continues to report chest pain. Eliminate.

(4) "Document the vital signs and continue to closely monitor the client." This is the correct choice. You identified it by recognizing the client's response as normal, thus eliminating the other three answer choices.

The correct answer is (4). You would expect a client's blood pressure to decrease after administration of nitroglycerin. The key to this question is to understand how the medication works and to correctly identify the expected outcome.

Read Answer Choices to Obtain Clues

Because the NCLEX-RN® exam is testing your critical thinking, the topic of the questions may be unstated. You may see a question that concerns a disease process or procedure with which you are unfamiliar. Most test takers who are "clueless" about a question will read the question and answer choices over and over again. They do this because they hope that:

- They will remember seeing the topic in their notes or on a textbook page.
- The light will dawn and they will remember something about the topic.
- They believe there is some clue in the question that will point them toward the correct answer.

What usually happens? Absolutely nothing! The student then randomly selects an answer choice. When you randomly select an answer, you have 1 chance in 4 of getting it right. You can better those odds, and here's how: When you encounter a question that deals with unfamiliar nursing content, look for clues in the answer choices instead of in the question stem.

If you find yourself "clueless" after you carefully read a question, follow these steps:

STEP 1. Resist the impulse to read and reread the question. Read the question only once. Identify the topic of the question. It is often unstated.

STEP 2. Read the answer choices, not to select the correct answer but to figure out, "What is the topic of the question?" or "What should I be thinking?" You are looking for clues from the answer choices.

STEP 3. After reading the answer choices, reword the question using the clues that you have obtained. Then use the strategies previously discussed to answer the question you have formulated.

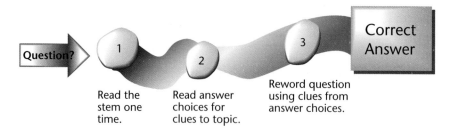

Question? → 1 — Read the stem one time. → 2 — Read answer choices for clues to topic. → 3 — Reword question using clues from answer choices. → Correct Answer

Let's try this strategy with a question.

> A client with type 1 diabetes contacts the home care nurse to report nausea and abdominal pain. What should the nurse advise the client to do?
>
> 1. "Hold your regular dose of insulin."
> 2. "Check your blood glucose level every 3 to 4 hours."
> 3. "Increase consumption of foods containing simple sugars."
> 4. "Increase your activity level."

STEP 1. Read the stem of the question. Can you identify the topic of the question? No, you can't. The nurse is telling the client to do something, but about what topic? The topic is unstated in the question.

STEP 2. Read the answer choices to obtain clues about the topic of the question. Each answer choice deals with ways to maintain a normal blood glucose.

STEP 3. Reword the question: "What does the nurse tell the client about 'sick day rules'?"

ANSWERS:

(1) "Hold your regular dose of insulin." This is an implementation that would increase the blood glucose level. The nurse should assess first. Eliminate.

(2) "Check your blood glucose level every 3 to 4 hours." This is an assessment. Before you can advise the client, you must identify whether the client is hypoglycemic or hyperglycemic. Keep this answer for consideration.

(3) "Increase your consumption of foods containing simple sugars." This is an implementation and would increase the client's blood glucose level. The nurse should assess first. Eliminate.

(4) "Increase your activity level." This is an implementation that would decrease the client's blood glucose level. The nurse should assess first. Eliminate.

The nurse should always assess before implementing nursing care. The correct answer is (2).

No matter how much you prepare for the NCLEX-RN® exam, there may be topics you see on your test with which you are unfamiliar. Reading the answer choices for clues will increase your chances of selecting a correct answer. Remember, you do have a body of knowledge. You just have to be calm and access this knowledge.

Read this question.

> A client is being treated for Addison disease. The primary health care provider prescribes cortisone 25 mg PO daily. The nurse should explain to the client that a dosage adjustment may be required in which situation?
>
> 1. Dosage is increased when the blood glucose level increases.
> 2. Dosage is decreased when dietary intake is increased.
> 3. Dosage is decreased when infection stimulates endogenous steroid secretion.
> 4. Dosage is increased relative to an increase in the level of stress.

Not sure what Addison disease is? Not sure how to adjust the dose of cortisone?

STEP 1. Read the question once. Resist the impulse to reread the question.

STEP 2. Read the answer choices. What should you be thinking? The question concerns cortisone. If the client is receiving cortisone, Addison disease must be something that requires cortisone, a hormone from the adrenal glands. You notice that dosages are both increased and decreased.

STEP 3. Use these clues to reword the question: "What is true about adjusting cortisone dosage?" Consider each answer choice. Does it answer THE REWORDED QUESTION?

(1) "Dosage is increased when the blood glucose level increases." Is this true about cortisone? No. This sounds like insulin. Eliminate.

(2) "Dosage is decreased when dietary intake is increased." Is this true about cortisone? No. Cortisone requirements are not related to diet. Eliminate.

(3) "Dosage is decreased when infection stimulates endogenous steroid secretion." Endogenous means "synthesized within the client." If receiving cortisone for Addison disease, the client must have adrenal insufficiency. Therefore, infection can't stimulate steroid secretion. Eliminate.

The correct answer is (4) because it is the only choice remaining. Even if you are not confident that cortisone is increased during periods of stress, you can conclude that this is the correct answer because the other choices have been eliminated.

If you're not sure about the topic of the question, read the answer choices for clues.

Let's look at another critical thinking path.

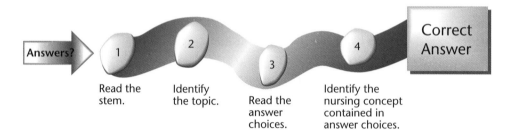

In some questions, the NCLEX-RN® exam asks you to figure out the topic of the question. In other questions you are required to use critical thinking skills to figure out what the answer choices *really* mean. The NCLEX-RN® exam can take a concept with which you are very familiar and make it difficult to recognize. The following question illustrates this point.

> A client with a history of heart failure visits the clinic. The client states, "I have not been feeling like my old self for about 2 weeks." It would be **most** important for the nurse to ask which question?
>
> 1. "Do your ankles swell at the end of the day?"
> 2. "How do you position yourself for sleep?"
> 3. "How do you feel after you eat dinner?"
> 4. "Do you have chest pain when you inhale?"

It is not difficult to identify the topic of this question, "What is a priority for a client with heart failure?" Many students get tripped up on this question by not thinking through the answers as carefully as they should. In some questions, you have to figure out the topic of the question. In this question, you have to figure out what the answer choices mean.

STEP 1. Read the stem of the question.

STEP 2. Reword the question in your own words.

STEP 3. Read the answer choices.

STEP 4. Think: "What nursing concept should I identify in the answer choices?"

THE REWORDED QUESTION: "What is a priority for a client with heart failure?"

ANSWERS:

(1) "Do your ankles swell at the end of the day?" Why would you ask a client this question? Because edema is a symptom of right-sided heart failure. Is right-sided failure your priority? No, left-sided failure takes priority because it affects the lungs. Eliminate this answer.

(2) "How do you position yourself for sleep?" Why would you ask a client this question? If the client sleeps flat in bed, breathing is not compromised. If the client sleeps in a recliner, the client experiences orthopnea, a symptom of left-sided failure. This would be a priority. Keep this answer for consideration.

(3) "How do you feel after you eat dinner?" Why would you ask a client this question? Bloating after meals is a symptom of right-sided failure. This is not as important as breathing problems. Eliminate this answer.

(4) "Do you have chest pain when you inhale?" Why would you ask a client this question? It does indicate a breathing problem. The student who reacts rather than thinks may select this answer. Pain on inspiration may indicate irritation of the parietal pleura of the lung, which is not associated with heart failure. Eliminate this answer.

The correct answer is (2). In order to select this answer, you must recognize that "How do you position yourself for sleep?" represents orthopnea. The NCLEX-RN® exam can take important concepts such as this, and "hide" the concept in some fairly simple behaviors.

Let's try another question where you have to figure out what the answer choices really mean.

> The nurse is caring for a client immediately after a paracentesis. It is **most** important for the nurse to ask which question?
>
> 1. "Do your clothes feel tight?"
> 2. "Do you need to void?"
> 3. "Are you feeling dizzy?"
> 4. "Do you have any pain?"

STEP 1. Read the stem of the question.

STEP 2. Reword the question in your own words.

STEP 3. Read the answer choices.

STEP 4. Think: "What nursing concept should I identify in the answer choices?"

THE REWORDED QUESTION: "What is the highest priority for a client after a paracentesis?"

ANSWERS:

(1) "Do your clothes feel tight?" Why would you ask a client this question? Clothes should fit looser because the abdominal girth has decreased after fluid has been removed with a paracentesis. This is an expected outcome. Eliminate.

(2) "Do you need to void?" Why would you ask a client this question? It is imperative to empty the bladder prior to the procedure, not after the procedure. There is no compelling reason to ask the client this question. Eliminate.

(3) "Are you feeling dizzy?" What makes a client dizzy? One of the causes is a decrease in cerebral perfusion due to a fall in blood pressure. Could this client have a decreased blood pressure? Yes. Hypotension and hypovolemic shock are complications of a paracentesis due to removal of a large volume of fluid. Keep this answer for consideration.

(4) "Do you have any pain?" You ask this question to assess pain level. This client may have discomfort where the paracentesis was performed, but this is an expected outcome. Eliminate.

The correct answer is (3).

Strategy Recap

These questions illustrate why knowing nursing content is not enough to answer application/analysis-level questions. You must be able to effectively use the information you learned in nursing school to answer NCLEX-RN® exam-style test questions.

Review the strategies that you learned in this chapter:

- Reword the question.
- Eliminate answer choices you know to be incorrect.
- Don't predict answers.
- Recognize expected outcomes.
- Read answer choices to obtain clues.

CHAPTER 3

NCLEX-RN® EXAM STRATEGIES

Now that you understand what kind of questions the NCLEX-RN® exam is going to ask, you need to learn more specific strategies for success on the NCLEX-RN® exam.

The NCLEX-RN® Exam Versus Real-World Nursing

Some of you are LPNs or LVNs completing your RN studies, while others are EMTs. Some of you worked during school as student techs. All of you, however, spent time in a clinical setting during your nursing education. All of this adds up to a significant amount of experience. Experience will help you get a job, but answering questions based on your experience can be dangerous on the NCLEX-RN® exam.

Look at the following question.

> On admission to the hospital, an elderly client is confused and appears disheveled and restless. During the client's second day on the unit, a nurse approaches the client to administer medication. The nurse is unable to identify the client because the identification band is missing. Which action by the nurse is **best**?
>
> 1. Have the roommate identify the client.
> 2. Ask the client to state the full name.
> 3. Ask another nurse to visually identify the client.
> 4. Look at photograph in client's medical record.

Let's see how someone using real-world experience would approach this question:

(1) "The roommate is never involved in identification of a client."

(2) "A confused client cannot be relied on for an accurate identification."

(3) "Sounds reasonable. I have seen this done in some circumstances."

(4) "A photograph? What photograph? I've never seen a photograph of a client in a medical record!"

Possible conclusions drawn by this person would include: *"OK, I've seen one nurse ask another for information so (3) must be the answer,"* or *"Well, maybe the client isn't all that confused, so I'll select (2)."*

According to nursing textbooks, asking another health care professional is not the correct way to identify a client. Many acute-care settings now include a photograph of the client in the medical record for just this type of situation. The correct answer to this question is (4). Many students reject this answer because they rarely see photographs of clients in medical records. Real-world experience doesn't count, though; in this case, the client does have a photograph in the medical record.

The NCLEX-RN® exam is a standardized exam administered by NCSBN. Because the NCLEX-RN® exam is a national exam, students should be aware that in some parts of the country, nursing is practiced slightly differently. However, to ensure that the test is reflective of national trends, questions and answers are all carefully documented. The test makers ensure that the correct answers are documented in at least two standard nursing textbooks, or in one textbook and one nursing journal.

When you are unsure of an answer choice, don't ask yourself, "What do they do on my floor?" but "What does the medical/surgical textbook writer Brunner say?" or "What do Potter and Perry say to do?" This test does not necessarily reflect what happens in the real world, but is based on textbook nursing.

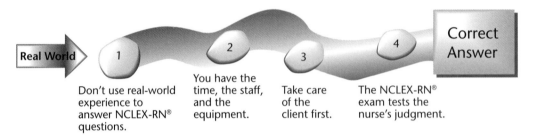

Remember the following when taking the NCLEX-RN® exam:

- You have all of the time and resources you need to provide appropriate care to your client. (Checking for bowel sounds for 5 minutes in all four quadrants, no problem!)
- You have all of the equipment you need. (Remember the bath thermometer you learned to use in the nursing lab? For the NCLEX-RN® exam, you will have one available to test the temperature of bath water.)
- There are no staffing problems on the NCLEX-RN® exam. You are caring only for the client described in the question, and that person is your only concern.
- All care given to clients is "by the book." No shortcuts are used. (You would not turn off an IV solution, flush the line, give another IV solution, flush the line, and then restart the original IV solution that was prescribed to be run continuously.)

Answer the following question.

> A client with a 5-year history of alcohol abuse is treated in the emergency department for acute alcohol intoxication. The client becomes agitated and verbally abusive. Admission prescriptions include chlordiazepoxide 50 mg IM or PO every 4 to 6 hours, as needed for agitation. The nurse should take which precaution after chlordiazepoxide administration?
>
> 1. Restrain the client with the help of a coworker.
> 2. Leave client alone until the sedative takes effect.
> 3. Assign an LPN/LVN to remain with the client.
> 4. Ask the security guard to remain with the client.

Let's look at this using real-world logic.

(1) "Restrain the client with the help of a coworker." Yes, that is done in the real world.

(2) "Leave the client alone until the sedative takes effect." Yes, that is done in the real world, but most students recognize that it is not the best answer.

(3) "Assign an LPN/LVN to remain with the client." Sounds good, but what if you don't have enough staff to assign an LPN/LVN to remain with this client?

(4) "Ask the security guard to remain with the client." Yes, in the real world, security is called when clients are agitated and jeopardize the safety of others.

According to real-world logic, the correct answer must be (1) or (4). However, textbook theoretical nursing practice states that this client should not remain alone while in an agitated state. A professional should remain with the client. Therefore, the correct answer is (3).

Use your real-world experience to help you visualize the client described in the test question, but select your answers based on what is found in nursing textbooks.

Your nursing faculty has probably been conscientious about instructing you in the most up-to-date nursing practice. According to the National Council, the primary source for documenting correct answers is in nursing textbooks, and the most up-to-date practice might not always agree with the textbooks. When in doubt, always select the textbook answer!

The next question illustrates this point.

> A client is admitted to the hospital in active labor. After delivery of a healthy newborn, the client decides to bottle-feed. Which statement by the client after a teaching session indicates to the nurse that the client needs further instruction?
>
> 1. "I'll pump my breasts and use warm packs to relieve breast pain."
> 2. "I'll wear a tight bra and apply ice packs to relieve engorgement discomfort."
> 3. "I'll take the prescribed pain medicine when I have pain or discomfort."
> 4. "I'll take the prescribed pills to help stop the production of milk."

Let's look at these answers more closely.

(1) Pumping the breasts will stimulate milk production. This is clearly wrong.

(2) Wearing a tight bra and applying ice packs are appropriate interventions for a nonbreastfeeding mother.

(3) Taking a medication (mild analgesic) is an appropriate intervention for a nonbreastfeeding mother.

(4) Medication to prevent lactation is not frequently prescribed because of potentially dangerous side effects. However, a medication may be prescribed to prevent lactation. This would be considered an appropriate intervention.

The correct answer is (1).

First Take Care of the Client, Then the Equipment

The NCLEX-RN® exam tests your ability to use critical thinking skills to make nursing judgments. It is very important that you remember to:

- Take care of the client first.
- Take care of the equipment second.

Look at the following question.

A client who sustained a fractured left femur in a car accident is placed in balanced suspension skeletal traction using a Thomas splint and a Pearson attachment. The client reports "terrible" pain in the left thigh. Which should the nurse do **first**?

1. Determine that the traction apparatus weights and ropes are aligned and hanging free.
2. Ask the client about characteristics and location of the pain.
3. Check the Thomas splint and Pearson attachment to ensure proper positioning.
4. Explain to the client that pain in the affected leg is expected.

Let's review the answers:

(1) Check the traction apparatus for correct positioning. While weights should be hanging free in balanced suspension skeletal traction, this answer choice has you checking the equipment. Your first concern should be the client, not the traction.

(2) Ask the client to describe the pain. All reports of pain should be thoroughly investigated by the nurse. Keep this option for consideration.

(3) Confirm proper positioning of the Thomas splint and Pearson attachment. This answer choice also has you checking the equipment. Your first concern should be the client.

(4) Explain that pain in the affected leg is expected. This response is incorrect. Any reports of pain are considered abnormal, and you should investigate them thoroughly.

The nurse should focus on assessing the client and the reported problem before assessing the function of the equipment. The correct answer is (2).

Laboratory Values

Answering questions about laboratory values is another example of how the real world does not work on the NCLEX-RN® exam. In nursing school, you learned laboratory values for a specific test and you may not have remembered them after the test. While you were in the clinical setting, the emphasis was on interpretation of laboratory values. Because most laboratory slips contained a listing of normal values, you were able to compare the client's results to the normal values. Questions on the NCLEX-RN® exam will not provide you with a listing of normal laboratory values.

To answer questions on the NCLEX-RN® exam, you must:

- Know normal laboratory test results.
- Correctly interpret normal or abnormal laboratory test results.

Compare the following two questions.

> A client is admitted to the hospital with influenza-like symptoms. When taking the history, the nurse learns that the client has been taking digoxin 0.125 mg PO daily and furosemide 40 mg PO daily for 3 years. Last month the primary health care provider changed the prescription for digoxin to 0.25 mg PO daily. The nurse would expect the primary health care provider to prescribe which laboratory tests?
>
> 1. Serum electrolyte and digoxin levels.
> 2. White blood cell count and hemoglobin level.
> 3. Cardiac enzymes and arterial blood gas analysis.
> 4. Blood culture and sensitivity and urinalysis.

You are probably familiar with the concepts presented in this question. The primary health care provider has increased the client's dose of digoxin. Furosemide, a loop diuretic, inhibits resorption of sodium and chloride; side effects include hypotension, hypokalemia, GI upset, and weakness. Hypokalemia may increase the client's risk of digitalis toxicity. Serum electrolyte and digoxin levels (1) is the correct answer.

Now look at this question.

> The nurse is planning care for a client admitted with fever, vomiting, and diarrhea. The nurse identifies the nursing diagnosis: "fluid volume deficit" in the client's plan of care. Which of the following changes in laboratory values would demonstrate an improvement in the client's condition?
>
> 1. Urine specific gravity, 1.015; hematocrit, 37%.
> 2. Urine specific gravity, 1.020; hematocrit, 45%.
> 3. Urine specific gravity, 1.032; hematocrit, 52%.
> 4. Urine specific gravity, 1.025; hematocrit, 35%.

In order to correctly answer this question, you must know:

- The specific gravity of urine (1.010–1.030) and the normal levels of hematocrit (male 42–50%, female 40–48%)
- How the specific gravity and hematocrit levels are affected by a fluid volume deficit

Fluid volume deficit occurs when water and electrolytes are lost in the same proportion as they exist in the body. When a client becomes dehydrated, both the specific gravity of urine and the hematocrit become elevated. The correct answer is (2).

Answer the following question.

> A client is hospitalized with a diagnosis of atrial fibrillation. The primary health care provider prescribes heparin 5,000 units every 12 hours by subcutaneous injection and daily partial thromboplastin times (PTT). The result of the client's most recent PTT is 55 seconds. Which action should be taken by the nurse?
>
> 1. Document the results and administer the heparin.
> 2. Withhold the heparin.
> 3. Notify primary health care provider of test results.
> 4. Have the test repeated.

In order to answer this question you need to know:

- Normal PTT ranges 20–45 seconds.
- The therapeutic range for a client receiving heparin, an anticoagulant, is 1.5–2 times the control or normal level.
- To calculate the therapeutic range, take the lower number for the normal range for a PTT (20) and multiply it by 1.5. The result is 30. Multiply the higher number (45) by 2. The result is 90. Any result that falls within 30 to 90 seconds is considered therapeutic. The goal is to keep the PTT within this range.

Evaluate the answer choices:

(1) "Document the results and administer the heparin." The client's most recent PTT is 55 seconds. This falls within the therapeutic range of 30 to 90 seconds, so the nurse should administer the medication.

(2) "Withhold the heparin." A side effect of heparin is bleeding. If the PTT is greater than 90 seconds, the nurse should notify the primary health care provider.

(3) "Notify primary health care provider of test results." There is no reason to notify the primary health care provider, since the PTT falls within therapeutic range.

(4) "Have the test repeated." There is no reason to have the test repeated.

The correct answer is (1).

Medication Administration

An important function in providing safe and effective care to clients is the administration of medications. Because this is one of the responsibilities of a beginning practitioner, questions about medications are often an important part of the NCLEX-RN® exam. The nurse who is minimally competent is knowledgeable about medications and uses the "rights" of medication administration.

In nursing school, most questions about medication followed the same pattern. You were told the client's diagnosis and the name of the medication, and then were asked a question. Even if you didn't know the information about the medication, sometimes you were able to select the correct answer by knowing the diagnosis.

The NCLEX-RN® exam does not give you any clues from the context of the question. The questions on this exam include the name of the medication, generally identifying it by generic name only. Most of the time, you will not be given the reason the client is receiving the medication.

Let's look at some medication questions.

> The primary health care provider prescribes furosemide and spironolactone for a client. Prior to administering the medications, the nurse determines that the client's potassium level is 3.2 mEq/L (3.2 mmol/L). In addition to notifying the primary health care provider, the nurse should anticipate taking which action?
>
> 1. Hold both the furosemide and spironolactone.
> 2. Administer the spironolactone only.
> 3. Administer the furosemide only.
> 4. Administer the furosemide and spironolactone.

This is a typical exam-style medication question. The question concerns the side effects and nursing implications of furosemide and spironolactone.

(1) "Hold both the furosemide and spironolactone." The potassium level falls below normal (3.5–5 mEq/L [3.5 –5 mmol/L]). Furosemide is a potassium-wasting diuretic and spironolactone is a potassium-sparing diuretic. There is no reason to hold the spironolactone because the client has a low potassium level. Eliminate this answer.

(2) "Administer the spironolactone only." The spironolactone should be administered.

(3) "Administer the furosemide only." The client's potassium level is already low, and furosemide is a potassium-wasting diuretic. Do not administer furosemide. Eliminate.

(4) "Administer the furosemide and spironolactone." Do not administer the furosemide. Eliminate.

The correct answer is (2).

Let's try this next question.

> A client returns to the clinic 2 weeks after being started on allopurinol 200 mg PO daily. The nurse reviews information about this medication with the client. Which statement by the client indicates that the teaching was effective?
>
> 1. "I should take my medication on an empty stomach."
> 2. "I should take my medication with orange juice."
> 3. "I should increase my intake of protein."
> 4. "I should drink at least 8 glasses of water every day."

To answer this question you need to know information about allopurinol, an antigout agent that reduces uric acid.

(1) "I should take my medication on an empty stomach." Allopurinol is best tolerated with or immediately after meals to reduce gastrointestinal (GI) irritation. Eliminate.

(2) "I should take my medication with orange juice." Orange juice makes the urine acidic. Allopurinol is more soluble in alkaline urine. Eliminate.

(3) "I should increase my daily intake of protein." It is not necessary to increase the intake of protein when taking allopurinol. Eliminate.

(4) "I should drink at least 8 glasses of water daily." Allopurinol can cause renal calculi. The client should drink 3,000 mL/day to reduce the risk of renal calculi formation.

The correct answer is (4). You must know the side effects and nursing implications of medications for the NCLEX-RN® exam.

Notify the Primary Health Care Provider

Another behavior that commonly occurs in the real world is calling the primary health care provider. In nursing school you were encouraged to notify your instructor of changes in your client's condition. Be very careful how you handle this on the NCLEX-RN® exam. More often than not, the answer choice that states "notify the primary health care provider," "contact the social worker," or "refer to the chaplain" is the WRONG answer. Usually there is something you need to do first before you make that call. The NCLEX-RN® exam does not want to know what the primary health care provider is going to do. The NCLEX-RN® exam wants to know what you, the registered professional nurse, will do in a given situation.

Answer this question.

A client is receiving a unit of red blood cells. Several minutes after the start of the infusion, the client reports itching and develops hives on the chest and abdomen. Which action should the nurse take **first**?

1. Slow the transfusion rate.
2. Call primary health care provider for an antihistamine prescription.
3. Mix IV fluid with the red blood cells to dilute the unit of blood.
4. Stop the transfusion.

THE REWORDED QUESTION: "What should you do *first* for a client experiencing symptoms of an allergic reaction during a transfusion?

It sounds like the client is having an allergic reaction to the transfusion. If this is what's going on, what should you do?

(1) "Slow the transfusion rate." If the client is experiencing a transfusion reaction, slowing the rate of the transfusion is not the right action.

(2) "Call primary health care provider for an antihistamine prescription." Antihistamines are given for allergic reactions. The primary health care provider needs to be notified. This answer might be a possibility, but is there something you should do first?

(3) "Mix IV fluid with the red blood cells to dilute the unit of blood." Mixing IV fluids with blood helps decrease the viscosity of red blood cells. This doesn't have anything to do with an allergic transfusion reaction. Eliminate.

(4) "Stop the transfusion." If the client was experiencing a transfusion reaction, the best action is to stop the transfusion. This is the correct action to take first, before calling the primary health care provider.

The correct answer is (4). After the transfusion is stopped, you will contact the primary health care provider and an antihistamine will probably be prescribed.

Before you want to choose the answer choice that involves "notify the primary health care provider," look at the other answer choices very carefully. Make sure that there isn't an answer that contains an assessment or action you should do before notifying the primary health care provider. The test makers want to know what you would do in a situation, not what the primary health care provider would do!

Here is one more real-world question.

> While returning from lunch, the nurse is approached in the elevator by an employee from another unit. The employee states that a close friend is a client on the nurse's unit. The employee asks about the friend's condition and if all tests were normal. How should the nurse respond?
>
> 1. Answer the employee's questions softly to prevent others from overhearing.
> 2. Refuse to discuss the friend's medical condition.
> 3. Refer the employee to the client's primary health care provider for information.
> 4. Tell the employee the client's normal test results.

THE REWORDED QUESTION: "What should a nurse do when asked about a client by a hospital employee?"

(1) Answer softly. Discussing client information in a public place is a breach of confidentiality. Eliminate.

(2) Refuse to discuss. Refusing to discuss a client's medical condition does not violate the client's right to privacy and confidentiality. Keep in consideration.

(3) Refer to the client's provider. Providing any information about a client to someone not directly involved in the client's care is a breach of privacy. Eliminate.

(4) Share the normal test results. It is a breach in the client's right to privacy to share information with others without the client's permission. Eliminate.

The correct answer is (2).

Expect to see real-world situations on your NCLEX-RN® exam, but make sure that you do not choose real-world answers! These strategies should help you use your previous nursing experience without encountering any pitfalls.

Strategies for Priority Questions

You will recognize priority questions on the NCLEX-RN® exam because they will ask you what is the "best," "most important," "first," or "initial response" by the nurse.

Take a look at this sample question.

> An hour after admission to the nursery, the nurse observes a newborn having spontaneous, jerky limb movements. The newborn's mother had gestational diabetes mellitus (GDM) during the pregnancy. Which action should the nurse take **first**?
>
> 1. Administer dextrose water.
> 2. Call primary health care provider immediately.
> 3. Determine the blood glucose level.
> 4. Observe the client for associated symptoms.

As you read this question you are probably thinking, "All of these look right!" or "How can I decide what I will do first?" The panic sets in as you try to decide what the best answer is when they all seem "correct."

As a registered nurse, you will be caring for clients who have multiple problems and needs. You must be able to establish priorities by deciding which needs take precedence over the other needs. You probably recognized the newborn's spontaneous, jerky limb movements as a sign of hypoglycemia. Don't forget that an important part of the assessment process is *validating* what you observe. You must complete an assessment before you analyze, plan, and implement nursing care. The correct answer is (3).

The following situation might sound familiar: You are called to a client's room by a family member and find the client lying on the floor. The client is bleeding from a wound on the forehead, and the indwelling urinary catheter is dislodged and hanging from the side of the bed. Where do you begin? Do you call for help? Do you return the client to bed? Do you apply pressure to the cut? Do you reinsert the catheter? Do you notify the primary health care provider? What do you do *first*? This is why establishing priorities is so important.

Your nursing faculty recognized the importance of teaching you how to establish priorities. They required you to establish priorities both in clinical situations and when answering test questions. These are the type of questions that nursing students find most controversial.

Here is an example of a nursing school test question:

> Which of the following would most concern the nurse during a client's recovery from surgery?
>
> 1. Safety.
> 2. Hemorrhage.
> 3. Infection.
> 4. Pain control.

A conversation in class with your instructor may then go something like this:

INSTRUCTOR: "The correct answer is (2)."

STUDENT: "Why isn't infection the correct answer? It says right here" [pointing to textbook] "that infection is a major complication after surgery."

INSTRUCTOR: "Yes, infection is an important concern after surgery. But if the client has a life-threatening hemorrhage, then the fact that the wound is infected is immaterial."

STUDENT: "But you can't count this answer wrong!"

In some situations, the faculty member will give you partial credit for your answer, or will "throw the question out" because there is more than one right answer. But you won't get the opportunity to argue about questions on the NCLEX-RN® exam. You either select the answer the test makers are looking for, or you get the question wrong. In the question given, all of the answers listed are important when caring for a postoperative client, but only one answer is the *best*.

The critical thinking required for priority questions is for you to recognize patterns in the answer choices. By recognizing these patterns, you will know which path you need to choose to correctly answer the question. There are three strategies to help you establish priorities on the NCLEX-RN® exam:

- Maslow strategy
- Nursing process strategy
- Safety strategy

We will outline each strategy, describe how and when it should be used, and show you how to apply these strategies to exam-style questions. By using these strategies, you will be able to eliminate the second-best answer and correctly identify the highest priority.

Strategy One: Maslow

Maslow's hierarchy of needs (Figure 3.1) is crucial to establishing priorities on the NCLEX-RN® exam. Maslow identifies five levels of human needs: physiological, safety or security, love and belonging, esteem, and self-actualization.

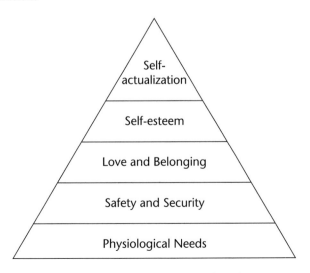

Figure 3.1 Maslow's Hierarchy of Needs

Because *physiological needs* are necessary for survival, they have the highest priority and must be met first. Physiological needs include oxygen, fluid, nutrition, temperature, elimination, shelter, rest, and sex. If you don't have oxygen to breathe or food to eat, you really don't care if you have stable psychosocial relationships!

Safety and security needs can be both physical and psychosocial. Physical safety includes decreasing what is threatening to the client. The threat may be an illness (myocardial infarction), accidents (a parent transporting a newborn in a car without using a car seat), or environmental threats (the client with COPD who insists on walking outside in 10° F [−12° C] temperatures).

To attain psychological safety, the client must have the knowledge and understanding about what to expect from others in the environment. For example, it is important to teach the client and family what to expect after a stroke. It is also important that you allow a client preparing for a mastectomy to verbalize her concerns about changes that might occur in her relationship with her partner.

To achieve *love and belonging,* the client needs to feel loved by family and accepted by others. When a client feels self-confident and useful, that client will achieve the need of *self-esteem* as described by Maslow.

The highest level of Maslow's hierarchy of needs is *self-actualization.* To achieve this level, the client must experience fulfillment and realize their potential. In order for self-actualization to occur, all of the lower-level needs must be met. Because of the stresses of life, lower-level needs are not always met, and many people never achieve this high level of functioning.

The Maslow Four-Step Process

The first strategy to use in establishing priorities is a four-step process, beginning with Maslow's hierarchy. To use the Maslow strategy, you must first recognize the pattern in the answer choices.

STEP 1. Look at your answer choices.

Determine if the answer choices are both physiological and psychosocial. If they are, apply the Maslow strategy detailed in Step 2.

STEP 2. Eliminate all psychosocial answer choices. If an answer choice is physiological, don't eliminate it yet. Remember, Maslow states that physiological needs must be met first. Though pain has a physiologic component, reactions to expected pain are considered "psychosocial" on this exam and given lower priority. However, pain that is acute, severe, or not relieved as expected with treatment requires immediate assessment.

STEP 3. Look at each of the answer choices that you have not yet eliminated and ask yourself if the answer choice makes sense with regard to the disease or situation described in the question. If it makes sense as an answer choice, keep it for consideration and go on to the next choice.

STEP 4. Can you apply the ABCs?

Look at the remaining answer choices. Can you apply the ABCs? The ABCs stand for airway, breathing, and circulation. If there is an answer that involves maintaining a patent airway, it will be correct. If not, is there a choice that involves breathing problems? It will be correct. If not, go on with the ABCs. Is there an answer pertaining to the cardiovascular system? It will be correct. What if the ABCs don't apply? Compare the remaining answer choices and ask yourself, "What is the highest priority?" This is your answer.

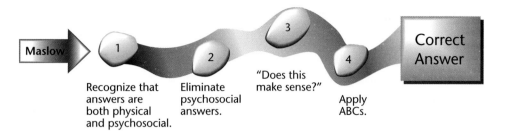

Let's apply this technique to a few sample exam-style test questions.

A client is admitted to the hospital with a ruptured ectopic pregnancy. A laparotomy is scheduled. Preoperatively, which intervention is **most** important for the nurse to include on the client's plan of care?

1. Fluid replacement.
2. Therapeutic communication.
3. Emotional support.
4. Oxygen therapy.

Look at the stem of the question. The words *most important* mean:

- This is a priority question.
- There probably will be more than one answer choice that is a correct nursing action, but only one will be the most important or highest priority action.

STEP 1. Look at the answer choices.

You see that both physical and psychosocial interventions are included. Apply Maslow.

STEP 2. Eliminate all psychosocial answer choices.

Answer choice (2), which is therapeutic communication, should be discarded. Remember, therapeutic communication falls under psychosocial interventions on the NCLEX-RN® exam. Answer choice (3), emotional support, is also a psychosocial intervention. Eliminate this answer. You have now eliminated two of the possible choices.

STEP 3. Now look at the remaining answer choices and ask yourself if they make sense.

Answer choice (1), fluid replacement, makes sense because this client has a ruptured ectopic pregnancy. An ectopic pregnancy is implantation of the fertilized ovum in a site other than the endometrial lining, usually the fallopian tube. Initially, the pregnancy is normal; but as the embryo outgrows the fallopian tube, the tube ruptures, causing extensive bleeding into the abdominal cavity. Answer choice (4), oxygen therapy, doesn't make sense with a ruptured ectopic pregnancy. The obstetrical client is not likely to need respiratory care prior to surgery. Eliminate this answer choice.

You are left with the correct answer, (1). After reading this question, many students select answer choice (2) or (3) as the correct answer. They justify this by emphasizing the importance of managing this client's emotional distress, or addressing her grief about losing the pregnancy. Neither answer choice takes priority over the physiological demand of fluid replacement prior to surgery.

Ready for another question? Try this one.

> The nurse obtains a diet history from a pregnant 16-year-old client. The client tells the nurse that a typical daily diet includes cereal and milk for breakfast, pizza and soda for lunch, and a cheeseburger, milk shake, fries, and salad for dinner. Which is the **most** accurate nursing diagnosis based on this data?
>
> 1. Impaired nutrition: more than body requirements related to high-fat intake.
> 2. Deficient knowledge: nutrition in pregnancy.
> 3. Impaired nutrition: less than body requirements related to increased nutritional demands of pregnancy.
> 4. Potential for injury: fetal malnutrition related to poor maternal diet.

The first thing you should notice about this question stem is the phrase *"most accurate."* This alerts you that there may be more than one answer choice that could be considered correct.

STEP 1. Look at the answer choices.

You will see that both physical and psychosocial interventions are included. Apply the Maslow strategy.

STEP 2. Eliminate all psychosocial answer choices. In this case, that means answer choice (2). Deficient knowledge is a psychosocial need.

STEP 3. Ask yourself whether the remaining answer choices make sense.

(1) "Impaired nutrition: more than body requirements related to high-fat intake" does make sense. This diet is high in fat.

(3) "Impaired nutrition: less than body requirements related to increased nutritional demands of pregnancy" also makes sense. This diet has an adequate number of calories, but it is deficient in the needed vitamins and minerals.

(4) "Potential for injury: fetal malnutrition related to poor maternal diet" does not make sense. There is an adequate number of calories to support fetal growth. Eliminate this choice.

You have now eliminated two of the choices. Let's go on.

STEP 4. Answer choices (1) and (3) remain. Can you apply the ABCs to these choices? No. So compare the answer choices. Which is higher priority: the fact that this pregnant 16-year-old client's diet contains too much fat, or that the diet does not have enough nutrients? Insufficient nutrients is a higher priority, so the correct answer is (3).

Many students, when they first read this question, choose (2), deficient knowledge. According to Maslow, physiological needs always take priority over psychosocial needs. Using this strategy on the NCLEX-RN® exam will enable you to choose the correct answer.

Now, let's try another question.

> The nurse plans care for an adolescent client admitted with anorexia nervosa. On admission, the client weighs 82 lb (37 kg) and is 5'4" (162 cm) tall. Laboratory test results indicate severe hypokalemia, anemia, and dehydration. The nurse should give which nursing diagnosis the **highest** priority?
>
> 1. Body image disturbance related to weight loss.
> 2. Self-esteem disturbance related to feelings of inadequacy.
> 3. Impaired nutrition: less than body requirements related to decreased intake.
> 4. Deficient cardiac output related to the potential for dysrhythmias.

The first thing you should notice in this question stem is the phrase *"highest priority."* This alerts you that there may be more than one answer that could be considered correct.

STEP 1. Look at the answer choices.

Both physical and psychosocial interventions are included. Apply the Maslow strategy.

STEP 2. Eliminate all psychosocial answer choices.

It is easy to see that answer choice (1), body image disturbance, is a psychosocial concern. The same is true of answer choice (2), self-esteem disturbance. Answer choices (3) and (4) are physiological. You have now eliminated all but two answer choices.

STEP 3. Ask yourself whether the remaining answer choices make sense.

Answer choice (3), "Impaired nutrition: less than body requirements related to decreased intake," does make sense. Remember, the client has anorexia nervosa, is 5'4" tall (162 cm), and weighs 82 lb (37 kg). Answer choice (4), "Deficient cardiac output related to the potential for dysrhythmias," also makes sense. Dysrhythmias are a concern for a client with severe hypokalemia, which often occurs with anorexia nervosa.

You still have work to do.

STEP 4. Can you apply the ABCs? Yes.

Deficient cardiac output is a higher priority than altered nutrition. One answer choice remains: (4).

When you first read this question, you probably identified each of the answer choices as appropriate for a client with anorexia nervosa. Only one nursing diagnosis can be the highest priority. By using strategies involving Maslow and the ABCs, you will choose the correct answer on your NCLEX-RN® exam.

Strategy Two: Nursing Process (Assessment versus Implementation)

A second strategy that will assist you in establishing priorities involves the assessment and implementation steps of the nursing process. As a nursing student, you have been drilled so that you can recite the steps of the nursing process in your sleep—assessment, analysis, planning, implementation, and evaluation. In nursing school, you did have some test questions about the nursing process, but you probably did not use the nursing process to assist you in selecting a correct answer on an exam. On the

NCLEX-RN® exam, you will be given a clinical situation and asked to establish priorities. The possible answer choices will include both the correct assessment and implementation for this clinical situation. How do you choose the correct answer when both the correct assessment and implementation are given? Think about these two steps of the nursing process.

Assessment is the process of establishing a data profile about the client and their health problems. The nurse obtains subjective and objective data in a number of ways: talking to clients, observing clients and/or significant others, taking a health history, performing a physical examination, evaluating laboratory results, and collaborating with other members of the health care team.

Once you collect the data, you compare it to the client's baseline or normal values. On the NCLEX-RN® exam, the client's baseline may not be given, but as a nursing student you have acquired a body of knowledge. On this exam, you are expected to compare the client information you are given to the "normal" values learned from your nursing textbooks.

Assessment is the first step of the nursing process and takes priority over all other steps. It is essential that you complete the assessment phase of the nursing process before you implement nursing activities. This is a common mistake made by NCLEX-RN® exam takers: don't implement before you assess. For example, when performing cardiopulmonary resuscitation (CPR), if you don't access the airway before performing mouth-to-mouth resuscitation, your actions may be harmful!

Implementation is the care you provide to your clients. Implementation includes: assisting in the performance of activities of daily living (ADLs), counseling and educating the client and the client's family, giving care to clients, and supervising and evaluating the work of other members of the health team. Nursing interventions may be independent, dependent, or interdependent. Independent interventions are within the scope of nursing practice and do not require supervision by others. Instructing the client to turn, cough, and breathe deeply after surgery is an example of an independent nursing intervention. Dependent interventions are based on the written orders of a primary health care provider. On the NCLEX-RN® exam, you should assume that you have an order for all dependent interventions that are included in the answer choices.

This may be a different way of thinking from the way you were taught in nursing school. Many students select an answer on a nursing school test that is later counted wrong because the intervention requires a primary health care provider's order. Everyone walks away from the test review muttering, "Trick question." It is important for you to remember that there are no trick questions on the NCLEX-RN® exam. You should base your answer on an understanding that you have a primary health care provider's order for any nursing intervention described.

Interdependent interventions are shared with other members of the health team. For instance, nutrition education may be shared with the dietitian. Chest physiotherapy may be shared with a respiratory therapist.

The following strategy, utilizing the assessment and implementation phases of the nursing process, will assist you in selecting correct answers to questions that ask you to identify priorities.

STEP 1. Read the answer choices to establish a pattern.

If the answer choices are a mix of assessment/validation and implementation, use the Nursing Process (Assessment vs. Implementation) strategy.

STEP 2. Refer to the question to determine whether you should be assessing or implementing.

STEP 3. Eliminate answer choices, and then choose the best answer.

If after Step 2 you find that, for example, it is an assessment question, eliminate any answers that clearly focus on implementation. Then choose the best assessment answer.

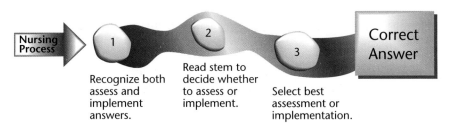

Try this strategy on the next question.

> The parent of a client with type 1 diabetes calls the primary health care provider's office to discuss the child's self-monitoring blood glucose (SMBG) home reading. The client's blood glucose level is being tightly regulated with a combination of NPH and regular insulin before breakfast and supper. The past two mornings the blood glucose levels were 220 mg/dL (12.2 mmol/L) and 210 mg/dL (11.7 mmol/L). Which of the following should the nurse tell the client's parent?
>
> 1. "Continue with the current medication regimen."
> 2. "Check blood glucose level during the night."
> 3. "Administer NPH insulin later in the evening."
> 4. "Serve the bedtime snack earlier in the evening."

THE REWORDED QUESTION: "What advice should the nurse give the parent about their diabetic child who is hyperglycemic in the morning?"

STEP 1. Read the answer choices to establish a pattern.

There is one assessment answer, (2), and three implementation answers, (1), (3), and (4). You can use the Nursing Process (Assessment vs. Implementation) strategy.

STEP 2. Refer to the question to determine whether you should be assessing or implementing.

The client's parent tells you that blood glucose levels have been elevated the last 2 mornings. This indicates that there is a problem. According to the nursing process, you should assess first.

STEP 3. Eliminate answer choices, and then choose the best answer.

Eliminate answers (1), (3), and (4), which are implementation answers. You are left with only one answer choice, (2). This question is about the Somogyi effect, which is rebound hyperglycemia that occurs in response to a rapid decrease in blood glucose level during the night. Treatment includes adjusting the evening diet, changing the insulin dose, and altering the amount of exercise to prevent nocturnal hypoglycemia. Even if you've never heard of the Somogyi effect, you are still able to correctly answer this question using the Nursing Process (Assessment vs. Implementation) strategy.

Let's look at another question.

> A child biking to school hit the curb and then fell, injuring the leg. The school nurse was called and found the child alert and conscious, but in severe pain with a possible right femur fracture. Which is the **first** action that the nurse should take?
>
> 1. Immobilize the affected limb with a splint and ask the client not to move.
> 2. Assess the circumstances surrounding the accident.
> 3. Place the client in semi-Fowler position for comfort.
> 4. Assess the neurovascular status of both legs and compare the findings.

The words *"first action"* tell you that this is a priority question.

THE REWORDED QUESTION: "What is the highest priority for a fractured femur?"

STEP 1. Read the answer choices to establish a pattern.

The answer choices are a mix of assessment and implementation. Use the Nursing Process (Assessment vs. Implementation) strategy.

STEP 2. Refer to the question to determine whether you should be assessing or implementing.

According to the question, the nurse has determined that the child has a possible femur fracture. This implies that the nurse has completed the assessment step. It is now time to implement.

STEP 3. Eliminate answer choices, and then choose the best answer.

Eliminate answers (2) and (4) because they are assessments. This leaves you with choices (1) and (3). Which takes priority: immobilizing the affected limb, or placing the client in a semi-Fowler position to facilitate breathing? The question does not indicate any respiratory distress. The correct answer is (1), immobilize the affected limb.

Some students will choose an answer involving the ABCs without thinking it through. Students, beware. Use the ABCs to establish priorities, but make sure that the answer is appropriate to the situation. In this question, breathing was mentioned in one of the answer choices. If you had chosen the ABCs immediately without looking at the context of the question, you would have answered this question incorrectly.

Look at this question in another form.

> A child biking to school hit the curb and then fell. The child tells the school nurse, "I think my leg is broken." Which is the **first** action the nurse should take?
>
> 1. Immobilize the affected limb with a splint and ask the client not to move.
> 2. Ask the client to explain what happened.
> 3. Place the client in semi-Fowler position to facilitate breathing.
> 4. Check the appearance of the client's leg.

In this question, the client has stated, "My leg is broken." This statement is not the nurse's assessment. This alerts the nurse that there is a problem, and the nurse should begin the steps of the nursing process. The first step is assessment, so eliminate answers (1) and (3); these are implementations. So what takes priority? Assessment of the injured leg takes priority over an assessment of what happened to cause the accident. The correct answer is (4).

Strategy Three: Safety

Nurses have the primary responsibility of ensuring the safety of clients. This includes clients in health care facilities, in the home, at work, and in the community. Safety includes: meeting basic needs (oxygen, food, fluids, etc.), reducing hazards that cause injury to clients (accidents, obstacles in the home), and decreasing the transmission of pathogens (immunizations, sanitation).

Remember that the NCLEX-RN® exam is a test of minimum competency to determine that you are able to practice safe and effective nursing care. Always think *safety* when selecting correct answers on the exam. When answering questions about procedures, this strategy will help you to establish priorities.

STEP 1. Are all the answer choices implementations? If so, use the Safety strategy illustrated here.

STEP 2. Can you answer the question based on your knowledge? If not, continue to Step 3.

STEP 3. Ask yourself, "What will cause the client the least amount of harm?" and choose the best answer.

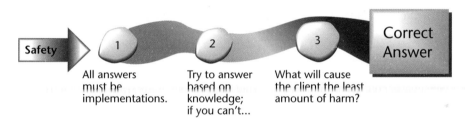

Apply this strategy to the following question.

> A pediatric client undergoes a tonsillectomy for treatment of chronic tonsillitis unresponsive to antibiotic therapy. After surgery, the client is brought to the postanesthesia care unit. Which action should the nurse include in the client's plan of care?
>
> 1. Institute measures to minimize crying.
> 2. Perform postural drainage every 2 hours.
> 3. Cough and deep-breathe hourly.
> 4. Provide ice cream as tolerated.

THE REWORDED QUESTION: What should you do after a tonsillectomy?

STEP 1. Are all the answer choices implementations? Yes.

STEP 2. Can you answer the question based on your knowledge of a tonsillectomy? If not, continue to Step 3.

STEP 3. Ask yourself, "What will cause the client the least amount of harm?"

(1)   Minimizing crying will help prevent bleeding. Keep in consideration.

(2)   Postural drainage may cause bleeding. Eliminate.

(3)   Coughing and deep-breathing may cause bleeding. Eliminate.

(4)   Providing ice cream may cause the client to clear the throat, causing bleeding. Eliminate.

The correct answer is (1). The nurse must prevent postoperative hemorrhage, a complication seen after this type of surgery. Crying would irritate the client's throat and increase the chance of hemorrhage.

Let's try another question.

> A client is receiving intravenous cimetidine. After 20 minutes of the infusion, the client reports a headache and dizziness. Which action should the nurse take **first**?
>
> 1. Stop the infusion.
> 2. Assess vital signs.
> 3. Reposition the client.
> 4. Call the pharmacist.

THE REWORDED QUESTION: What should you do if a client experiences side effects to a medication being administered?

STEP 1. Are all answers implementations? Yes.

STEP 2. Can you answer this question based on your knowledge? If not, proceed to Step 3.

STEP 3. Ask yourself, "What will cause the client the least amount of harm?"

(1)   Stopping the infusion would not harm the client. If the symptoms described are due to a side effect of the medication, this action would help the client. Retain this choice.

(2)   Assessing vital signs would not harm the client. Retain it for consideration.

(3)   Repositioning the client would not harm the client, but would not help the client. Eliminate.

(4)   Calling the pharmacist would not harm the client, but would not help the client. Eliminate.

Choices (1) and (2) are left to consider. The infusion may be the cause of the client's reported symptoms. The client's vital signs can be taken after the infusion is stopped. Choice (1) is the correct answer.

Let's look at one more question.

A client admitted with a diagnosis of dementia attempts several times to remove the nasogastric tube. The nurse receives a prescription for wrist restraints. Which action by the nurse is **most** appropriate?

1. Attach the ties of the wrist restraints to the client's bed frame.

2. Perform daily range-of-motion exercises to the restrained extremities.

3. Remove the restraints when the client is out of bed in a wheelchair.

4. Explain restraint need to the family only, because the client is confused.

THE REWORDED QUESTION: What is the safest way to apply restraints?

STEP 1. Are all answers implementations? Yes.

STEP 2. Can you answer based on your knowledge? If not, proceed to Step 3.

STEP 3. Ask yourself, "What will cause the client the least amount of harm?"

(1) Attaching the restraint ties to the client's bed frame will not harm the client. Retain this answer.

(2) Performing daily range-of-motion exercises will not harm the client. However, they should be performed more frequently. Retain this answer.

(3) Removing the restraints when the client is out of bed in a wheelchair will be harmful to the client. Restraints should not be removed when the client is unattended. Eliminate.

(4) Explaining the need for restraints only to the family can cause harm to the client. Restraints can increase the confusion or combativeness of the client. Even though confused, the client needs to receive an explanation. Eliminate.

You are now considering answer choices (1) and (2). What will cause the least amount of harm to the client—attaching the ties of the restraint to the bed frame, or performing daily range-of-motion exercises to the extremities? Range-of-motion exercises should be performed every 2 to 4 hours to prevent loss of joint mobility. Eliminate (2). The correct answer is (1). Attaching the ties of the restraints to the bed frame will allow the nurse to raise and lower the side rail without injury to the client.

Priority questions are an important component of the NCLEX-RN® exam. To help you select correct answers, think:

- Maslow
- The Nursing Process
- Safety

Answer the following three questions using the appropriate priority strategy. The explanations follow the questions.

Question 1

> The nurse is caring for a client with a diagnosis of stroke. The nurse is feeding the client in a chair when the client suddenly begins to choke. Which action should the nurse take **first**?
>
> 1. Assess the client for breathlessness.
> 2. Leave the client in the chair and apply vigorous abdominal or chest thrusts.
> 3. Ask the client, "Are you choking?"
> 4. Return the client to the bed and apply vigorous abdominal or chest thrusts.

Question 2

> A client with a history of bipolar disorder is admitted to the psychiatric hospital. The client was found by the police attempting to climb onto the wing of a plane at the airport. A family member reports that the client has not eaten or slept in 2 days, and suspects the client has stopped taking lithium. On admission, the nurse should place the **highest** priority on which client care need?
>
> 1. Teaching the client about the importance of taking lithium as prescribed.
> 2. Providing the client with a safe environment with few distractions.
> 3. Arranging for food and rest for the client.
> 4. Setting limits on the client's behavior.

Question 3

> The primary health care provider prescribes a nasogastric (NG) tube insertion to low intermittent suction for a client diagnosed with an intestinal obstruction. Two hours after NG tube insertion, the client vomits 200 mL. While irrigating the NG tube, the nurse notes resistance. Which action should the nurse take **first**?
>
> 1. Replace the NG tube with a larger one.
> 2. Turn the client on the left side.
> 3. Implement continuous NG tube suction.
> 4. Continue NG tube irrigation.

Let's see if you were able to correctly identify which strategy you should use to determine priorities.

Question 1

The answer choices include both assessments and implementations. Use the Nursing Process strategy to select the correct answer.

STEP 1. Read the answer choices to establish a pattern.

Choices (1) and (3) are assessments; choices (2) and (4) are implementations.

STEP 2. Refer to the question to determine whether you should be assessing or implementing. According to the situation, the client has begun to choke. This alerts the nurse that there is a problem. The first step of the Nursing Process is to assess.

STEP 3. Eliminate answer choices, and then choose the best answer.

Eliminate answer choices (2) and (4) because they are implementations. Now choose the best answer from the remaining answer choices, (1) and (3).

What takes priority—assessing for breathlessness or assessing the client by asking, "Are you choking?" Inability to speak or cough indicates airway obstruction. Breathlessness should be assessed only in an unconscious client. The correct answer is (3).

Question 2

Look at the answer choices. They include both physiological and psychosocial interventions. Apply the Maslow strategy.

STEP 1. Look at the answer choices and identify which are physiological—choices (2) and (3)—and which are psychosocial—choices (1) and (4).

STEP 2. Eliminate all psychosocial answer choices—(1) and (4).

STEP 3. Ask yourself if the remaining answer choices make sense. Choice (2), providing the client with a safe environment, does make sense. Retain this answer. Choice (3), arranging for food and rest, also makes sense. Retain this answer.

STEP 4. Can you apply the ABCs to the remaining answer choices? No; neither choice refers to airway, breathing, or circulation. Since the ABCs don't apply, ask yourself "What is the highest priority—providing for a safe environment, or providing for food and rest?" According to Maslow, food and rest take highest priority. The correct answer is (3).

Question 3

This question is about a procedure: What should the nurse do when resistance is met while irrigating an NG tube? If you are unsure about a procedure, think *safety*.

STEP 1. Are all the answer choices implementations? Yes.

STEP 2. Can you answer the question based on your knowledge? If not, continue to Step 3.

STEP 3. Ask yourself, "What will cause the client the least amount of harm?"

(1) Replacing the NG tube with a larger one could harm the client by damaging the mucosa. Eliminate.

(2)   Turning the client to the left side would not hurt the client. Retain this answer.

(3)   Changing the NG tube suction from intermittent to continuous is never done because it will erode the mucosa. Eliminate.

(4)   Continuing the irrigation when there is resistance might be harmful. Never force an irrigation. Eliminate.

The correct answer is (2). The tip of the tube may be against the stomach wall. Repositioning the client might allow the tip to lie unobstructed in the stomach.

Using these critical thinking strategies will help you unlock the secrets of correctly answering priority questions. Now let's look at some strategies for answering another type of question, Management of Care.

Strategies for Management of Care Questions

Every three years, the National Council conducts a job analysis study to determine the activities required of a newly licensed registered nurse. Based on this study, the National Council adjusts the content of the test to accurately reflect what is happening in the workplace. This ensures that the NCLEX-RN® exam tests what is needed to be a safe and effective nurse.

The role of the nurse has expanded in today's health care environment. In addition to providing quality client care, the nurse is also responsible for coordination and supervision of care provided by other health care workers. Many health care settings are staffed by registered nurses, licensed practical nurses/licensed vocational nurses (LPN/LVNs), and unlicensed assistive personnel (UAPs) such as nursing assistants and support staff. It is the responsibility of the registered nurse to coordinate the efforts of these health care workers to provide affordable quality client care. Appropriate supervision of LPN/LVNs and/or UAPs by the registered professional nurse is essential for safe and effective client care.

To reflect these changes, the NCLEX-RN® exam contains questions about delegation and assignment of client care. There are several reasons why you may find these questions difficult to answer correctly on the NCLEX-RN® exam:

- Many nursing schools test the content presented in the management course with essay questions rather than multiple choice questions.

- You may have received lectures regarding management of care, but your clinical rotation in management may have been less than ideal. Regardless, do not choose answers based on decisions you may have observed during your clinical experience in the hospital or clinic setting. Remember, the NCLEX-RN® exam is ivory-tower nursing. Always ask yourself, "Is this textbook nursing care?"

- Your experience may have been restricted to caring for one or two clients without any opportunity to supervise others, or you may have spent time on a hospital unit providing client care under the supervision of a preceptor.

Even if you have no direct experience in these areas, the Rules of Management will get you through the test. They will help you choose more right answers when answering management questions on the NCLEX-RN® exam.

Rule #1: Do not delegate the functions of assessment, evaluation, and nursing judgment.

During your nursing education, you learned that assessment, evaluation, and nursing judgment are the responsibility of the registered professional nurse. You *cannot* give this responsibility to someone else.

Rule #2: Delegate activities for stable clients with predictable outcomes.

If the client is unstable, or the outcome of an activity not assured, it should not be delegated.

Rule #3: Delegate activities that involve standard, unchanging procedures.

Activities that frequently reoccur in daily client care can be delegated. Bathing, feeding, dressing, and transferring clients are examples. Activities that are complex or complicated should not be delegated.

Rule #4: Remember priorities!

Remember Maslow, the ABCs, and "stable versus unstable" when determining which client the RN should attend to first. Keep in the mind that you can see only one client or perform one activity when answering questions that require you to establish priorities.

The Rules of Management

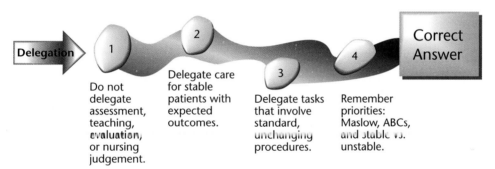

Let's use the Rules of Management to eliminate answer choices in exam-like Management of Care questions.

> A client with a compound fracture of the left femur is being admitted to a pediatric unit. Which action is **best** for the nurse to take?
>
> 1. Ask the unlicensed assistive personnel (UAP) to obtain the client's vital signs while the nurse obtains a history from the parents.
> 2. Ask the LPN/LVN to assess the peripheral pulses of the client's left leg while the nurse completes the admission forms.
> 3. Ask the LPN/LVN to stay with the client and parents while the nurse obtains phone orders from the primary health care provider.
> 4. Ask the UAP to obtain equipment for the client's care while the nurse talks with the child and the parents.

STEP 1. Reword the question in your own words.

The question asks what the nurse should do when a pediatric client with a fractured femur is first admitted. That question is very broad. To establish *exactly* what is being asked, you must read the answer choices. In each answer, the RN is delegating tasks to the LPN/LVN or UAP. The real question is, "What is appropriate delegation?"

STEP 2. Eliminate answer choices based on the Rules of Management.

(1)   Obtaining vital signs is an important part of assessment. According to Rule #1, the registered nurse cannot delegate assessment. Eliminate this answer choice.

(2)   Checking the peripheral pulses is an important assessment for this client because of the diagnosis of a fractured left femur. The nurse needs to assess the client before delegating activities to someone else. Assessment of the client is much more important than completing paperwork. Eliminate.

(3)   The LPN/LVN is with the client and parents while the nurse phones for provider orders. There is no assessment, evaluation, or nursing judgment involved in this option, so leave it in for consideration.

(4)   The nurse is with the client and the parents while the UAP obtains needed equipment. There is no assessment, evaluation, or nursing judgment when gathering equipment, so leave this choice in for consideration.

STEP 3. Select an answer from the remaining choices.

You are left with answer choices (3) and (4). You are halfway to the correct answer!

Answer (3) indicates that the nurse is on the phone and the LPN/LVN is with the client. Have you seen this done in the real world? Probably. Is this what nursing textbooks and journals say should be done in this situation? Probably not. Eliminate this answer. Remember, on the NCLEX-RN® exam, emphasis is placed on providing care to clients according to how nursing care is defined in textbooks and journals.

The correct answer is (4). The nurse is caring for the client and the parents while delegating tasks to the UAP.

Let's look at another Management of Care question.

Which task is appropriate for the nurse to delegate to an experienced UAP?

1.   Obtain a 24-hour diet recall from a client recently admitted with anorexia nervosa.

2.   Obtain a clean-catch urine specimen from a client with suspected urinary tract infection.

3.   Observe the characteristics of the continuous bladder irrigation returns for a client after a transurethral resection.

4.   Observe a client newly diagnosed with diabetes mellitus practice injection techniques using an orange.

STEP 1. Reword the question.

"What task will you assign to a UAP?" The fact that the UAP is "experienced" is a distracter.

STEP 2. Eliminate answer choices based on the Rules of Management.

(1)   Obtain 24-hour diet recall from a client with anorexia nervosa. Some students may consider this answer choice because eating is certainly a recurring daily activity, but this answer isn't about feeding a client. Eating has special significance for a client with anorexia nervosa. An important assessment that the nurse must make is the quantity of food consumed by this client. The nurse cannot delegate assessment. Eliminate.

(2)   Obtain a clean-catch urine specimen from a client with suspected urinary tract infection. Rule #4 states, "Delegate activities that involve standard, unchanging procedures." There is no indication that the client has a catheter, so this is a routine procedure. Keep for consideration.

(3)   Observe bladder irrigation returns after a transurethral resection. The color of the fluid needs to be assessed to determine if hemorrhage is occurring. This is an assessment. Eliminate.

(4)   Observe a client newly diagnosed with diabetes mellitus practicing injection techniques. This answer choice involves the evaluation of client teaching. According to Rule #1, the nurse cannot delegate evaluation of client care. Eliminate.

STEP 3. Select an answer from the remaining choices.

That leaves only answer choice (2), the correct answer.

Let's look at one more question.

Which client should the nurse on a pediatric unit assign to an LPN/LVN?

1. A toddler-age client admitted yesterday with laryngotracheobronchitis who has a tracheostomy.

2. A preschool-age client admitted after gastric lavage for acetaminophen ingestion.

3. A school-age client admitted for a fracture of the femur, in balanced suspension traction.

4. A school-age client admitted for observation after an acute asthma attack.

STEP 1. Reword the question.

The question is asking for the appropriate assignment for an LPN/LVN.

STEP 2. Eliminate answer choices based on the Rules of Management.

After reading the answer choices, you may have already seen that Rule #3 (Delegate activities for stable clients with predictable outcomes) will be particularly helpful.

(1)   "A toddler-age client admitted yesterday with laryngotracheobronchitis who has a tracheostomy." Ask yourself, is this a stable client with a predictable outcome? A 3-year-old child with a new tracheostomy is not stable or predictable. Eliminate this answer choice.

(2) "A preschool-age client admitted after gastric lavage for acetaminophen ingestion." This child may be unstable and the outcome of a poisoning is unpredictable. Eliminate this answer choice.

(3) "A school-age client admitted for a fracture of the femur, in balanced suspension traction." This child has a problem that has a predictable outcome. No information is provided in the choice to lead you to believe that this child is unstable at this time. Keep this answer choice in consideration.

(4) "A school-age client admitted for observation after an acute asthma attack." Because of the narrow airway of a child, this child may be unstable and the outcome is unpredictable. Eliminate this answer choice.

STEP 3. Select an answer from the remaining choices.

Answer choice (3) is the correct answer.

Strategies for Positioning Questions

Because many illnesses affect body alignment and mobility, you must be able to safely care for these clients in order to be an effective nurse. These topics are also important on the NCLEX-RN® exam. The successful test taker must correctly answer questions about impaired mobility and positioning.

Immobility occurs when a client is unable to move about freely and independently. To answer questions on positioning, you need to know the hazards of immobility, normal anatomy and physiology, and the terminology for positioning.

Many graduate nurses are not comfortable answering these questions because:

- They don't understand the "whys" of positioning.
- They don't know the terminology.
- They have difficulty imagining the various positions.

If you have difficulty answering positioning questions, the following strategy will assist you in selecting the correct answer.

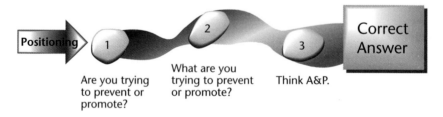

STEP 1. Decide if the position for the client is designed to prevent something or promote something.

STEP 2. Identify what it is you are trying to prevent or promote.

STEP 3. Think about anatomy, physiology, and pathophysiology ("A&P").

STEP 4. Which position best accomplishes what you are trying to prevent or promote?

Does this sound a little confusing? Hang in there. Let's walk through a question using this strategy.

> Immediately after a percutaneous liver biopsy, the nurse should place the client in which position?
>
> 1. Supine.
> 2. Right side-lying.
> 3. Left side-lying.
> 4. Semi-Fowler.

Before you read the answers, let's go through the four steps.

STEP 1. By positioning the client after a liver biopsy, are you trying to prevent something or promote something? Think about what you know about a liver biopsy. You position a client after this procedure to prevent something.

STEP 2. What are you trying to prevent? The most serious and important complication after a percutaneous liver biopsy is hemorrhage.

STEP 3. Think about the principles of anatomy, physiology, and pathophysiology. What do you do to prevent hemorrhage? You apply pressure. Where would you apply pressure? On the liver. Where is the liver? On the right side of the abdomen under the ribs.

STEP 4. How should the client be positioned to prevent hemorrhage from the liver, which is on the right side of the body? Look at your answer choices.

(1) Supine. If you lay the client flat on the back, no pressure will be applied to the right side. Eliminate.

(2) Right side-lying. If you lay the client in a right side-lying position, will pressure be applied to the right side? Yes. Keep it in for consideration.

(3) Left side-lying. No pressure is applied to the right side. Eliminate.

(4) Semi-Fowler. If you lay the client on the back with the head partially elevated, no pressure is applied to the right side. Eliminate.

The correct answer is (2). Some students select (3) because they don't know normal anatomy and physiology. Some students select (4) because semi-Fowler position is used for so many different reasons.

Things to Remember

- Even if you didn't memorize what position to use before, during, and after a procedure, think about the question for a moment. You can figure out what position is needed.

- You cannot figure out the correct position if you do not know what the terms (such as *supine* or *Fowler*) mean.

- You cannot figure out a correct position if you do not know anatomy and physiology. If you think the liver is on the left side of the body, you are in trouble!

- You cannot figure out a correct position if you do not know what you are trying to accomplish. If you couldn't remember that a complication after a liver biopsy is hemorrhage, you will simply be taking a random guess at the correct answer.
- If you think in images, you should form a mental image of each position. Picture yourself placing the client in each position, and then see if the position makes sense.

Let's try another question using the strategies for positioning.

> An angiogram is scheduled for a client with decreased circulation to the right leg. After the angiogram, the nurse should place the client in which position?
>
> 1. Semi-Fowler with right leg bent at the knee.
> 2. Side-lying with a pillow between the knees.
> 3. Supine with right leg extended.
> 4. High-Fowler with right leg elevated.

Let's go through the steps.

STEP 1. By positioning the client after an angiogram, are you trying to prevent something or promote something? You are trying to promote something.

STEP 2. What are you trying to promote? Adequate circulation of the right leg.

STEP 3. Think about the principles of anatomy, physiology, and pathophysiology. What promotes adequate circulation in the right leg? Keeping the leg at or below the level of the heart so blood flow is not constricted.

STEP 4. How will the client be positioned after an angiography to prevent constriction of vessels and keep the right leg at or below the level of the heart? Look at the answer choices.

(1) "Semi-Fowler with right leg bent at the knee." The head of the bed is elevated 30–45 degrees in this position. The leg is lower than the heart. If the right leg is bent at the knee, this could constrict arterial blood flow. Eliminate.

(2) "Side-lying with a pillow between the knees." Use of a pillow in this position could create pressure points in the right leg. You don't want the knees bent. Eliminate.

(3) "Supine with right leg extended." In this position, the leg is at the level of the heart. Circulation will not be constricted because the leg is straight. Keep for consideration.

(4) "High-Fowler with right leg elevated." The head of the bed is elevated 60–90 degrees in this position. Elevating the leg promotes venous return. Eliminate.

The correct answer is (3). The client is on bed rest for 8–12 hours in a supine position after an angiogram.

If you didn't know the specific positioning needed after an angiogram, you can apply your knowledge to select the correct answer by just thinking about it.

Let's look at another question.

> The nurse is caring for a client after a lumbar laminectomy. Which statement **best** describes the method of turning a client following lumbar laminectomy?
>
> 1. The head of the bed is elevated 30 degrees; the client locks the knees when turning.
> 2. A pillow is placed between the client's legs; the body is turned as a unit.
> 3. The client straightens the back and grasps the side rail on the opposite side of the bed.
> 4. The head of the bed is flat; the client bends the knees and rolls to the side.

This question isn't about positioning after a procedure. It asks how to turn the client after surgery.

STEP 1. When turning the client after a laminectomy, are you trying to prevent or promote something? Promote.

STEP 2. What are you trying to promote? A straight back. The client can't bend or twist the torso.

STEP 3. Think about the principles of anatomy, physiology, and pathophysiology. A laminectomy is removal of one or more vertebral laminae. After a laminectomy, the back should be kept straight.

STEP 4. How should the client be turned in order to keep the back straight?

(1) If the head of the bed is elevated 30 degrees, the back will not be straight. Eliminate.

(2) If a pillow is placed between the legs and the body is rolled as a unit, the client's back will be kept straight. Keep in for consideration.

(3) If the client grabs the opposite side rail, the client's torso will twist. The back will not be straight even though the client straightened the back before turning and twisting. Eliminate.

(4) If the head of the bed is flat, the client's back will be straight. If the client bends the knees and rolls to the side, the back will not be kept straight. Eliminate.

The correct answer is (2). That is a textbook description of log-rolling. But if you didn't recall log-rolling, you were able to select the correct answers by thoughtfully considering each answer choice.

Sometimes a positioning question will be difficult to identify, such as in the following example.

> The nurse is caring for a client after an appendectomy. The client continues to report discomfort to the nurse shortly after receiving an analgesic. Which measure by the nurse would be **most** appropriate?
>
> 1. Notify the primary health care provider.
> 2. Place the client in Fowler position.
> 3. Gently massage the client's abdomen.
> 4. Provide the client with reading material.

As you can see, not all of the answer choices involve positioning! How should you approach this question?

First, reword the question so you know what to focus on in the answer choices. The question really being asked is, "What should the nurse do to help this client with pain relief?" Let's look at the answer choices.

(1)   Calling the primary health care provider, as you know, is almost never the right answer. See if another answer choice is more appropriate.

(2)   Fowler position. Why change this client's position? To promote pain relief. Will Fowler position decrease the client's pain? Yes, by relieving pressure on the client's abdomen. This answer is a possibility.

(3)   Massaging the client's abdomen will increase the client's pain. Eliminate.

(4)   Providing the client with reading materials might distract the client from the discomfort, but this is not an appropriate intervention for a client in pain. Eliminate.

The correct answer is (2).

Positioning is an important part of the NCLEX-RN® exam. You must be able to answer these questions correctly in order to prove your competence. If you use the strategies just discussed, you will be thinking about nursing principles and you will select correct answers!

Essential Positions to Know for the NCLEX-RN® Exam

POSITION	THERAPEUTIC FUNCTION
Flat (supine)	Avoids hip flexion, which can compress arterial flow
Dorsal recumbent	Supine with knees flexed; more comfortable
Side lateral	Allows drainage of oral secretions
Side with leg bent (Sims)	Allows drainage of oral secretions; used for rectal exam
Head elevated (Fowler) • High-Fowler: 60–90 degrees • Fowler: 45–60 degrees • Semi-Fowler: 30–45 degrees • Low-Fowler: 15–30 degrees	Increases venous return; allows maximal lung expansion
Feet and leg elevated	Increases blood return to heart
Feet elevated and head lowered (Trendelenburg)	Used to insert central venous pressure (CVP) line, or for treatment of umbilical cord compression
Feet elevated 20 degrees, knees straight, trunk flat, and head slightly elevated (modified Trendelenburg)	Increases venous return; used for shock; may be used to prevent shock

POSITION	THERAPEUTIC FUNCTION
Elevation of extremity	Increases venous return; decreases blood volume to extremity
Flat on back, thighs flexed, legs abducted (lithotomy)	Increases vaginal opening for examination
Prone	Promotes extension of hip joint; not well tolerated by persons with respiratory or cardiovascular difficulties
Knee-chest	Provides maximal visualization of rectal area

Strategies for Communication Questions

Communication is emphasized on the NCLEX-RN® exam because it is critical to your success as a beginning practitioner. Therapeutic communication means listening to and understanding the client while promoting clarification and insight. It enables the nurse to form a working relationship with both the client and the health care team, using both verbal and nonverbal communication. Remember that nonverbal communication is the most accurate reflection of attitude. Therapeutic responses include the following:

RESPONSE	GOAL/PURPOSE
Using silence	Allows the client time to think and reflect; conveys acceptance. Allows the client to take the lead in conversation
Using general leads or broad opening	Encourages the client to talk. Indicates your interest in the client. Allows the client to choose the subject.
Clarification	Encourages recall and details of a particular experience. Encourages description of feelings. Seeks explanation; pinpoints specifics.
Reflecting	Paraphrases what the client says. Reflects on what client says, especially the feelings conveyed.

There are many questions on the NCLEX-RN® exam that require you to select the correct therapeutic communication response. As with other NCLEX-RN® exam questions, one of the biggest errors that test takers commit when trying to answer this type of question is to look for the correct answer. Remember, you are selecting the *best* answer from the four possible answers that you are given.

To select the best answer, you must eliminate answer choices. Let's look at some different answer choices you can eliminate:

- **"Don't worry" answers:** Eliminate answer choices that offer false reassurance. This type of response discourages communication between the nurse and the client by not allowing the client to explore their own ideas and feelings. False reassurance also discounts what the client is feeling. Examples include:
  - "It's going to be OK."
  - "Don't worry. Your doctors will do everything necessary for your care."

- ***"Let's explore" answers:*** Another incorrect answer choice that many graduate nurses select is the choice that includes the word "explore." On the NCLEX-RN® exam, avoid being a junior psychiatrist. It isn't the nurse's role to delve into the reasons why the client is feeling a particular way. The client must be allowed to verbalize the fact that they are sad, angry, fearful, or overwhelmed. Examples include:
  - "Let's talk about why you didn't take your medication."
  - "Tell me why you really injured yourself."

- ***"Why" questions:*** Eliminate answer choices that include "why" questions: ones that seek reasons or justification. "Why" questions imply disapproval of the client, who may become defensive. A "why" question can come in many forms, and need not always begin with "why." Any response that puts the client on the defensive is nontherapeutic and therefore incorrect. Examples include:
  - "What makes you think that?"
  - "Why do you feel this way?"

- ***Authoritarian answers:*** Eliminate answer choices in which the nurse is telling the client what to do without regard for the client's desires or feelings. Examples include:
  - Insisting that the client follow unit rules
  - Insisting that the client do what you command immediately

- ***Nurse-focused answers:*** Eliminate answer choices in which the focus of the comment is on the nurse. Be careful, because these answer choices may sound very empathetic. The focus of your communication should always be on the client. Examples include:
  - "That happened to me once."
  - "I know from experience this is hard for you."

- ***Closed-ended questions:*** Eliminate answer choices that include closed-ended questions that can be answered with the words yes, no, or another monosyllabic response. Closed-ended questions discourage the client from sharing thoughts and feelings. Examples include:
  - "Are you feeling guilty about what happened?"
  - "How many children do you have?"

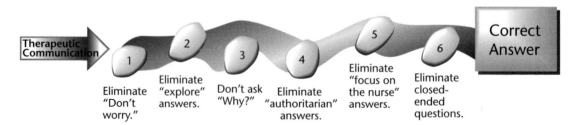

Eliminating these types of nontherapeutic responses that appear as answer choices is an effective strategy when answering therapeutic communication questions. Don't simply look for the specific words that you see here; you may need to "translate" the answer choices into the above errors of therapeutic communication.

So how do you select the correct response? By choosing from the answer choices that are left! The correct response will usually contain one or both of the following elements:

- *Gives correct information:* Offering information encourages further communication from the client. Examples of giving correct information include:
  - "You are experiencing acute alcohol withdrawal; you may see and feel things that aren't real."
  - "There are many reasons for memory loss; tell me more about what you have noticed."

- *Is empathetic and reflects the client's feelings: Empathy* is the ability to perceive what another person experiences using that person's frame of reference. *Reflection* communicates to the client that the nurse has heard and understands what the client is trying to communicate. When reflecting feelings, the nurse focuses on the feelings and not the content of what is said. Examples of empathetic, reflective statements include:
  - "I can see that you are frightened about being here."
  - "You seem very upset. Tell me how you're feeling."

Let's practice therapeutic communication with a few exam-style questions.

> A client is admitted to the emergency department with a diagnosis of acute myocardial infarction. The client tells the nurse, "I'm scared. I think I'm going to die." Which response by the nurse would be **most** appropriate?
>
> 1. "Everything is going to be fine. We'll take good care of you."
> 2. "I know what you mean. I thought I was having a heart attack once."
> 3. "I'll call your primary health care provider so you can discuss it."
> 4. "It's normal to feel frightened. We're doing everything we can for you."

STEP 1. Eliminate incorrect answer choices.

(1) "Everything is going to be fine. We'll take good care of you." This is a "don't worry" response. There is no acknowledgment of the client's fears. Eliminate.

(2) "I know what you mean. I thought I was having a heart attack once." The focus of this response is on the nurse, not the client. Eliminate.

(3) "I'll call your primary health care provider so you can discuss it." It is within the scope of nursing practice for the nurse to respond to the client's feelings. Don't pass the responsibility to the primary health care provider. Eliminate.

(4) "It's normal to feel frightened. We're doing everything we can for you." This answer choice responds to feelings and provides information. Keep it in consideration.

STEP 2. Select an answer from the remaining choices.

One answer was not eliminated: (4). This is the correct answer. The nurse is empathetic, acknowledging that the client feels frightened, and provides information.

Let's look at another question.

> A client is to undergo a breast biopsy. The client tells the nurse, "If I lose my breast, I know my husband will no longer find me attractive." Which response by the nurse would be **most** appropriate?
>
> 1. "You don't know if you are going to lose your breast. They are just doing the biopsy now."
> 2. "You should focus on your children. They are young and they need you."
> 3. "You seem to be concerned that your relationship with your husband might change."
> 4. "Why don't you wait and see what your husband's reaction is before you get upset."

STEP 1. Eliminate answer choices.

(1) "You don't know if you are going to lose your breast. They are just doing the biopsy now." This response gives false reassurance and discounts the client's feelings. Eliminate it.

(2) "You should focus on your children. They are young and they need you." This response is authoritarian: the nurse tells the client what to do. Eliminate it.

(3) "You seem to be concerned that your relationship with your husband might change." This response reflects the fears of the client. The response is open-ended and allows the client to express personal feelings. Keep it in for consideration.

(4) "Why don't you wait and see what your husband's reaction is before you get upset." This response dismisses the client's feelings and gives advice. Eliminate it.

STEP 2. Select an answer from the remaining choices.

You have eliminated three of the four answer choices. The correct answer is the only answer choice remaining, (3).

Let's look at one more question.

> A client in the psychiatric unit asks the nurse, "Am I in a special radioactive shelter? When was it last checked for radioactivity?" Which response by the nurse would be **most** appropriate?
>
> 1. "This is a hospital, and we do not have a nuclear medicine department here."
> 2. "Don't worry, you're safe. There's no radioactivity here."
> 3. "I'm sure your safety is of concern to you, but this is a hospital."
> 4. "Please share with me what makes you think there is radioactivity here."

STEP 1. Eliminate answer choices.

(1) "This is a hospital, and we do not have a nuclear medicine department here." This response provides information. Leave it in for consideration.

(2)   "Don't worry, you're safe. There's no radioactivity here." This response offers false reassurances. Eliminate it.

(3)   "I'm sure your safety is of concern to you, but this is a hospital." This response reflects the client's concern about safety and provides information. Keep it in for consideration.

(4)   "Please share with me what makes you think there is radioactivity here." This response allows the client to verbalize, but you don't want to encourage a client with psychological problems to talk about hallucinations or delusions. Rather, you want your discussion to focus on the feelings that accompany them. Eliminate this choice.

STEP 2. Select an answer from the remaining choices.

You have more than one possible answer choice: (1) and (3). Look for the answer choice that reflects feelings and gives information. The correct answer is (3).

Your NCLEX-RN® Exam Study Plan

Now that you've read about the various Kaplan test taking strategies, you are probably thinking, "Wow! This is great!" Most of you have started identifying why you are having difficulty answering application/analysis-level test questions. Some of you have already formulated a plan to master your NCLEX-RN® exam questions using the strategies outlined in this book, and are confident that you will pass the exam. Others are thinking, "This sounds great, but can I really answer questions using these strategies?"

The authors of this book work for Kaplan, the oldest test prep company in the nation. We have been preparing graduate nurses and international nurses for the NCLEX-RN® exam for more than 40 years. We know what works to prepare for the exam and what doesn't work.

Ineffective Ways to Prepare

Here are a few of the biggest mistakes some NCLEX-RN® exam test takers make before Test Day.

Relying on False Hopes

Some students use what is known as the "hope" method of study. "I hope that I don't have questions about chest tubes on the test." "I hope that I don't have questions about medication on my test." "I hope that I have questions about ABGs because I did great on that test in school." The "hope" method usually doesn't work very well. The test pool contains thousands of questions. How many topics do you "hope" won't be on your test?

Lacking Respect for the Exam

Many candidates for the NCLEX-RN® exam are good students in school. Because of their school success, they expect to pass the exam with minimal preparation. After all, it's just a test of minimum competency. These students do some studying, but they really believe there is no chance they might fail this exam. You might think that you can't possibly fail, but if you do not respect this exam and prepare for it correctly, you run the risk of failure.

All students know why they take the NCLEX-RN® exam. However, after interviewing hundreds of students, we have discovered that many graduate nurses have no idea what the exam content is. How can you effectively study for a test if you don't know what content the exam tests? Learn what is on the NCLEX-RN® exam, and then you will realize that preparation with a review course or a planned method of study is essential.

Cramming

Some students completed nursing school with a minimal understanding of nursing content. These students studied long and hard on the night before a nursing school test, cramming as many facts into their heads as they could remember. Because the test questions primarily involved recognition and recall, cramming worked for tests in nursing school. But as we said earlier, the NCLEX-RN® exam is not an exam about facts. It tests your ability to apply the knowledge that you have learned and to think critically. Recognition and recall will not work!

Planning Poorly

As with all standardized exams, you must work on your areas of weakness. This is hard to do because there's usually a reason you're weak in an area. Some graduate nurses, for example, profess a weakness in or dislike for obstetrical nursing. Some students didn't understand the theory, while other students had a poor clinical experience or didn't get to see many deliveries; still other students simply didn't like this rotation. Whatever the reason, it causes them to have a weakness in this particular area. In order to pass a standardized test, you must work on your areas of weakness.

Some students don't establish a plan of study. Other students establish a plan of study but don't follow it. You can enroll in a review course or buy review books, but if you don't apply yourself, they will do you no good.

Effective Methods of Preparation

To pass the NCLEX-RN® exam, you not only need to know nursing content, you also need to be able to apply the critical thinking skills we've just reviewed. Next, you need to be an expert on the content of the exam. What topics are usually included on the NCLEX-RN® exam? How is the content organized? And finally, you need to create a study plan, and make sure that you are able to cope with the testing experience.

So let's start by talking about some of the issues that you may be asking yourself.

QUESTION: "I'm terrible at standardized tests. Is this really going to help me?"

ANSWER: Yes, these strategies will help you choose more correct responses when you take the NCLEX-RN® exam. Read this book—more than once if necessary—to review the content being tested on the exam and learn the strategies. Then practice, practice, practice. Use the strategies to answer many, many practice test questions, and you will find yourself answering more and more questions correctly. Tear out the Summary of Critical Thinking Paths in Appendix A and consult it while you are answering practice test questions. This will help you become more comfortable with putting the strategies into practice. As you answer more and more questions, put the diagram aside and rely on your memory to identify and implement a critical thinking strategy.

QUESTION: "Am I going to have enough time when I take the NCLEX-RN® exam to figure out which strategy to use?"

ANSWER: Timing is a concern on the NCLEX-RN® exam. You need to maximize your efforts on each test question. Practice answering test questions using the various strategies we've outlined. As you get more proficient, you will discover that it takes you less time to identify the strategy or path that will lead you to the correct answer.

QUESTION: "I don't have to use these strategies on every question, do I? I think I'll use them only when I can't figure out the correct answer on my own."

ANSWER: Wrong! You should use critical thinking to answer every question on the NCLEX-RN® exam to make sure that you pass. Go through the steps that we have outlined for every practice question that you answer as you prepare for the exam. If you practice these steps, you will not need to randomly guess the correct answer on the NCLEX-RN® exam.

QUESTION: "So all I have to do is memorize the strategies, right?"

ANSWER: Just memorizing the various strategies will not ensure your success on the NCLEX-RN® exam. Remember, the exam does not test your ability to memorize either critical thinking strategies or nursing content. The NCLEX-RN® exam tests your ability to think critically and use the nursing knowledge that you have. It's relatively easy to just memorize nursing content. The hard part is to figure out how to use this knowledge to make nursing judgments. It's relatively easy to memorize the critical thinking strategies. The hard part is to figure out which strategy to use on each and every question. That takes practice.

QUESTION: "What if I use the strategies but still can't figure out the correct answer?"

ANSWER: It's not unusual that students will read a question, read the answers, and think "Huh? Something is missing!" If you feel like something is missing, reread the question to determine if you have correctly identified what the question is asking. If you have identified the question correctly, then read the answer choices to make sure you haven't missed the nursing concept contained in the answer choices.

QUESTION: "Will these strategies work on every practice question that I answer?"

ANSWER: The critical thinking strategies discussed in this book will enable you to answer all kinds of multiple choice test questions. The critical thinking strategies apply to test questions written at the application/analysis level and do not work with knowledge-based test questions. If you feel that the strategies don't work with the practice questions you are answering, determine the level of difficulty of the questions you are working with. Are the practice questions knowledge-based, or are they at the application/analysis level of difficulty? Remember, the majority of questions that are of a passing level of difficulty on the NCLEX-RN® exam are at the application/analysis level of difficulty.

It's time for you to start your successful preparation for the NCLEX-RN® exam! Begin by identifying your strengths and weaknesses, as follows:

- Take as many diagnostic exams as you can.
- Identify your weaknesses in nursing content.
- Identify your weaknesses in test taking skills.

Next, decide if you need to take a review course. If you decide that this is the best way for you to prepare, ask yourself these questions:

- Is the course mainly a review of nursing content or memory techniques? This type of review won't help you put it all together on Test Day. You can know everything about heart failure, but if you don't know how to use this information to answer a question about heart failure correctly on the NCLEX-RN® exam, you will have difficulty on the exam. Are the strategies specific for the NCLEX-RN® exam?

- Are there plenty of opportunities for practice testing? You need to prove your competence by answering NCLEX-RN® exam-style test questions, so you should practice answering these questions. If the exam were about opening a sterile pack, what would you spend your time doing to prepare for the exam? Reading about opening a sterile pack or practicing opening a sterile pack? Are there exam-style questions included in the course? Do the questions require recall and recognition of facts or application of nursing care principles? Remember, your NCLEX-RN® exam will consist mainly of application-level questions.

- What do students who have taken the course have to say about how it helped them prepare for the exam? If a review course boasts of a particularly high pass rate, ask to see their statistics. Be an informed consumer.

- Is there a guarantee? There are guarantees and there are empty promises. Make sure the course you are considering puts the guarantee in writing. Study the small print. Is your total tuition refunded? Do you have to fail the exam more than once?

- How much does it cost? This sounds easy, but "extras" can add up. Are there additional charges for books? Software? Registration fees?

- Is this course right for me?

And finally, create a realistic study schedule that works for you. Then make a vow to stick to that plan and reward yourself when you do. Spend at least 3 weeks before your exam date preparing. Don't cram! Your content focus should be in understanding the principles of nursing care, not memorizing facts.

Stay away from people who are "prophets of doom." You know the type. With the proper preparation you can and will pass the NCLEX-RN® exam. Keep a positive attitude.

You may need to consider some techniques for battling stress and managing the Test Day experience. Do any of these statements apply to you?

"I always freeze up on tests."

"I need to pass to get my new job/promotion/commission."

"My best friend/girlfriend/sister/brother did really well, but I won't."

"My hospital/family/parents paid for my test prep course. They won't like it if I fail."

"I'm afraid of losing concentration."

"I'm afraid I'm not spending enough time preparing."

If these sound familiar, you may want to mentally prepare yourself by understanding ways to manage test stress. Forcing yourself to identify and face fears may make you edgy at first, but will significantly alleviate test stress in the long run by adding another dimension to your preparation.

Mental Preparation*

1. Visualize

You have probably learned how to do this with clients; now it's your turn. Sit back and let your shoulders and arms relax. Close your eyes and imagine yourself in a relaxing situation—it can be fictional, but a real-life memory is best. Make it as detailed as possible. Think about the sights, the sounds, the smells, even the tastes that you associate with the relaxing situation. Keep your eyes shut; keep sinking back into your chair. Now that you're in that situation, start bringing your test in—think about the experience of taking the test while *in* that relaxing situation. Imagine how much easier it would be if you could take your test in that situation. Notice how much easier your test seems in that situation.

Here's another variation. Close your eyes and think about a situation in which you did well on a test. If you can't come up with one, pick a situation in which you did some good academic work that you were really proud of, or some other kind of genuine accomplishment. Not a fiction, mind you: it has to be from real life. Make it as detailed as possible. Think about the sights, the sounds, the smells, and even the tastes that you associate with this experience of academic success. Now think about your test in line with that experience. Don't make comparisons between them. Just imagine taking your test with that same feeling of relaxed control.

2. Exercise

Whether it be jogging, walking, yoga, push-ups, or a pickup basketball game, physical exercise is a great way to stimulate the mind and body and improve one's ability to think and concentrate. A surprising number of those who prepare for standardized tests don't exercise regularly because they spend so much time preparing. Sedentary people—this is a medical fact—get less oxygen in the blood, and therefore to the brain, than active people.

3. Do the Following on Exam Day

- *Disregard negative words and behaviors.* Don't be distracted by the ignorant babble or the behavior of other, less-prepared, less-skilled candidates around you. Negative thoughts lead to negative feelings and may interfere with performing your best on Test Day.

- *Ignore the pace of other test takers.* Don't be anxious if others seem to be working harder or answering questions more quickly. Continue to spend your time patiently but persistently thinking through your answers; it's going to lead to higher-quality test taking and better results. Set your own pace and stick to it.

- *Keep moving forward.* You can achieve the the ability to keep moving forward by doing enough preparation with practice questions by Test Day that it becomes an instinct to move on instead of getting bogged down by one difficult question. You don't need to get everything right to pass, so don't linger on a question that is going nowhere. The best test takers don't get bothered by difficult questions because they accept that everyone encounters them on the NCLEX-RN® exam.

- *Keep breathing!* Weak standardized test takers tend to share one major trait: forgetting to breathe steadily as the test proceeds. They do not know the value of proper breathing. They start holding

---

* Some of these methods were originally conceptualized by Dr. Émile Coué, who in the 1920s told everyone that the key to a happy life was to constantly repeat the phrase, "Every day in every way I am getting better and better." As advice to test takers, that isn't bad at all!

their breath without realizing it, or begin breathing erratically or arrhythmically. This can hurt confidence and accuracy. Do what you can to instill an awareness of proper breathing before and during each study or testing session.

- ***Do some quick isometrics during the test.*** This is especially helpful if your concentration is wandering or energy is waning. For example, put your palms together and press intensely for a few seconds.

Strategy Recap

Here is a brief review of the various strategies that you have learned in this chapter:

- The NCLEX-RN® exam isn't the real world, so don't rely on your real-world experience to answer NCLEX-RN® exam questions.
- To answer priority questions correctly, think Maslow, the nursing process, and safety.
- The Rules of Management will help you answer questions about delegation and assignment of client care.
- Use the Positioning strategy when you encounter questions about positioning and mobility.
- The Therapeutic Communication strategy will help you eliminate incorrect answer choices in communication questions.
- Identify your strengths and weaknesses, and choose an effective method of study that works for you.
- Use mental preparation techniques to reduce stress and manage your Test Day experience.

PART TWO

NCLEX-RN® EXAM CONTENT REVIEW AND PRACTICE

CHAPTER 4

SAFE AND EFFECTIVE CARE ENVIRONMENT: MANAGEMENT OF CARE

One of the most important parts of your job in client care is keeping the care environment safe for all involved. In addition, it's also important to provide care effectively. Providing a safe and effective care environment involves both proper management of care, and safety and infection control.

Management of care refers specifically to the way nursing care is provided and directed so that the client receives proper treatment, and so that health care personnel remain safe. It also covers management, delegation, and other skills you are expected to have, as well as your ethical and legal obligations regarding client care.

On the NCLEX-RN® exam, you can expect approximately 18 percent of the questions to relate to Management of Care. Exam content related to this subcategory includes, but is not limited to, the following areas:

- Advance directives/self-determination/life planning
- Advocacy
- Assignment, delegation, and supervision
- Case management
- Client rights
- Collaboration with interdisciplinary teams
- Concepts of management
- Confidentiality/information security
- Continuity of care
- Delegation
- Establishing priorities
- Ethical practice
- Information technology
- Informed consent
- Legal rights and responsibilities
- Organ donation
- Performance improvement (quality improvement)
- Referrals

Now let's review the most important concepts covered by the Management of Care subcategory on the NCLEX-RN® exam.

Advance Directives/Self-Determination/Life Planning

An advance directive is a legal document, such as a living will, a health care proxy, or a Durable Power of Attorney for Health Care (DPAHC). Advance directives provide guidance to caregivers about the client's wishes and are followed if a client's decision-making powers become impaired. The 1990 Client Self-Determination Act requires that upon admission to hospitals, long-term care facilities, and home health agencies, clients be informed that they have the right to accept or refuse medical care, as well as to specify in advance (through advance directives) what their wishes are.

Advance directives document clients' self-determined wishes regarding life planning and end-of-life care in a formal way and enhance the likelihood that health care professionals follow clients' wishes. An advance directive spells out the client's health care goals and instructions and, in the event of incapacity, appoints an agent or proxy decision-maker.

Your role as a nurse is to integrate advance directives into the client care plan. To accomplish this, evaluate client status regarding advance directives, and help to determine whether family members and/or significant others should be involved in conversations and decision-making. If the client, a family member, significant other, or staff member is not familiar with the details of advance directives, provide the information as needed.

You must also ensure that copies of advance directives are placed in the client's medical record. This includes information on organ or tissue donation for clients over 18 years of age. The Uniform Anatomical Gift Act, for example, governs organ donations for transplantation and how to donate one's cadaver as an anatomical gift.

Advocacy

Client advocacy—promoting your clients' rights and interests—is an important part of nursing. Discuss treatment options with clients, including what the options are, how they work, and what the side effects may be, so the client understands all available choices. You must respect client decisions even if you do not agree with them. You may need to provide information regarding these discussions to other staff members so you can advocate for your client. When necessary, use an interpreter or translator for non-English-speaking clients. Know when it is appropriate to engage others higher in the chain of command or with different areas of expertise, such as a social worker, on your client's behalf.

Assignment, Delegation, and Supervision

Delegation is a crucial skill. You must be able to identify an appropriate person to carry out a specific task or set of tasks, explain the tasks clearly, and make sure you are understood. It is also your responsibility to make sure the person to whom you are delegating a task has the authority to do the job. Good delegators provide support and monitoring, provide sufficient time to complete the task, retain responsibility for knowing the outcome, and praise and acknowledge a job well done.

Do not delegate the following to nonprofessional staff:

- Nursing assessments
- Diagnosis, care goals, or progress plans
- Interventions that require professional knowledge and skill

Remember the five "rights" of delegation:

- **Right task:** Can the task be safely delegated?
- **Right circumstance:** Is the client stable, and is the outcome predictable?
- **Right person:** Does the person to whom the task will be delegated have the necessary knowledge and appropriate skills?
- **Right direction/communication:** Has the nurse communicated appropriate instructions for accomplishing the task?
- **Right supervision:** Will the delegating nurse remain responsible for the task and outcomes?

You can delegate activities for stable clients with predictable outcomes, and activities that involve standard, unchanging procedures, such as bathing, feeding, dressing, and transferring clients. Do not delegate an activity if the client is unstable, if the outcome of the activity is not assured, or if the activity is complex or complicated.

Leadership will be critical to your success. You should be able to create a common vision for staff, and promote a sense of urgency. This helps connect daily activities to a larger strategic plan, and keeps nursing activities in line with the overall goals of the institution.

A supervisor is someone who has authority to manage other employees. Supervision includes guidance and direction, evaluation, and follow-up to ensure tasks are accomplished. A good supervisor provides the following:

- Clear direction and communication
- Timely follow-up
- Active listening
- Complete technical knowledge of supervised work
- Feedback and resolution of problems and conflicts

As a supervisor, you are expected to select and implement strategies for interventions with staff members as necessary, to report staff member performance, and to evaluate the skills and abilities of staff members, particularly as they relate to time management.

Types of staff members you might be called upon to supervise include other RNs, licensed practical nurses (LPNs), licensed vocational nurses (LVNs), and unlicensed assistive personnel (UAPs).

Case Management

It is important to assist your clients in achieving and/or maintaining their independence by identifying and utilizing the resources available to them. The individualized care plan you develop for each client should be aimed at providing safe, cost-effective care for the client. The plan is based on your assessment of client needs as well as goals, such as providing self-care. You should also incorporate evidence-based research from medical literature and other resources, where applicable, into the care plan. In addition to initiating the care plan for each client, you are expected to evaluate and revise that plan, as needed.

When a client leaves the hospital, provide the client with information on discharge procedures to home, hospice, or community living, whichever may be relevant to the client's situation. This includes information about medications the client should be taking, follow-up visits, future lab tests, and so on.

Client Rights

Part of your job as a health care provider is to discuss treatment options and decisions with your clients, and educate them about client rights and responsibilities. As noted previously, the Client Self-Determination Act requires that upon admission to hospitals, long-term care facilities, and home health agencies, clients be informed that they have the right to accept or refuse medical care. At times, you may need to recognize the client's right to refuse treatment. The Health Insurance Portability and Accountability Act (HIPAA) protects personally identifying information, such as the client's name, social security number, date of birth, and information about diagnosis and treatment. HIPAA provides that such information should only be shared with individuals directly involved in the client's care, the payment of care, and/or the management of the client's care.

The Clients' Bill of Rights, adopted by the President's Advisory Commission on Consumer Protection and Quality in the Health Care Industry, is a statement about the rights to which individuals are entitled as recipients of health care, and their responsibilities. It covers the following areas:

- **Information disclosure:** The client has a right to accurate and easily understood information about health plans, health care professionals, and health care facilities.
- **Choice of providers and plans:** The client has the right to choose health care providers who can provide high-quality health care when needed.
- **Access to emergency services:** The client has the right to be screened and stabilized using emergency services whenever and wherever the client needs them, without having to wait for authorization, and without any financial penalty.
- **Participation in treatment decisions:** The client has the right to know about treatment options and take part in decisions about care. Parents, guardians, family, and significant others can represent the client if the client cannot make their own decisions.
- **Confidentiality of health information:** The client has the right to talk privately with health care providers and have health care information protected; it also includes the right to read and copy one's own medical records.
- **Complaints and appeals:** The client has the right to a fair, fast, and objective review of any complaint against a health plan, a physician, other health care personnel, or a hospital.
- **Consumer responsibilities:** This includes, among other things, a client's responsibility to provide information about medications and past illnesses.

Evaluate the client's understanding of their rights and responsibilities, including the right to informed consent and the difference between privileged communication and the duty to disclose, as well as staff understanding of client rights.

Collaboration with Interdisciplinary Teams

The term *interdisciplinary* or *multidisciplinary* refers to situations in which health care professionals from various disciplines are involved in reaching a common goal, with each contributing their specific expertise. The interdisciplinary interaction between different branches of health care such as nursing, medicine, and social work is known as *collaboration*. Such collaboration in the management of a particular disorder enables caregivers to provide a more comprehensive and individualized approach. Collaboration with an interdisciplinary team requires cooperation, integration, and teamwork.

Because nurses are often the caregivers that clients see most often, be prepared to identify the need for interdisciplinary conferences regarding a client, and know how to initiate such conferences. This includes identification of significant information to report to other disciplines, including health care providers, pharmacists, social workers, and respiratory therapists.

You should be ready to act as the point person to review the care plan and ensure continuity across disciplines, and to collaborate with health care members in other disciplines to provide efficient and effective client care.

Concepts of Management

It's important to identify the roles and responsibilities of all members of the health care team. You'll often need to act as the liaison between those team members and the client to coordinate and manage care.

As issues arise regarding client treatment, apply the principles of conflict resolution, as needed, when working with health care staff. You should also be able to plan overall strategies to address client problems. Know how to supervise care provided by others (see the "Delegation" and "Supervision" sections later in this chapter), and know which staff members can perform particular procedures related to client care.

Confidentiality/Information Security

Like all health care providers, you should maintain client confidentiality and take the necessary steps to ensure that client information security is not breached. An individual not involved in the care of the client does not have a legitimate need to access the client's medical record. Know the provisions of HIPAA (summarized in the Client Rights section of this chapter) and protect the client's right to privacy. Ensure that only authorized individuals access medical records, that no medical records are viewable by the general public, and that no conversations about client information can be overheard by unauthorized persons.

You may need to intervene when confidentiality is breached by other staff members. You'll also be expected to assess staff members' and your clients' understanding of confidentiality requirements, such as those governed by HIPAA.

Continuity of Care

Continuity of care is the process by which a client and health care providers are cooperatively involved in the ongoing health care management of the client, with the goal of providing high-quality and cost-effective health care. Ideally, all people involved in a client's health care, including the client, communicate with one another to coordinate care, as well as agree and understand the goals of health care for the client.

To help ensure continuity of care, know the proper procedures to admit, transfer, and discharge a client. This includes maintaining continuity of care between/among health care agencies when clients are transferred or handed off from one department to another, or from one agency to another. It also includes using documents and proper forms to enter client information into medical records or on transfer/referral forms. You may also need to follow up on unresolved issues regarding client care (such as laboratory results and client requests) and provide reports on assigned clients.

Establishing Priorities

There are several other frameworks for establishing the priority of client care. They include:

- ABCs (airway, breathing, circulation/cardiovascular system)
- Maslow's hierarchy of needs (physiological needs, safety and security, love and belonging, self-esteem, and self-actualization)
- Agency policies and procedures
- Time
- Client and family preferences
- Care related to client activity
- Priorities in medication therapy

Assess/triage (French for *sort*) clients to prioritize order of care delivery, and focus on the least stable clients first. Use your knowledge of pathophysiology when establishing priorities for interventions with multiple clients. Once you have provided care to multiple clients, evaluate and adjust your care plans as needed.

The following general problems indicate priority needs:

- Postoperative clients just out of surgery
- Clients whose status has deteriorated from their normal baseline
- Clients exhibiting signs of shock
- Clients with allergic reactions
- Clients with chest pain
- Postdiagnostic-procedure clients who require temporary monitoring
- Clients who tell you they have unusual symptoms
- Clients with malfunctioning equipment or tubing

Ethical Practice

Ethical principles help you determine whether an action is right or wrong. In addition to understanding basic ethics and morals, you should be familiar with the American Nurses Association (ANA) Code of Ethics for Nurses. These guidelines delineate values and standards for professional practice.

Make sure you understand the following ethical principles:

- **Autonomy:** The right of individuals to make decisions for themselves
- **Beneficence:** A nurse's duty to do what is in the best interests of the client
- **Justice:** A fair, equitable, and appropriate treatment
- **Nonmaleficence:** A nurse's duty to do no harm
- **Fidelity:** Keeping faithful to ethical principles and the ANA Code of Ethics for Nurses
- **Virtues:** Compassion, trustworthiness, integrity, and veracity (truthfulness)
- **Confidentiality:** Maintaining the client's privacy by not disclosing personal information about the client
- **Accountability:** Responsibility for one's actions

You should be able to identify ethical issues affecting staff or clients, provide information on ethics, and intervene appropriately to promote ethical practice. You'll also be expected to review outcomes of interventions to promote ethical practice.

Information Technology

An electronic health record (EHR) is a digital version of a client's paper chart that makes information available instantly and securely to authorized users. Included in this information are client demographics, progress notes, problems, medications, vital signs, past medical history, immunizations, laboratory data, and radiology reports. The EHR has the ability to generate a complete record of a clinical client encounter as well as supporting other care-related activities directly or indirectly (via interface, including evidence-based decision support, quality management, and outcomes reporting). The use of information technology should always be centered on client safety and improved outcomes. With EHRs, information is available whenever and wherever it is needed. Likewise, electronic medication administration records (eMARs) have proven to reduce medication administration errors.

You must know how to use information technology and information systems to enter computer documentation in a client's medical record in a timely and accurate manner. You must also understand the principles of privacy, confidentiality, and security in accessing client records. Whenever you access a client record, apply your knowledge of the facility's specific regulations.

You should also know how to use information technology (such as website resources or videos) to enhance the care provided to a client. Telehealth, for example, uses transmissions via telecommunications technology to transmit health information remotely.

Informed Consent

Informed consent is the right of clients to be adequately informed of the risks and benefits of a proposed procedure or treatment before determining whether or not to consent to that procedure or treatment. The components of informed consent include an explanation of the following:

- Details of the procedure or treatment
- Risks and benefits of the procedure or treatment, including the potential for serious injury or death
- Alternative procedures or treatments
- Potential consequences of refusing the procedure or treatment

Typically, the health care provider who is performing the procedure or providing the treatment (usually the physician) is responsible for obtaining the client's informed consent. One of your roles in the process is to advocate for the client by ensuring that the client has been provided the necessary information to make an informed decision. In cases where the client does not speak English, provide written materials in the client's native language, when possible. Another one of your roles is to ensure that a client has actually given informed consent for treatment before that treatment occurs. One way to do so is to act as a witness to the informed consent. As a witness, you confirm that the client gave informed consent voluntarily, the client's signature is authentic, and the client is competent to give consent. You may be called upon to evaluate clients to determine whether they are capable of providing informed consent, and identify an appropriate person to do so, such as a parent or legal guardian, if the client is a minor.

If the client waives consent, ensure it is documented in the medical record. If the client is deemed incompetent to give informed consent, a court-appointed guardian may do so on the client's behalf.

The requirement to obtain the client's informed consent can be waived in an emergency situation in which the client is incapacitated and the situation requires immediate treatment.

Legal Rights and Responsibilities

Know the confines of applicable laws and understand the parameters of your nursing license. Legal limits and the scope of practice for nursing are dictated by federal and state laws, such as the Nurse Practice Acts (NPAs) and related guidelines, and are regulated by each state's board of nursing/regulatory body. Nurses are accountable and responsible for incorrect or inappropriate actions or inactions. These may include negligence, malpractice, or other legal charges. Negligence involves the unintentional failure to act as a reasonable person would in similar circumstances that results in an injury to the client. Elements include a breach of a duty of care, with a resultant injury that has been proximately caused (i.e., there is reasonably close connection between the nurse's actions and the resulting injury), and actual damages to the injured party. Malpractice involves the failure by a medical professional to carry out or perform their duties such that injury to the client results. The specific requirements for malpractice are typically defined by the statutes and rules/regulations of each state.

There are specific areas with which you should be familiar. They include:

- Identifying legal issues affecting clients (such as refusing treatment) and knowing how to respond appropriately
- Recognizing tasks and assignments you are not prepared to perform and seeking assistance
- Identifying and managing clients' valuables according to facility or agency policy
- Educating clients and staff on legal and ethical issues
- Complying with state and/or federal regulations for reporting client conditions (such as abuse or neglect, communicable disease, gunshot wound, or dog bite)
- Reporting unsafe practices of health care personnel to internal or external entities
- Intervening appropriately when you observe unsafe practices by staff members

Organ Donation

Organ donation takes healthy organs and tissues from one person for transplantation into another. Organs that can be donated include internal organs (kidneys, liver, pancreas, intestines, and lungs), skin, bone and bone marrow, and corneas. Most organ and tissue donations occur after the donor has died, but some organs and tissues can be donated while the donor is alive, such as kidneys and bone marrow.

Nurses play several roles in the field of organ donation. Specialist nurses known as procurement nurses coordinate the harvesting and collection of organs; the Federal Conditions of Participation (§42 CFR 482.45) require that those making request of families for organ donation receive specific training. Other nurses work with clients waiting for transplant or with individuals who have already received organ transplants. For the NCLEX-RN®, you should understand the role of the entry-level nurse in interacting with clients and their families facing decisions related to organ donation.

You must ensure that copies of advance directives, which include information on organ or tissue donation for clients age 18 years or older, are placed in the client's medical record.

Performance Improvement (Quality Improvement)

Each institution may define it differently, but a standard definition of quality involves meeting or exceeding the expectations of customers and standards, and achieving planned outcomes. Quality management principles include total quality management (TQM), continuous quality improvement (CQI), and evidence-based decision making, among others. Quality improvement includes activities such as identifying opportunities and developing policies for improving the quality of nursing practice. Methods include establishing a comprehensive quality management plan, establishing benchmarks, completing performance appraisals, performing intradisciplinary and interdisciplinary assessments, performing nursing audits, conducting peer reviews and utilization reviews, and managing outcomes. Mock codes can improve performance by encouraging teamwork, improving communication and skill building, and enhancing confidence of caregivers.

You must report identified client care issues or problems to appropriate personnel (such as the nurse manager or risk manager). A nurse is also expected to participate in the performance improvement and quality assurance process, which may include data collection or participation on a team.

You may be asked to utilize research and other references when determining how best to improve performance, and you will be expected to evaluate the impact of performance improvement measures on client care and resource utilization using a variety of specific indicators.

Nurse-sensitive indicators are measurements of client care that are impacted by nursing interventions. Examples include maintenance of skin integrity, pressure ulcer prevalence and incidence, fall injury rate, medication incident rate, restraint utilization rate, client satisfaction with pain management, client satisfaction with overall nursing care, and nurse satisfaction.

Referrals

Nurses often have a role to play in assisting and coordinating client care that requires referrals. There are different types of referrals: authorization for care or a service, recommendation of a specific provider, referral to specialists, and referral to a different facility for care. Some of these may require specific approvals, although in some cases you can refer a client directly to a dietary or wound care specialist.

Assess the need to refer clients for assistance with actual or potential problems (physical therapy, speech therapy), and match community resources to the client's needs (respite care, social services, shelters). In all referral situations, you need to know which documents to include when referring a client, such as a medical record or referral form.

Chapter Quiz

1. An adolescent client newly diagnosed with diabetes mellitus (DM) is preparing for discharge. Which activity **best** describes the nurse's role as a client advocate?

    1. Arranging for a visit with a home health nurse.
    2. Providing written medication instructions to the client's parents.
    3. Instructing the client to follow up with the provider in 4 weeks.
    4. Teaching the client how to administer insulin injections.

2. A client is seen for an outpatient appointment. The client asks the nurse to obtain a copy of the client's medical record. The nurse knows that the client's right to read and obtain a copy of the medical record is guaranteed by virtue of which regulation?

    1. The Client Self-Determination Act.
    2. The Health Insurance Portability and Accountability Act (HIPAA).
    3. The Uniform Anatomical Gift Act.
    4. The Americans with Disabilities Act.

3. After receiving report at the start of the shift, which client should the nurse attend to **first**?

    1. A client being treated for non-Hodgkin lymphoma with a potassium level of 7.5 mEq/L (7.5 mmol/L).
    2. A client with sickle-cell anemia with pain of 6 on a scale of 1–10.
    3. A client with ovarian cancer waiting to be discharged home.
    4. A client with chronic obstructive pulmonary disease (COPD) and an oxygen saturation of 96% on room air.

Refer to the Case Study to answer the next six questions.

The charge nurse on an adult medical surgical unit is working with a team of RNs, LPNs, and unlicensed assistive personnel (UAP). The charge nurse is reviewing staff documentation in the medical records.

Medical Records

Team Member	Record Entry
RN #1	Client reports leg incision pain 7/10. Incision slightly pink, 12 staples intact. No drainage noted. Morphine sulfate 2 mg IV given per order.
RN #2	Physician notified of cloudy, foul-smelling urine. Orders received. Obtained mid stream urine specimen and sent to lab.
LPN/LVN #1	Taught client and spouse how to perform simple dressing change in preparation for discharge. Removed client's anti-embolic stockings, as directed by RN. Abdomen soft with positive bowel sounds × 4 quadrants.
LPN/LVN #2	Vital signs: Temp 98.2° F (36.6° C) BP 130/78 HR 78 RR 14 SpO$_2$ 98% on room air. Ambulated client to bathroom. Client denies dizziness. Finger stick blood glucose reading 118 mg/dL (6.55 mmol/L).
UAP #1	Urine output measured and recorded on flow sheet. Client's nasogastric tube flushed with 30 mL normal saline.
UAP #2	Client's left hand dressing wet. Removed wet dressing and reapplied 4×4 gauze with tape over hand wound. Wound clean with well approximated edges and sutures intact. Reported observation of wound to RN.

4. For each documentation entry, highlight tokenized findings that are concerning to the nurse. Tokenized options are enclosed in boxes.

Team Member	Record Entry
RN #1	Client reports leg incision pain as sharp and intermittent 7/10. Incision slightly pink, 12 staples intact. No drainage noted. Morphine sulfate 2 mg IV given per order.
LPN/LVN #1	Physician notified of cloudy, foul-smelling urine. Orders received. Obtained mid stream urine specimen and sent to lab.
LPN/LVN #2	Taught client and spouse how to perform simple dressing change in preparation for discharge. Removed client's anti-embolic stockings, as directed by RN. Abdomen soft with positive bowel sounds × 4 quadrants.
UAP #1	Urine output measured and recorded on flow sheet. Client's nasogastric tube flushes easily with 30 mL normal saline.
UAP #2	Client's left hand dressing wet. Removed wet dressing and reapplied 4×4 gauze with paper tape over hand wound. Wound edges appear dry and wound bed dark pink.

5. For each task, specify which team member is legally permitted to complete the task. **Each task may be completed by more than 1 team member.**

Task	RN	LPN/LVN	UAP
Obtain vital signs.	☐	☐	☐
Assess a wound.	☐	☐	☐
Administer insulin.	☐	☐	☐
Ambulate a client.	☐	☐	☐
Assess characteristics of pain.	☐	☐	☐

6. The charge nurse recognizes which team member is out of compliance with scope of practice and must be corrected **immediately**? **(Select all that apply.)**

   1. RN #1
   2. LPN #1
   3. LPN #2
   4. UAP #1
   5. UAP #2

7. The charge nurse develops a plan to intervene with team members.

   For each potential intervention, specify whether the intervention is appropriate or not appropriate.

Intervention	Appropriate	Not appropriate
Shares concerns with friend who is a charge nurse on another unit in the same facility.	○	○
Discusses findings with Nurse Manager.	○	○
Meets with each individual privately to discuss concerns.	○	○
Notifies the state Board of Nursing.	○	○
Conducts a unit wide education session, reviewing scope of practice for each team member.	○	○

8. The charge nurse and the nurse manager conduct individual meetings with the staff members.

   Which statement is correct for the Nurse Manager to make when discussing scope of practice? **(Select all that apply.)**

   1. "LPN/LVNs do not conduct initial client teaching but can reinforce teaching done by RN."
   2. "UAPs do not obtain pulse oximetry reading."
   3. "LPN/LVNs are not allowed to administer narcotics."
   4. "Only LPN/LVNs and RNs can assess wounds."
   5. "UAPs cannot flush nasogastric tubes or drains."
   6. "LPN/LVNs and UAPs can collaborate with the RN to implement a plan of care."

9. Three weeks later, the charge nurse reviews staff documentation on the unit.

For each type of staff listed, specify the documentation entry that indicates **further** teaching is necessary. Each staff member supports 1 documentation entry.

Staff Member	Documentation Entry
LPN/LVN	Select... ▾
	Client expectorating thick yellow sputum. Sputum specimen collected and sent to lab.
	Sterile wet to dry dressing applied to abdominal wound.
	20g peripheral IV started in left forearm × 2 attempts.
UAP	Select... ▾
	Client turned to left side and head of bed elevated 30 degrees.
	Indwelling urinary catheter not draining. Irrigated with 30 mL sterile water.
	Client states having increased chest pain. RN notified.

10. A client who developed Stevens-Johnson syndrome is being transferred in stable condition from the intensive care unit (ICU) to the medical unit. Which client would be the **best** choice as a roommate for the client with Stevens-Johnson syndrome?

    1. A client with methicillin-resistant *Staphylococcus aureus* (MRSA).
    2. A client admitted for diarrhea.
    3. A client with fever of unknown origin.
    4. A client with atrial fibrillation.

11. A client who had a stroke is being transferred from a medical unit to a rehabilitation center. The nurse case manager is assisting in the process. The nurse knows that which of these is a goal of case management? **(Select all that apply.)**

    1. Improving the coordination of care.
    2. Increasing referrals to local organizations.
    3. Reducing the fragmentation of care.
    4. Discharging clients quickly.
    5. Training the client's home attendant.

12. An client with acute lymphocytic leukemia is admitted to the bone marrow transplantation unit. The client's family is having difficulty dealing with the emotional and financial pressures of the client's condition. The nurse, case manager, health care provider, and social worker meet to discuss the plan of care. This interdisciplinary interaction is **best** referred to as which concept?

    1. Case management.
    2. Collaboration.
    3. Cooperation.
    4. Collegiality.

13. A pregnant client at 15 weeks' gestation is scheduled for an amniocentesis. As the client is being prepped for the procedure, it becomes clear to the nurse that the client doesn't fully understand the risks and benefits associated with the procedure. Which action describes the nurse's role in obtaining informed consent? **(Select all that apply.)**

    1. Explain the risks and benefits associated with the procedure.
    2. Describe alternatives to the amniocentesis procedure.
    3. Inform the client examples of successful amniocentesis.
    4. Witness the client's signature on the consent form.
    5. Advocate for the client in making an informed decision.

14. The nurse noticed an increase in the prevalence of pressure injury among clients in an intensive care unit (ICU). The nurse documented the findings and worked with the manager to develop and implement a new policy addressing the consistent use of pressure injury risk assessment scale. Which term **best** describes the nurse's actions?

    1. Quality improvement.
    2. Collaboration.
    3. Advocacy.
    4. Case management.

15. The nurse is working on a surgical unit. Which task would be appropriate for the nurse to delegate to an unlicensed assistive personnel (UAP)?

    1. Assist a new postoperative client to the bathroom.
    2. Set up the clients' lunch trays.
    3. Change a central line dressing.
    4. Teach a client how to administer discharge medications.

16. A client with leukemia has consented to a blood transfusion against the wishes of the client's family, who are all Jehovah's Witnesses. The nurse knows that which ethical principle **best** supports the client's decision?

    1. Autonomy.
    2. Beneficence.
    3. Nonmaleficence.
    4. Justice.

17. The nurse wants to delegate the task of showering an elderly client in a wheelchair to the unlicensed assistive personnel (UAP). Before delegating a task to the UAP, the nurse should **first** ensure which is accomplished?

    1. The UAP is supervised at all times.
    2. The UAP demonstrated competency for the task during orientation.
    3. The UAP has performed the task before.
    4. The UAP has received the assignment during report.

18. A well-known actor has been admitted to an ambulatory surgical unit. The nurse notices a staff member who is not involved in the client's care reading the actor's medical record. Which is the **most** appropriate action to do next?

    1. Nothing. The staff member has a hospital ID badge and is authorized to read the medical record.
    2. Inform the staff member that without a legitimate need for the information, staff should not be reading the medical record.
    3. Tell the client an unauthorized individual has read the client's medical records.
    4. Page the health care provider and ask if it's acceptable for the staff member to access the medical records.

19. The nurse is learning how to use the hospital's new electronic medication administration record. The nurse knows this tool has the potential to achieve which goal? **(Select all that apply.)**

    1. Reduce medication administration errors.
    2. Improve access to information at the point of care.
    3. Eliminate the need for the nurse to document medication.
    4. Eliminate the need for the nurse to verify dose calculations.
    5. Allow the client to verify which medications are prescribed.

20. The nurse uses the Internet to receive electrocardiogram results from a client living in a nursing home. The nurse knows this type of information technology is **best** described as which of these?

    1. Encryption.
    2. Telecommunications.
    3. Telehealth.
    4. Nursing informatics.

Refer to the Case Study to answer the next question.

The nurse is caring for an older adult client on the medical telemetry unit.

| History and Physical | Nurse's Notes | Vital Signs |

1000: Emergency Department

The client has a history of heart failure, hypertension, type 2 diabetes, and depression. The client's spouse brought the client to the Emergency Department (ED) this morning due to increased difficulty breathing with wheezing and coughing, and increased edema in the lower extremities. The client gained 7 pounds over the past week. An electrocardiogram (ECG), chest x-ray, arterial blood gases (ABGs), and lab work were completed in the ED. Results are significant for elevated B-type natriuretic peptide (BNP) and hypoxemia with an oxygen saturation of 86% on room air. The client was given diuretics and placed on oxygen at 3 L/min per nasal cannula. The client was admitted to the medical telemetry unit for further treatment. This is the client's third hospital admission this year for an exacerbation of heart failure.

Body System	Assessment Findings ED
General	Well developed, slightly overweight, sitting up on side of bed. Temp 98.8° F (37.1° C)
Neurologic	Awake and alert, oriented × 4. Answers appropriately. Appears anxious. Moving all extremities, grasps equal bilaterally.
Cardiovascular	Skin pale, warm, dry. HR 106. S3 auscultated. Rhythm sinus tachycardia. Client denies chest pain. BP 168/92. Bilateral 3+ pitting ankle and foot edema. Faint dorsalis pedis pulses auscultated with doppler.
Respiratory	RR 22. Faint crackles auscultated in bilateral lung bases. Faint expiratory wheezing throughout. Client sitting up on side of bed and states, "I feel like I am smothering when I lie down." SpO$_2$ 90% on O$_2$ 3 L/min per nasal cannula.
Gastrointestinal	Abdomen soft and protuberant. Bowel sounds present × 4 quadrants. Denies nausea. Last bowel movement yesterday.
Genitourinary	Client able to void per urinal with assistance. Voiding pale light yellow urine.
IV	IV 0.9% normal saline (NS) infusing at 30 mL/hour to right forearm. Dressing dry and intact.

| History and Physical | Nurse's Notes | Vital Signs |

Medical ICU

1300: Client admitted to unit with spouse present. Fowler position. Awake and alert × 4. Responds to questions appropriately. Placed on continuous cardiac monitor. Client in sinus rhythm in 90s. Client denies pain, but states, "I feel heavy in my chest and I can't take a good breath." Lungs with faint wheezes throughout and coarse crackles present in bases bilaterally. Client on O$_2$ at 3 L/minute per nasal cannula. Client's spouse leaving unit to go home to pack toiletries.

1345: Client's heart monitor alarming. Heart rate 116–128 with 2–3 beat runs of ventricular tachycardia (VT). Client awake but not speaking, appears anxious, holding chest, and grunting. Skin dusky, cool, clammy. Respirations shallow and rapid. SpO$_2$ 78% on O$_2$ 3L/min per nasal cannula.

History and Physical	Nurse's Notes	Vital Signs

Vital Signs	1300	1345
BP	146/88	88/64
HR	94	118
RR	20	28
SpO$_2$ (O$_2$ 3 L/min per NC)	92%	78%
Temperature (oral)	98.4° F (36.9° C)	N/A

21. The nurse responds to the client's telemetry alarm and assesses the client.

   Complete the diagram by choosing from the choices below to specify what condition the client is most likely experiencing, 2 actions the nurse **immediately** takes to address that condition, and 2 **priority** parameters the nurse monitors to assess the client's progress.

Action to Take	→	Condition Most Likely Experiencing	←	Parameter to Monitor
Action to Take				Parameter to Monitor

Actions to Take	Potential Conditions	Parameters to Monitor
Notify the client's spouse.	Sepsis.	Bowel sounds.
Apply oxygen 15 L/min per non rebreather face mask.	Pneumonia.	Intake and output.
Administer epinephrine.	Stroke.	Vital signs.
Place the client in Trendelenburg position.	Cardiogenic shock.	Level of consciousness.
Notify the rapid response team.		Skin temperature.

22. The nurse prepares to transfer a client to the operating room. The nurse knows that adhering to the hospital policy for client hand-off communication **best** ensures which aspect of care management?

    1. Case management.
    2. Continuity of care.
    3. Confidentiality protection.
    4. Collaboration.

23. The nurse prepares to perform an admission assessment on a client admitted for Crohn disease. The nurse knows that according to the Clients' Bill of Rights, the client is responsible for which of these? **(Select all that apply.)**

    1. Consenting to treatment.
    2. Providing information about medications.
    3. Providing proof of insurance.
    4. Providing information about past illnesses.
    5. Respect and consideration.

24. The nurse cares for a client with a newly created colostomy. As part of the care planning for this client, the nurse knows a referral to which staff member will be the **priority**?

    1. A certified wound, ostomy, and continence nurse (CWOCN).
    2. Social services.
    3. Physical therapy.
    4. Occupational therapy.

25. A registered nurse (RN) is in charge of a team on a medical-surgical unit that includes a licensed practical nurse (LPN). The RN understands that which is an activity that falls within the scope of practice of an LPN?

    1. Administer oral medications to a client.
    2. Collaborate with social services to plan care.
    3. Formulate a nursing diagnosis.
    4. Develop an institutional policy.

26. The nurse in a maternity unit cares for a client who has just given birth to twins. The client voices concern about her ability to manage when she gets home. Which statement **best** illustrates quality care delivery by the nurse? **(Select all that apply.)**

    1. "Just focus on how lucky you are to have two healthy babies."
    2. "We can arrange for follow-up visits with a home health nurse."
    3. "Here is information on support groups for parents of multiples."
    4. "You will find it easier to formula-feed your babies at home."
    5. "Right now your priority is to sign these discharge documents."

27. After responding to a "code," several staff nurses express concerns over their confidence levels and performance to the nurse in charge of the hospital's performance improvement program. The nurse in charge knows the **best** way to evaluate and improve performance is to implement which of these?

    1. Analyze performance data.
    2. Mock codes.
    3. Inservice training.
    4. Written competency exams.

28. A client is being treated for uncontrolled hypertension. The nurse knows that the involvement of nursing, pharmacy, cardiology, and nutritional services is an example of which approach?

    1. Managed care.
    2. Multidisciplinary.
    3. Case management.
    4. Performance improvement.

29. The nurse caring for a client who is newly diagnosed with diabetes mellitus performs the following tasks. Place the tasks the nurse would perform in the appropriate order. **All options must be used.**

    1. The nurse establishes a goal with the client to be able to self-administer insulin injections.
    2. The nurse assesses the client's level of knowledge about how to administer insulin injections.
    3. The nurse evaluates the client while self-administering insulin injections.
    4. The nurse establishes the diagnosis of knowledge deficit.

30. The nurse administers the first dose of chemotherapy to a client. The nurse knows that which activity is appropriate to delegate to the licensed practical nurse (LPN)?

    1. Obtain the client's blood pressure (BP).
    2. Teach about the side effects of chemotherapy.
    3. Administer the second dose of chemotherapy.
    4. Flush the client's central line with heparin.

Chapter Quiz Answers and Explanations

1. The answer is 4

An adolescent client newly diagnosed with diabetes mellitus (DM) is preparing for discharge. Which activity **best** describes the nurse's role as a client advocate?

Category: Advocacy

(1) Arranging for a visit with a home health nurse may be important in the overall management of this client's care, but does not directly assist in teaching the client the necessary skills to manage the client's DM.

(2) Providing written medication instructions to the client's parents may be important in the overall management of this client's care, but does not directly assist in teaching the client the necessary skills to manage the client's DM.

(3) Instructing the client to follow up with the provider in 4 weeks may be important in the overall management of this client's care, but does not directly assist in teaching the client the necessary skills to manage the client's DM.

(4) CORRECT: Teaching the client how to administer own medication is the best example of the nurse's role as a client advocate, because this action directly helps the client develop self-advocacy skills.

2. The answer is 2

A client is seen for an outpatient appointment. The client asks the nurse to obtain a copy of the client's medical record. The nurse knows that the client's right to read and obtain a copy of the medical record is guaranteed by virtue of which regulation?

Category: Client rights

(1) The 1990 Client Self-Determination Act was passed by Congress to ensure that upon admission to hospitals, long-term care facilities, and home health agencies, clients are informed that they have the right to accept or refuse medical care, as well as to specify in advance (through advance directives) what their

wishes are. It does not address whether clients may read and obtain a copy of their medical records.

(2) CORRECT: HIPAA protects the clients' right to review, copy, and request amendments to their medical records.

(3) The Uniform Anatomical Gift Act governs organ donations for transplantation and how to donate one's cadaver as an anatomical gift. It does not address whether clients may read and obtain a copy of their medical records.

(4) The Americans with Disabilities Act does not address whether clients may read and obtain a copy of their medical records.

3. The answer is 1

After receiving report at the start of the shift, which client should the nurse attend to **first**?

Category: Establishing priorities

(1) CORRECT: Hyperkalemia is a potentially serious condition that, in a client undergoing treatment for non-Hodgkin lymphoma, could indicate tumor lysis syndrome. Tumor lysis syndrome occurs when tumor cells release their contents into the bloodstream, either spontaneously or in response to chemotherapy, leading to the characteristic findings of hyperkalemia, hyperphosphatemia, and hypocalcemia.

(2) A client with sickle-cell anemia with pain of 6 on a scale of 1–10 should be attended to, but the condition is not as urgent as the client's with a serum potassium level of 7.5 mEq/L (7.5 mmol/L) (normal range: 3.5–5 mEq/L [3.5-5 mmol/L]).

(3) A client with ovarian cancer waiting to be discharged should be attended to but does not require immediate attention.

(4) A client with COPD and an oxygen saturation of 96% on room air does not require immediate attention.

4. See explanation for answers

For each documentation entry, highlight tokenized findings that are concerning to the charge nurse. Tokenized options are enclosed in boxes.

Team Member	Record Entry
RN #1	Client reports leg incision pain as sharp and intermittent 7/10. Incision slightly pink, 12 staples intact. No drainage noted. Morphine sulfate 2 mg IV given per order.
LPN/LVN #1	Physician notified of cloudy, foul-smelling urine. Orders received. Obtained mid stream urine specimen and sent to lab.
LPN/LVN #2	Taught client and spouse how to perform simple dressing change in preparation for discharge. Removed client's anti-embolic stockings, as directed by RN. Abdomen soft with positive bowel sounds × 4 quadrants.
UAP #1	Urine output measured and recorded on flow sheet. Client's nasogastric tube flushes easily with 30 mL normal saline.
UAP #2	Client's left hand dressing wet. Removed wet dressing and reapplied 4×4 gauze with paper tape over hand wound. Wound edges appear dry and wound bed dark pink.

CORRECT OPTIONS: In this situation, the **LPN/LVN will report abnormal findings and concerns to the RN, who will notify the physician and obtain orders**. Educational preparation and professional licensing prepares the **RN to conduct initial client teaching**. However, LPN/LVNs can reinforce teaching that was previously taught by the RN. **Flushing a nasogastric tube, changing a dressing, and assessing a wound require assessment and judgement by the UAP, which is beyond the scope of practice.**

INCORRECT OPTIONS: The remaining documentation facts are appropriate to the designated role of the health care team member. The RN has the educational preparation, skill, and licensing to perform the listed tasks needed to provide care for the client.

5. See explanation for answers

For each task, specify which team member is legally permitted to complete the task. **Each task may be completed by more than 1 team member.**

While Nurse Practice Acts may vary slightly from state to state and within acute care settings versus long term care settings, the American Nurse's Association indicates the guidelines for scope of practice. Keep in mind the principles of appropriate delegation not only includes scope of practice but also clear communication, surveillance, supervision, evaluation, and feedback.

RN: The scope of practice for an RN is much broader than that of an LPN/LVN and a UAP. RNs can independently assess, plan, evaluate, and use nursing judgement. It is within the scope of practice for the RN to **obtain vital signs, assess a wound, administer insulin, ambulate the client**, and **assess the character of a client's pain.**

LPN/LVN: The LPN/LVN's scope of practice includes administering non-IV medications, performing dressing changes, and monitoring an IV and the client's condition. The LPN/LVN must report abnormal findings to an RN. The LPN/LVN can **obtain VS, administer insulin,** and **ambulate the client.**

UAP: UAPs perform routine, uncomplicated tasks such as taking VS, obtaining finger stick blood glucose readings, and assisting with activities of daily living, including feeding and bathing. The UAP reports to the RN or LPN/LVN. The UAP can **obtain vital signs** and **ambulate the client.**

6. The answer is 2, 3, 4, and 5

CORRECT OPTIONS: **LPN/LVN #1** directly notified the physician of a change in client condition. In this setting, the LPN/LVN will report findings to the RN. **LPN/LVN #2** conducted initial teaching to the client on a simple dressing change, which is outside the scope of practice of the LPN/LVN. **UAP #1** flushed a nasogastric tube and **UAP #2** changed a dressing and assessed a wound, which are both outside the scope of practice of a UAP.

INCORRECT OPTION: The RN demonstrates appropriate scope of practice.

7. See explanation for answers

APPROPRIATE: When managing employee performance issues, the **nurse manager of the unit needs to be informed** because the manager is responsible for employee practice and client outcomes on that specific unit. Having a **one-on-one discussion with each employee** helps the employee to understand any actions which need to be addressed. Meeting with the employee helps the Charge Nurse determine and implement a plan for behavior change and evaluate changed behavior. A **unit wide education session** would be helpful to review and clarify roles and responsibilities for all team members.

NOT APPROPRIATE: **Sharing concerns with a friend** does not address the incorrect scope of practice of the staff. **Notifying the State Board of Nursing** occurs when there is a more serious infraction such as working while impaired, gross negligence, or fraud. It would not be the initial action the Charge Nurse would take. Usually the Nurse Manager is the one who reports issues to the State Board of Nursing.

8. The answer is 1, 5, and 6

CORRECT OPTIONS: When practice issues arise on a nursing unit, the standard of practice, at the least, is for management to meet with individuals and review correct practice. **LPN/LVNs do not conduct initial client teaching but can reinforce teaching done by RN**. In addition, **UAPs cannot flush nasogastric tubes** nor assess wounds. Flushing nasogastric tubes and wound assessment is within the scope of practice of the RN. **LPN/LVNs and UAPs can work with the RN to implement a client plan of care.** Developing the plan of care is the role of the RN.

INCORRECT OPTIONS: A UAP is trained to obtain all vital signs, and is taught how to use a pulse oximeter to obtain readings. LPN/LVNs can administer non-IV medications. So PO, IM, and subcutaneous administration of narcotics is allowed. While an LPN/LVN may have a very important role in wound care, assessment of the wound is the responsibility of the RN.

9. See explanation for answers

LPN/LVN: It is **out of the scope of practice for the LPN/LVN to initiate an intravenous catheter**. In some facilities, LPN/LVNs with documented, specific training are able to perform skills involving intravenous therapy. All other entries indicate teaching has been successful.

UAP: The **UAP cannot irrigate drains or tubes**. The RN or LPN/LVN could irrigate an indwelling urinary catheter. All other entries indicate teaching has been successful.

10. The answer is 4

A client who developed Stevens-Johnson syndrome is being transferred in stable condition from the intensive care unit (ICU) to the medical unit. Which client would be the **best** choice as a roommate for the client with Stevens-Johnson syndrome?

Category: Concepts of management

(1) A client with MRSA may be an infection risk for an individual with altered skin integrity.

(2) A client with diarrhea may be an infection risk for an individual with altered skin integrity.

(3) A client with fever of unknown origin may be an infection risk for an individual with altered skin integrity.

(4) CORRECT: A client with Stevens-Johnson syndrome is likely to have severe skin integrity issues, including blistering and skin shedding, which can place the client at high risk for infection. Atrial fibrillation is not an infectious process.

11. The answer is 1 and 3

A client who had a stroke is being transferred from a medical unit to a rehabilitation center. The nurse case manager is assisting in the process. The nurse knows that which of these is a goal of case management? **(Select all that apply.)**

Category: Case management

(1) CORRECT: One of the primary goals of case management is to improve the coordination of care and the transition of care.

(2) Although case managers do make referrals to local organizations, this is not a goal of case management.

(3) CORRECT: One of the primary goals of case management is to reduce fragmentation of care.

(4) Although case managers help to make discharges more efficient, discharging clients quickly, by itself, is not a goal of case management.

(5) Training the client's home attendant is not a goal of case management.

12. The answer is 2

An client with acute lymphocytic leukemia is admitted to the bone marrow transplantation unit. The client's family is having difficulty dealing with the emotional and financial pressures of the client's condition. The nurse, case manager, physician, and social worker meet to discuss the plan of care. This interdisciplinary interaction is **best** referred to as which concept?

Category: Interdisciplinary collaboration

(1) Case management refers to the coordination of care to reduce fragmentation and improve quality and outcomes, as well as to reduce costs.

(2) CORRECT: The interdisciplinary interaction between different health care professions, such as nursing, medicine, and social work, is known as collaboration.

(3) Although the health care team may have been cooperating, or operating as a team, the term "cooperation" does not specifically refer to the concept of interdisciplinary action.

(4) Although the health care team may have been operating in a collegial (cooperative and professional) manner, this term does not specifically refer to the concept of interdisciplinary action.

13. The answer is 4 and 5

A pregnant client at 15 weeks' gestation is scheduled for an amniocentesis. As the client is being prepped for the procedure, it becomes clear to the nurse that the client doesn't fully understand the risks and benefits associated with the procedure. Which action describes the nurse's role in obtaining informed consent? **(Select all that apply.)**

Category: Informed consent

(1) It is the primary health care provider's duty to provide information to the client related to risks and benefits.

(2) It is the primary health care provider's duty to provide information to the client related to alternatives.

(3) Informing the client of successful amniocentesis does not fully address the client's lack of understanding of the risks and benefits.

(4) CORRECT: One of the nurse's roles in the informed consent process is to witness the signature on the consent form.

(5) CORRECT: One of the nurse's roles in the informed consent process is to advocate for the client by ensuring she has been provided the necessary information to make an informed decision.

14. The answer is 1

The nurse noticed an increase in the prevalence of pressure injury among clients in an intensive care unit (ICU). The nurse documented the findings and worked with the manager to develop and implement a new policy addressing the consistent use of pressure injury risk assessment scale. Which term **best** describes the nurse's actions?

Category: Performance improvement (quality improvement)

(1) CORRECT: Quality improvement includes activities such as identifying opportunities and developing policies for improving the quality of nursing practice. Identifying an increase in pressure injuries and implementing a policy aimed at improving the assessment and prevention of pressure injuries best fits the definition of quality improvement.

(2) The nurse may have collaborated (or worked together) with colleagues, but the nurse's actions described are examples of quality improvement activities.

(3) Advocacy refers to the nurse's duty to act on behalf of the client. Although reducing pressure ulcers may indirectly advocate for the client, the nurse's actions described are examples of quality improvement activities.

(4) Case management refers to the coordination of care to reduce fragmentation and costs, as well as to improve quality and outcomes.

15. The answer is 2

The nurse is working on a surgical unit. Which task would be appropriate for the nurse to delegate to an unlicensed assistive personnel (UAP)?

Category: Delegation

(1) Assisting a new postoperative client to the bathroom is a task the registered nurse or another licensed individual, such as an LPN/LVN, should perform.

(2) CORRECT: Setting up the client's lunch trays is an appropriate task to delegate to the UAP.

(3) Changing a central line dressing is a task the registered nurse or another licensed individual, such as an LPN/LVN, should perform.

(4) Teaching a client how to administer discharge medications is a task the registered nurse or another licensed individual, such as a pharmacist, should perform.

16. The answer is 1

A client with leukemia has consented to a blood transfusion against the wishes of the client's family, who are all Jehovah's Witnesses. The nurse knows that which ethical principle **best** supports the client's decision?

Category: Ethical practice

(1) CORRECT: Autonomy refers to the right of individuals to make decisions for themselves.

(2) Beneficence refers to the nurse's duty to do what is good for the client.

(3) Nonmaleficence refers to the nurse's duty to do no harm.

(4) Justice refers to the concept of fair and equitable treatment.

17. The answer is 2

The nurse wants to delegate the task of showering an elderly client in a wheelchair to the unlicensed assistive personnel (UAP). Before delegating a task to the UAP, the nurse should **first** ensure which is accomplished?

Category: Delegation

(1) Supervising the UAP does not ensure that the UAP's competency has been verified.

(2) CORRECT: Prior to delegating a task appropriate for the UAP, the nurse should first ensure that competency has been verified during the UAP's orientation.

(3) The fact that the UAP has performed the task before does not ensure that the UAP's competency has been verified.

(4) The fact that the UAP has received the assignment during report does not ensure that the UAP's competency has been verified.

18. The answer is 2

A well-known actor has been admitted to an ambulatory surgical unit. The nurse notices a staff member who is not involved in the client's care reading the actor's medical record. Which is the **most** appropriate action to take next?

Category: Confidentiality and information security

(1) A staff member who is not involved in the client's care is not authorized to access protected health information.

(2) CORRECT: An individual not involved in the care of the client does not have a legitimate need to access the medical record. The nurse should protect the client's right to privacy by ensuring only authorized individuals access medical records.

(3) The nurse should do more than simply inform the client of the breach.

(4) The nurse should do more than simply ask a physician if it's acceptable for the staff member to access the client's medical records.

19. The answer is 1 and 2

The nurse is learning how to use the hospital's new electronic medication administration record. The nurse knows this tool has the potential to achieve which goal? **(Select all that apply.)**

Category: Information technology

(1) CORRECT: Electronic medication administration records have the potential to reduce medication administration errors.

(2) CORRECT: Electronic medication administration records have the potential to improve access to client information at the point of care.

(3) It is always the nurses' responsibility to document medication administration.

(4) It is always the nurses' responsibility to verify the doses of drugs being administered.

(5) Electronic medication administration records are not accessible to the client.

20. The answer is 3

The nurse uses the Internet to receive electrocardiogram results from a client living in a nursing home. The nurse knows this type of information technology is **best** described as which of these?

Category: Information technology

(1) Encryption refers to the conversion of information to code during transmission to keep the information secure.

(2) Telecommunications refers to the electronic transmission of data over phone-based lines.

(3) CORRECT: Telehealth uses transmissions via telecommunications technology to transmit health information remotely.

(4) Nursing informatics refers to a specialty of nursing that integrates nursing and computer science.

21. See explanation for answers

Condition Most Likely Experiencing	
Cardiogenic shock.	☑

CORRECT OPTION: The client's rapid deterioration with hypotension, tachycardia, and reports of chest pressure indicate the client has developed decreased myocardial perfusion. The client's history of heart failure with an acute exacerbation and the client's advanced age increase the client's risk of developing **cardiogenic shock**.

INCORRECT OPTIONS: There are no indications of infection or sepsis. Although the client is wheezing with coarse crackles in the lung fields, the client's history indicates heart failure with volume overload and pulmonary congestion. The client's symptoms do not suggest stroke. The decrease in speech and interaction the client is displaying is due to the client's distress and possible decreased cerebral perfusion due to hypotension.

Actions to Take	
Apply oxygen 15 L/min per non rebreather face mask.	☑
Notify the rapid response team.	☑

CORRECT OPTIONS: The client must receive immediate actions to restore oxygenation and circulation, or the client's condition will further deteriorate and the client may go into cardiopulmonary arrest. The nurse will immediately administer **high-flow oxygen** and **notify the rapid response team**. The client's plan of care requires collaboration with the interdisciplinary team and treatment with vasopressors, fluids, and positive inotropic medications.

INCORRECT OPTIONS: The client's spouse does need to be notified of the change in condition as soon as possible, but that action is not the priority in the current situation. Epinephrine would increase the heart rate and would not be given unless the client went into cardiopulmonary arrest. The client would not tolerate Trendelenburg position; due to respiratory distress, the client will need the head of bed elevated. Using positioning to increase blood pressure will not be effective for this client.

Parameters to Monitor
Vital signs. ☑
Level of consciousness. ☑

CORRECT OPTIONS: As treatment continues to stabilize the client, the nurse will monitor the **vital signs** and pulse oximetry, as well as the client's **level of consciousness**. The main goals of treatment are to improve oxygenation and restore blood flow to the myocardium. If the client becomes unresponsive, the course of action will be altered. The client may have already developed myocardial ischemia and may require intervention to restore myocardial circulation.

INCORRECT OPTIONS: The nurse will continue to monitor the client's bowel sounds, intake and output, and skin temperature as indicators of perfusion, but these parameters are not as critical as the client's blood pressure, heart rate, respiratory rate, oxygen saturation, and level of consciousness. The client's skin temperature is not the best indicator of peripheral perfusion.

22. The answer is 2

The nurse prepares to transfer a client to the operating room. The nurse knows that adhering to the hospital policy for client hand-off communication **best** ensures which aspect of care management?

Category: Continuity of care

(1) Case management does not address the issue of hand-off communication between caregivers.

(2) CORRECT: Improving hand-off communication allows each caregiver to communicate completely, effectively, and consistently as the client transitions to different departments in the hospital. This process improves the continuity of care.

(3) Confidentiality protection does not address the issue of hand-off communication between caregivers.

(4) Collaboration does not address the issue of hand-off communication between caregivers.

23. The answer is 2, 4, and 5

The nurse prepares to perform an admission assessment on a client admitted for Crohn disease. The nurse knows that according to the Clients' Bill of Rights, the client is responsible for which of these? **(Select all that apply.)**

Category: Client rights

(1) Consenting to treatment is not a client responsibility delineated in the Clients' Bill of Rights; it is a client right.

(2) CORRECT: According to the American Hospital Association, clients' responsibilities include (among other things) providing information about medications.

(3) Providing proof of insurance is not a client responsibility delineated in the Clients' Bill of Rights.

(4) CORRECT: According to the American Hospital Association, clients' responsibilities include (among other things) providing information about past illnesses.

(5) CORRECT: The client has the responsibility to be considerate and respectful of the rights of other clients.

24. The answer is 1

The nurse cares for a client with a newly created colostomy. As part of the care planning for this client, the nurse knows a referral to which staff member will be the **priority**?

Category: Referral

(1) CORRECT: A referral to a certified wound, ostomy, and continence nurse (CWOCN), if available, is important to the management of a client with a colostomy during and after hospitalization.

(2) Although a referral to social services might be necessary based on other factors, it is not the priority in the situation described.

(3) Although a referral to physical therapy might be necessary based on other factors, it is not the priority in the situation described.

(4) Although a referral to occupational therapy might be necessary based on other factors, it is not the priority in the situation described.

25. The answer is 1

A registered nurse (RN) is in charge of a team on a medical-surgical unit that includes a licensed practical nurse (LPN). The RN understands that which is an activity that falls within the scope of practice of an LPN?

Category: Supervision

(1) CORRECT: Administering oral medications is an appropriate activity for the LPN.

(2) Collaborating with social services to develop a care plan is an activity that falls within registered nurses' scope of practice.

(3) Formulating a nursing diagnosis is an activity that falls within registered nurses' scope of practice.

(4) Developing policies are activities that fall within registered nurses' scope of practice.

26. The answer is 2 and 3

The nurse in a maternity unit cares for a client who has just given birth to twins. The client voices concern about her ability to manage when she gets home. Which statement **best** illustrates quality care delivery by the nurse? **(Select all that apply.)**

Category: Referrals

(1) Saying to focus on the babies' health dismisses the new mother's concerns about her ability to cope.

(2) CORRECT: A referral to home health care provides the client with opportunities for support and assistance during this transition.

(3) CORRECT: A referral to support groups provides the client with opportunities for support and assistance during this transition.

(4) Recommending a feeding method for the twins ignores the new mother's concerns about her ability to cope.

(5) Filling in paperworks is not a priority concern of the client. This action dismisses the client's concerns.

27. The answer is 2

After responding to a "code," several staff nurses express concerns over their confidence levels and performance to the nurse in charge of the hospital's performance improvement program. The nurse in charge knows the **best** way to evaluate and improve performance is to implement which of these?

Category: Performance improvement (quality improvement)

(1) Although analyzing performance data can be helpful in understanding performance issues, it is not the best way to improve performance.

(2) CORRECT: Mock codes can improve performance by encouraging teamwork, improving communication and skill-building, and enhancing confidence of caregivers.

(3) Studies suggest that, although important for learning, training courses are not the best way to improve performance.

(4) A written competency exam is not the best way to evaluate and improve performance because it tests knowledge rather than performance.

28. The answer is 2

A client is being treated for uncontrolled hypertension. The nurse knows that the involvement of nursing, pharmacy, cardiology, and nutritional services is an example of which approach?

Category: Collaboration with interdisciplinary team

(1) The concept of managed care does not directly relate to multidisciplinary approach in care.

(2) CORRECT: A multidisciplinary approach involves members from nursing, medicine, and other health care teams in the management of a particular disorder, in order to provide a more comprehensive and individualized approach.

(3) The concept of case management does not directly relate to multidisciplinary approach in care.

(4) The concept of performance improvement is not related to a multidisciplinary approach.

29. The answer is 2, 4, 1, 3

The nurse caring for a client who is newly diagnosed with diabetes mellitus performs the following tasks. Place the tasks the nurse would perform in the appropriate order. **All options must be used.**

Category: Establishing priorities

(1) Establishing outcomes/planning is the third step in the nursing process.

(2) Assessment is the first step in the nursing process.

(3) Evaluation is the last step in the nursing process.

(4) Diagnosis is the second step in the nursing process.

30. The answer is 1

The nurse administers the first dose of chemotherapy to a client. The nurse knows that which activity is appropriate to delegate to the licensed practical nurse (LPN)?

Category: Delegation

(1) CORRECT: An LPN may obtain the client's blood pressure and other vital signs.

(2) Providing teaching about the side effects of chemotherapy is not an activity that should be performed by an LPN.

(3) Administering a dose of chemotherapy is not an activity that should be performed by an LPN.

(4) Flushing the client's central line is not an activity that should be performed by an LPN.

CHAPTER 5

SAFE AND EFFECTIVE CARE ENVIRONMENT: SAFETY AND INFECTION CONTROL

Safety and infection control are closely linked areas that are particularly important in keeping clients healthy or helping them get well. Both home safety and safety in a hospital setting are covered in this topic area. An important part of hospital safety is the control of infections that clients might acquire while they are in the hospital (called *nosocomial infections*). These infections might not be related to their original condition or reason for admission but may have tremendous impact on their ability to heal.

On the NCLEX-RN® exam, you can expect approximately 13 percent of the questions to relate to Safety and Infection Control. This subcategory focuses on protecting clients and health care personnel from health and environmental hazards.

Exam content related to the Safety and Infection Control subcategory includes, but is not limited to, the following areas:

- Accident/error/injury prevention
- Emergency response plan
- Ergonomic principles
- Handling hazardous and infectious materials
- Home safety
- Reporting of incident/event/irregular occurrence/variance
- Safe use of equipment
- Security plan
- Standard precautions/transmission-based precautions/surgical asepsis
- Use of restraints/safety devices

Safety Background

Begin your review of safety issues by making sure you understand the various elements that are involved in client safety and accident prevention, including developmental- or age-related risks specific to infants, toddlers, school-age children, adolescents, adults, and older adults (geriatric clients), as follows:

- **Infants:** Educate parents or caretakers regarding infant safety and their responsibility to take proper precautions to prevent injury. Infants should be placed on their backs after eating and while sleeping, and transported using car seats. This age group has a high risk for falls and burns.

- **Toddlers:** Mobility and curiosity create safety issues including poisoning, choking, and drowning. Keep medications, poisons, and cleaning supplies in locked cabinets. Toddlers should be transported only in car seats.

- **School-age children:** Time spent in school and playing with friends creates new safety risks. Emphasize traffic safety, water safety, fire safety, and the dangers of strangers. Car seats and/or booster seats should be used for children until adult seat belts fit correctly, which typically does not occur until the child reaches 4′9″, weighs at least 80 lb, and is between ages 8 and 12. (Age and height/weight requirements vary by state.)

- **Adolescents:** Their sense of independence and invincibility, and access to cars, creates risk. Emphasize driver education, alcohol and substance abuse education, and sexual health information.

- **Adults:** Safety risks for this age group include home, workplace, and leisure activities. Educate adults about motor vehicle, fire, and firearm safety.

- **Older adults:** Aging issues, both physical and cognitive, impact safety, particularly regarding falls and side effects of medication. Possibilities of elder abuse and motor vehicle accidents also increase for older adults.

You also need to understand the elements that are involved in client safety and accident prevention related to the care environment. For example, in a hospital setting, fall risks are most common in infants and geriatric clients. Know the elements of a fall prevention program, including the different steps taken based on the age of the client. Safety also involves the use of restraints to limit mobility, and taking proper seizure precautions. You should be able to explain these precautions, which include the use of physical restraints, and the need for suction and oxygen equipment.

Infection Control Background

To correctly answer questions about infection control, begin by making sure you understand some basic information about etiologic agents and the chain of infection.

An *etiologic agent* is any pathogen that can cause an infection. Etiologic agents include bacteria, fungi, protozoa, rickettsiae, and helminths.

There are six elements in the chain of infection:

(1) **Pathogen:** An infectious agent, like a bacteria or virus.

(2) **Reservoirs:** Any environment that is favorable for growth and reproduction of infectious agents. A reservoir may be animate or inanimate. Human systems that can act as reservoirs include blood, respiratory, gastrointestinal, reproductive, and urinary.

(3) **Portal of exit:** A place where the infectious organisms get out of a host. Any of the above-mentioned systems may be portals of exit.

(4) **Method of transmission:** The way an infectious organism is transferred from reservoir to host. This happens in one of three ways: direct contact, indirect contact via a vector, or through the air (airborne).

(5) **Portal of entry:** A place where an infectious agent enters the susceptible host. A portal of entry may also be through a system that can act as a reservoir.

(6) **Susceptible host:** A client, staff member, or other individual at risk for infection.

Now let's review the most important concepts covered by the Safety and Infection Control subcategory on the NCLEX-RN® exam.

Accident/Error/Injury Prevention

To help protect clients from accident and injury, you should assess risk factors upon the client's admission and identify appropriate methods to minimize risk of injury. This includes knowledge of the developmental stages mentioned previously in the Safety Background section, the client's lifestyle, and the client's knowledge of safety precautions.

You should know how to identify specific deficits, such as sight, hearing, and other sensory perceptions that may impact client safety. It's also important to be able to teach families how to properly install and use infant and child car seats.

Medication and allergies are primary areas for error. Error prevention, therefore, begins with proper identification of the client. You should be able to identify client allergies and intervene appropriately, know how to verify appropriateness and/or accuracy of a treatment or medication order, and be able to prevent treatment errors using critical thinking and by following policies.

Emergency Response Plan

The Joint Commission requires hospitals to have a disaster plan and periodically practice response to the plan. You are responsible for knowing your role in disaster response.

Know all of the steps involved in fire safety in a hospital setting. If a fire occurs, first get clients out of danger, then work to contain the fire, and finally determine the order in which to evacuate clients, including identification of clients who must be evacuated in beds or on stretchers (horizontally). You must also know how to teach clients about fire safety at home, such as knowing emergency numbers, installing and testing smoke alarms, acquiring fire extinguishers, and so on.

Ergonomic Principles

In order to protect not only the client but also yourself, you must understand ergonomic principles when caring for clients. This includes using assistive devices and proper lifting techniques. Assess a client's ability to balance and use assistive devices, such as crutches or a walker, and use that information to help develop an appropriate care plan.

For clients with repetitive stress injuries, provide instruction and information about body positions that can minimize or prevent these injuries. For clients with conditions that cause stress to specific skeletal or muscular groups, understand and educate the clients about necessary modifications. These may include changing positions frequently, and performing routine stretching exercises for the shoulders, neck, arms, hands, and fingers.

To protect yourself, you must not only use the proper lifting techniques when moving and transferring clients, but also use correct posture in carrying out your daily routines. Technology and technological devices (such as computer workstations, computers on wheels, monitors) add to the physical stress that nurses unconsciously put on their bodies—for instance, by overextending the wrists, slouching, sitting without foot support, or straining to look at poorly placed monitors. You must know how to correctly adjust workstations to minimize awkward and frequently performed movements.

Handling Hazardous and Infectious Materials

It is important to be aware of the elements of employee safety. These include the safe use of equipment, safe handling of hazardous chemicals, and the use of Material Safety Data Sheets (MSDS), which are Occupational Safety and Health Administration (OSHA)-required handouts that describe all chemical agents in an employment setting.

Know the standard precautions to protect against blood-borne pathogen exposure. (OSHA has written standards that include recommendations from the Centers for Disease Control and Prevention [CDC], including the use of gloves and face and eye protection.) You must know what to do in case of a needle-stick, the standards for environmental infection control, and necessary information related to latex allergies for both staff and clients. Be sure latex-free gloves and latex-free carts are available and used as necessary.

You also need to be able to identify biohazardous, flammable, and infectious materials; know how to control the spread of infectious agents; follow procedures for handling biohazardous materials; and be able to demonstrate safe handling techniques to staff and clients.

The Needlestick Safety and Prevention Act is significant legislation that was enacted to protect health care workers. Do not re-cap needles or bend or break them before disposal. Ensure that sharps containers are in each client room and medication area.

Home Safety

Home safety includes evaluating the client's home care environment for fire risk, environmental hazards, and other elements that present a risk of accident or injury to the client. It also involves working with the client and the client's family and significant others to recommend modifications, such as lighting or handrails.

Home safety also includes teaching clients self-care, and teaching parents how to care for children. It also includes teaching preventive measures for home care, such as encouraging the client to use protective equipment when using devices that can cause injury.

Reporting of Incident/Event/Irregular Occurrence/Variance

Incident reports are tools designed to provide information about potential areas of exposure to liability, and are also used to identify problems and develop solutions to prevent the same incident from happening again. Being able to accurately identify situations requiring completion of an incident or unusual occurrence report is an important skill. Although each hospital has its own procedures, the most important thing is to prevent further injury. In addition to reporting, you need to evaluate the response to the event to ensure it helped to correct the situation and to prevent further errors. Record the facts of the incident in the medical record, but do not include a copy of the incident report or make reference to its existence in the medical record.

Safe Use of Equipment

You must make sure that equipment needed to perform client care procedures and treatments is used safely and properly. This includes inspecting equipment to make sure it is safe to use. If a client needs to use equipment at home, you must teach the client how to use the equipment safely and properly.

If equipment is not safe, or if it malfunctions, you should stop using it, label it as broken, remove it from any possible use, put it in a designated area for broken equipment (if available), and report the problem to the appropriate person.

Security Plan

You may be asked to triage injured or ill clients in an emergency, and to identify those in need of urgent care. The exam focuses on airway, breathing, circulation, and neurological deficits.

The order is:

(1) Clear and open the airway.

(2) Assess for respiratory distress.

(3) Assess quality of breathing (rate, and color of skin, lips, and fingernails) and auscultate lungs.

(4) Check pulse.

(5) Assess for external bleeding.

(6) Take blood pressure.

(7) Assess the level of consciousness and pupillary response, and the weakness or paralysis of extremities.

You should also be aware of your facility's procedures and protocols during an evacuation, newborn nursery security event, and bomb threat. Nurses often participate in developing security and emergency plans, so you should be prepared to do so. Clinical decision-making skills and critical thinking are important components of the development and successful execution of a security plan.

Standard Precautions/Transmission-Based Precautions/Surgical Asepsis

There are a variety of different precautions that should be used to prevent the spread of infection. These include "standard" precautions that should always be used, precautions specifically aimed at the transmission of pathogenic microorganisms, and surgical asepsis (sterile techniques).

Standard Precautions

In addition to understanding the chain of infection, you should be able to apply standard precautions (such as handwashing, wearing gloves and gowns, and using face protection, such as masks, goggles, and face shields) with respect to hand hygiene, blood, bodily fluids, excretions, and secretions. These principles apply whether or not the skin and mucous membranes are intact, and should always be used in caring for clients across all diagnoses and all care settings.

Be aware of how, and in what order, to correctly put on and remove personal protective equipment (PPE). Perform hand hygiene first. Then before making contact with the client, and preferably outside the room, put on PPE: gown first, then the mask, then eye protection, and gloves last. The steps reverse for PPE removal are: remove gloves first, then eye protection, then gown, then mask, with hand hygiene coming last.

Transmission-Based Precautions

Transmission-based precautions limit the spread of pathogenic microorganisms. You should be able to compare and contrast airborne, droplet, and contact precautions; know when to use each; and know when multiple precautions may be needed. For example, when small (< 5 mcm) pathogen-infected droplets remain suspended in the air over time and travel distances greater than 3 feet, use airborne precautions. Pathogens may include measles (rubeola), chickenpox (varicella), and tuberculosis, among others. Use droplet precautions for larger (> 5 mcm) pathogen-infected droplets that travel 3 feet or less via coughing, sneezing, and so on. An example of this type of pathogen is *Haemophilus influenzae*. Use contact precautions with known or suspected microorganisms transmitted by direct hand-to-skin contact or indirect contact with surfaces (*Clostridium difficile*, herpes simplex, impetigo, etc.).

You should also be able to identify infectious agents that require transmission-based precautions, and specific precautions used in cases of drug-resistant infections.

Surgical Asepsis

You need to understand the principles of surgical asepsis—the practices necessary to maintain objects and areas free of microorganisms—also known as *sterile techniques*. Know how to use these techniques in implementing a variety of procedures, including IV therapy and urinary catheterization.

The basic principles of surgical asepsis are:

- Every object used in a sterile field must be sterile.
- If a sterile object touches an unsterile object, it is no longer sterile.
- If a sterile object is out of view, or below waist level, it is considered unsterile.

- A sterile object can become unsterile through exposure to airborne microorganisms.
- Fluids flow in the direction of gravity.
- Moisture passing through a sterile object can draw microorganisms from unsterile surfaces above or below through capillary action.
- The edges of a sterile field are unsterile.
- The skin cannot be sterilized.

Use of Restraints/Safety Devices

You need to understand the difference between chemical (medication) and physical restraints (bedside rails, jacket, and extremity strap restraints). In addition, you need to know how to utilize restraints safely, effectively, and only when necessary, as well as how and with what frequency to monitor clients who are restrained. It's also important to understand the legal implications of restraining clients, as well as agency-specific policies and procedures. This includes understanding that seizures may necessitate restraint.

Chapter Quiz

1. The provider prescribes a magnetic resonance imaging (MRI) of the brain for an adult client. Which finding in the client's history should the nurse report to the health care provider?

   1. Allergy to iodine-based contrast dye.
   2. Implanted cardiac pacemaker.
   3. Chronic obstructive pulmonary disease (COPD).
   4. Hernia repair.

2. The nurse develops a care plan for a client with hepatitis C. The nurse knows that the hepatitis C virus is primarily transmitted through which route?

   1. Contaminated food.
   2. Feces.
   3. Blood.
   4. Sputum.

3. The nurse prepares to discharge a client with rheumatic heart disease who is recovering from endocarditis. Which client statement indicates to the nurse that the client understands the teaching?

   1. "I'm so glad I don't need any more antibiotics now that I'm feeling better."
   2. "I can restart my exercise program in a day or two."
   3. "I will watch for signs of relapse the first few days after discharge."
   4. "I will inform my dentist should I ever need any dental work."

4. The nurse prepares a client with acquired immunodeficiency syndrome (AIDS) for discharge to home. Which instruction should the nurse include?

   1. "Avoid sharing articles such as razors and toothbrushes."
   2. "Do not share eating utensils with family members."
   3. "Limit the time you spend in public places."
   4. "Avoid eating food from serving dishes shared with others."

5. The nurse prepares to administer a tuberculin (Mantoux) skin test to a client suspected of having tuberculosis (TB). The nurse knows that the tuberculin test will reveal which of these?

   1. How long the client has been infected with TB.
   2. Active TB infection.
   3. Latent TB infection.
   4. Whether the client has been infected with TB.

Refer to the Case Study to answer the next six questions.

The nurse is caring for a middle-age adult client in a medical surgical unit.

Admission Notes	Nurse's Notes

The client is referred from a community health care clinic for evaluation of pulmonary symptoms and general debilitation. The client is experiencing a cough of four (4) months duration with productive sputum, night sweats, weight loss, and extreme fatigue. The client has human immunodeficiency virus (HIV) infection diagnosed three (3) years ago. The client tested positive for latent tuberculosis infection (LTBI) at the time of the HIV diagnosis but did not complete the recommended treatment. Various social and personal factors have also negatively impacted the client's adherence to antiretroviral therapy (ART) for HIV infection. Clinic records indicate the client had a positive reaction to the tuberculin skin test two (2) weeks ago.

Social History: The client is currently experiencing homelessness and has lived in numerous overcrowded housing and community homeless shelters for several years. The client admits to a "several year" history of smoking 1–2 packs of cigarettes per day, and has an uncertain history of substance use disorder (SUD).

Pending diagnostic studies:

- Tuberculosis (TB) blood test.

- Chest x-ray.

- Sputum for acid fast bacilli (AFB) smear and culture.

Admission Notes	Nurse's Notes

Admission Vital Signs	Results
BP	110/62 mmHg
Heart rate	106, irregular
Respiratory rate	24, regular
Temperature (oral)	99.6° F (37.5° C)
Pulse Oximetry	95% on room air
Body Mass Index (BMI)	17 kg/m^2, underweight

Assessment	Client Finding
General	Frail, appears undernourished
	Lethargy
Integument	Skin intact, pale, warm, and dry
	Dry oral mucous membranes
	Decreased turgor
Cardiovascular	S1 and S2 auscultated, irregular rhythm, no murmurs
	Capillary refill less than 2 seconds
	2+ radial pulses, equal
Respiratory	Crackles in bilateral lung bases
	Productive cough with discolored sputum
	No dyspnea or chest pain
Abdomen	Soft, flat, non tender
	Normoactive bowel sounds × 4 quadrants
Musculoskeletal	Moves all extremities
	Muscle wasting present
	Muscle strength 3/5 bilaterally

6. The nurse reviews the admission notes and performs an assessment.

The nurse is concerned with which client finding? **(Select all that apply.)**

1. Untreated latent tuberculosis infection (LTBI).
2. 2+ radial pulses, equal.
3. HIV infection.
4. Productive cough of four (4) months duration.
5. Night sweats.
6. Respiratory rate 24.
7. Pulse oximetry 95% on room air.
8. Heart rate 106, irregular.
9. Crackles in bilateral lung bases.

7. Complete the following sentence by choosing from the list of options.

The nurse recognizes the client's findings may indicate symptoms related to [Select from list 1] that is associated with risk factors of [Select from list 2] and [Select from list 3].

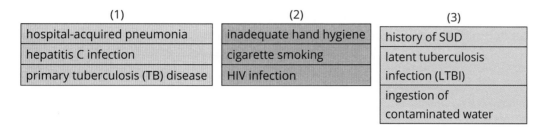

(1)	(2)	(3)
hospital-acquired pneumonia	inadequate hand hygiene	history of SUD
hepatitis C infection	cigarette smoking	latent tuberculosis infection (LTBI)
primary tuberculosis (TB) disease	HIV infection	ingestion of contaminated water

8. The client's AFB smear strongly indicates a diagnosis of TB. The health care team begins treatment while awaiting the finalization of sputum cultures.

To reduce transmission and prevent the spread of TB infection, which isolation precaution is a priority for the nurse to use?

1. Contact.
2. Droplet.
3. Protective environment.
4. Airborne.

9. Drag the choices below to fill in each blank in the following sentence. Each choice will only be used once.

When developing the plan of care, the nurse includes goals to _____ [Select from the list], _____ [Select from the list], and _____ [Select from the list].

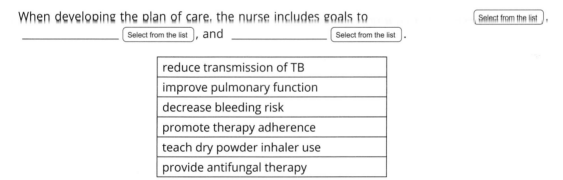

reduce transmission of TB
improve pulmonary function
decrease bleeding risk
promote therapy adherence
teach dry powder inhaler use
provide antifungal therapy

10. The nurse implements care related to infection control using standard precautions and airborne precautions for TB. Select **4** actions that are appropriate implementations of these precautions.

    1. Wear a surgical mask when within 3 to 6 feet of the client.

    2. Place client in a single room with negative pressure airflow.

    3. Put on shoe and hair coverings before entering the room.

    4. Wear a proper fitting high-efficiency particulate air (HEPA) mask when entering the room.

    5. Place client in a single room with positive pressure airflow.

    6. Close the door to the room to control the direction of airflow.

    7. Teach the client proper cough etiquette.

11. The client has responded clinically and is discharged to housing arrangements obtained by social services. The nurse provides discharge teaching about reducing transmission of TB in the community.

    For each client statement below, specify whether the statement indicates effective teaching or ineffective teaching.

Assessment Finding	Effective	Ineffective
"Taking my medicine is the best way to keep from spreading TB to my friends."	○	○
"I like to be outdoors by myself and won't mind not being around lots of people or riding the public bus."	○	○
"It's so good that I don't need to bother my close friends with being screened for TB since I'm taking my medications."	○	○
"I'll keep my clinic visits so that I can get my phlegm checked for TB to know how I'm doing."	○	○
"Once I feel pretty good, I'm looking forward to cutting back on my medicine."	○	○

12. The nurse has just administered insulin to a client. Which is the appropriate action to dispose the insulin syringe and needle?

1. Re-cap the needle and discard it in the nearest puncture-resistant container.

2. Re-cap the needle and discard it in the nearest biohazard container.

3. Discard the needle in a puncture-resistant container.

4. Break the needle and discard it in the nearest puncture-resistant container.

13. The nurse prepares to administer packed red blood cells (PRBCs) to a client. Arrange the following steps in the order the nurse should perform them. **All options must be used.**

1. Explain the procedure to the client.

2. Obtain the client's vital signs.

3. Assess that the client has a blood bank identification armband.

4. Obtain the PRBCs from the blood bank according to hospital policy and perform a visual check of the blood.

5. Perform a bedside identification and blood product verification by two licensed independent practitioners.

6. Verify the physician order.

7. Prime the transfusion tubing with a 0.9% sodium chloride solution.

14. Two nurses prepare to lift a client up in bed. Which precaution should the nurses take to help avoid injuring their backs?

1. Bend from the waist.

2. Lift with the back, not with the legs.

3. Lower the head of the bed to about 30 degrees, if the client can tolerate it.

4. Make certain the bed is in a reasonably high position.

15. In the emergency department (ED), the nurse assesses a child suspected of having measles. Which infection control precaution should the nurse initiate?

1. Contact precautions.

2. Droplet precautions.

3. Airborne precautions.

4. Reverse isolation.

16. A client presents to the emergency department reporting vaginal discharge, irritation of the vagina, and the need to urinate often. The nurse suspects a sexually transmitted infection (STI). The provider prescribes diagnostic testing of the vaginal discharge. Which STI must be reported to the local Department of Health in every state?

1. Genital herpes.

2. Human papillomavirus infection.

3. Gonorrhea.

4. Trichomoniasis.

17. A client who had a total hip replacement is disoriented to time, place, and person. The client is attempting to get out of bed and pull out the IV line that is infusing antibiotics. The client has bilateral soft wrist restraints and a vest restraint. Which intervention by the nurse are appropriate? **(Select all that apply.)**

1. Ask the client if he needs to use the bathroom, and provide range-of-motion exercises every 2 hours.

2. Document the type of restraint used and assess the need for continued use.

3. Tie the restraints to the side rails of the bed.

4. Obtain a new health care provider prescription for the restraint every 12 hours.

5. Observe for correct placement of restraints.

6. Tie the restraints in a quick-release knot.

Refer to the Case Study to answer the next question.

The nurse in the community clinic is caring for an older adult client.

History and Physical	Vital Signs

Client presents in clinic for follow up care for chronic human immunodeficiency virus (HIV) type-1. The client has been living with HIV for eight years and reports being healthy and having no symptoms during this time. The client has not been seen by a health provider for several years and was encouraged to return to care by a peer mentor at a veteran organization.

Two weeks ago, the client was seen in clinic with new onset of oral candidiasis, mild fever, fatigue, occasional night sweats, and diarrhea, along with 5% of body weight unintentional weight loss. The client's most recent CD4+ T-cell lymphocyte count is 323 cells/mm^3 (low) and HIV RNA (viral load) is high. At the time of HIV diagnosis, the client was not ready to start antiretroviral therapy (ART). Client now states, "I've thought about taking it, and want to learn about some of my options. I'm not as afraid of it as I once was."

Social History: The client has had inconsistent access to care, and poor coordination of care and retention in care. Uncertain history of substance abuse. Lives alone, and reports for some time unstable living arrangements due to economic barriers. Client has low health literacy and reports little social support.

Physical Exam: Pleasant and conversational, appears slightly anxious, appropriately groomed. Alert, oriented × 4, pupils equal, round, react to light (PERRL). White creamy patches on tongue and buccal surfaces. Skin pale, warm and dry, decreased turgor. Tender, swollen axillary nodes, bilaterally. Lungs clear bilaterally, breathing unlabored, dry cough. S1 and S2 auscultated, regular rhythm, no murmurs, 2+ radial pulses. Abdomen soft, rounded, positive bowel sounds × 4. Moves all extremities, no edema. Joint tenderness in elbows, hips, and knees bilaterally.

History and Physical	Vital Signs

Vital Signs	Results
BP	142/73 mmHg
Pulse	90, regular
Respiratory rate	20, regular
Temperature (oral)	99.8° F (37.66° C)
Pulse oximetry	97% on room air
Body Mass Index (BMI)	22 kg/m^2 (normal)

18. The nurse reviews the client's history and physical and provides care.

Complete the diagram by dragging from the choices below to specify the priority concern for the client, 2 actions the nurse takes to address that concern, and 2 parameters the nurse monitors to assess the client's progress.

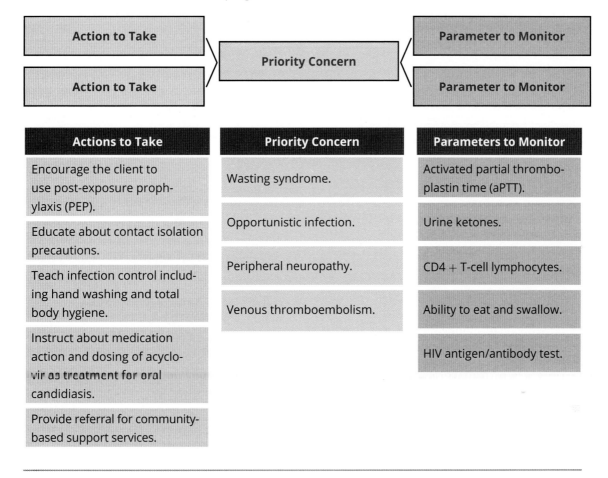

Actions to Take	Priority Concern	Parameters to Monitor
Encourage the client to use post-exposure prophylaxis (PEP).	Wasting syndrome.	Activated partial thromboplastin time (aPTT).
Educate about contact isolation precautions.	Opportunistic infection.	Urine ketones.
Teach infection control including hand washing and total body hygiene.	Peripheral neuropathy.	CD4 + T-cell lymphocytes.
Instruct about medication action and dosing of acyclovir as treatment for oral candidiasis.	Venous thromboembolism.	Ability to eat and swallow.
Provide referral for community-based support services.		HIV antigen/antibody test.

19. Which action does the nurse implement **first** before administering medications to a client?

    1. Scan the medication label and the client's wristband.

    2. Ask the client their name to properly identify this client as the one for whom the medications were prescribed.

    3. Match the client's date of birth and name on the client's wristband with the same information on the medication prescription.

    4. Match the client's name and room number with the medication prescription.

20. The health care provider verbally prescribes a medication for a client during an emergency. Which steps should the nurse take next?

    1. Repeat the prescription back to the provider for confirmation and administer it.

    2. Retrieve the medication and administer it.

    3. Write the prescription down, retrieve the medication, and administer it.

    4. Read the prescription to another nurse, have that nurse retrieve the medication, and stay with the client.

21. The client has a prescription for the placement of a urinary catheter due to urinary retention. What should the nurse do before starting the procedure? **(Select all that apply.)**

    1. Verify the client's identity using two identifiers.

    2. Confirm the client's medical record number via the wristband and prescription.

    3. Ask the client's name only, because this is a procedure and not a medication administration.

    4. Obtain a signed informed consent witnessed by another nurse.

    5. Confirm the client's name via the wrist ID band and provider prescription.

22. Which action by the nurse is the **most** effective means of preventing infection?

    1. When hands are visibly contaminated with body fluids, rub hands with Clorox wipes.

    2. Perform hand hygiene before reporting for work.

    3. Wear sterile gloves when giving IV medications.

    4. When hands are not visibly soiled, use an alcohol-based hand rub for routine hand decontamination.

23. The nurse cares for a client who is obese with pressure injuries. Treatment requires frequent turning and repositioning. The nursing unit has a special lift that allows for turning of clients and placement onto a bedpan without any lifting on the part of the staff. The client urgently requests the bedpan. Because the lift apparatus takes a few minutes to set up, which action should the nurse take?

    1. Quickly assist the client onto the bedpan without the lifting apparatus.

    2. Encourage the client to try to be patient, and set up the lifting apparatus.

    3. Get the assistance of an unlicensed assistive personnel (UAP) to help lift the client.

    4. Encourage the client to wear an incontinence brief while confined to bed.

24. The nurse cares for client who has experienced multiple episodes of hyperglycemia not manageable by subcutaneous insulin injections. The client is prescribed an insulin drip for glycemic management which will be discontinued at bedtime, after which the client is NPO. The client's most recent blood glucose level, taken at 1500, was 60 mg/dL (3.3 mmol/L). Which action by the nurse is **best**?

    1. Continue the current prescribed infusion until bedtime.

    2. Recheck the client's blood glucose level.

    3. Notify the provider about the client's blood glucose level and discuss stopping the infusion.

    4. Seek advice from other nurses.

25. The adult children of a hospice home care client inquire about whether it is safe to hug their mother, because she has had a methicillin-resistant *Staphylococcus aureus* (MRSA) infection in the past. Which statement by the children would indicate a need for further teaching by the nurse?

    1. "We should wash our hands frequently."
    2. "We should use alcohol-based hand sanitizer."
    3. "Those of us with poor immune systems should be extra careful when visiting our mother."
    4. "We should wear gowns and gloves at all times when having contact with our mother."

26. The hospitalized client is receiving an intravenous infusion and the pump has malfunctioned. Which action by the nurse is **best** once the infusion is restarted with a functioning pump?

    1. Place a "Broken" sticker on the malfunctioning pump, and place it in the designated area.
    2. Place the malfunctioning pump in the dirty utility room and call the manufacturer.
    3. Remove the malfunctioning pump from the client's room and place with other pumps.
    4. Place the malfunctioning pump to the side in the client's room and attach a "Do not use" sign.

27. The nurse completes a peripherally inserted central catheter (PICC) line dressing change. Which is the appropriate sequence when removing the personal protective equipment (PPE)?

    1. Remove the mask and then the gloves.
    2. Remove the gloves and then the mask.
    3. Remove the goggles and then the mask.
    4. Remove the gown and then the gloves.

28. A client is found on the floor by the UAP. Once the client is safe, which is the **most** appropriate action by the nurse?

    1. Document the event in the client's medical record and file an incident report.
    2. File an incident report as soon as possible.
    3. Document the event in the medical record and have the UAP file an incident report.
    4. Document the event in the client's medical record only.

29. The medical center encounters a bomb threat. The emergency response team informs the staff that the threat is legitimate and that clients should be evacuated. Which client should the nurse begin evacuating **first** to the safe designated area?

    1. Ambulatory clients.
    2. Bedridden clients.
    3. Intensive care unit clients.
    4. Pediatric clients.

30. The nurse discovers that a client received the wrong dose of intravenous antibiotic. Which is the most appropriate action by the nurse?

    1. Document the event in the client's medical record only.
    2. File an incident report, and document the event in the client's medical record.
    3. Document in the client's medical record that an incident report was filed.
    4. File an incident report, but do not document the event in the client's medical record, because information about the incident is protected.

Chapter Quiz Answers and Explanations

1. The answer is 2

The provider prescribes a magnetic resonance imaging (MRI) of the brain for an adult client. Which finding in the client's history should the nurse report to the health care provider?

Category: Accident/injury prevention; Safe use of equipment

(1) Allergy to iodine-based contrast dye is contraindicated in CT scans with contrast, not MRI.

(2) CORRECT: Metallic items, including metallic implants such as a cardiac pacemaker, are contraindicated in MRI. Other devices that are contraindicated in MRI include implanted pacemaker defibrillator, ferromagnetic aneurysm clips, cochlear implant, deep brain stimulation device, and metallic foreign bodies. Clients are advised to remove all jewelry, clothing, and other items that may contain metal before entering the MRI area.

(3) COPD is not a contraindication for MRI.

(4) Hernia repair is not a contraindication for MRI.

2. The answer is 3

The nurse develops a care plan for a client with hepatitis C. The nurse knows that the hepatitis C virus is primarily transmitted through which of these?

Category: Standard precautions/transmission-based precautions/surgical asepsis

(1) The hepatitis A (not hepatitis C) virus is transmitted through the fecal-oral route, primarily through ingestion of contaminated food.

(2) The hepatitis A (not hepatitis C) virus is transmitted through the fecal-oral route, primarily through ingestion of contaminated food.

(3) CORRECT: The hepatitis C virus is transmitted through blood and parenteral routes.

(4) The hepatitis C virus is not transmitted through sputum.

3. The answer is 4

The nurse prepares to discharge a client with rheumatic heart disease who is recovering from endocarditis. Which client statement indicates to the nurse that the client understands the teaching?

Category: Standard precautions/transmission-based precautions/surgical asepsis

(1) The client must take the full course of prescribed antibiotics even if feeling better.

(2) The client must restrict activity as directed by the provider.

(3) Relapse may occur, but not until about 2 weeks after treatment stops.

(4) CORRECT: Susceptible clients must understand the need for prophylactic antibiotics before, during, and after dental work. During dental work bacteria in the mouth may trigger endocarditis in people at higher risk.

4. The answer is 1

The nurse prepares a client with acquired immunodeficiency syndrome (AIDS) for discharge to home. Which instruction should the nurse include?

Category: Standard precautions/transmission-based precautions/surgical asepsis

(1) CORRECT: The human immunodeficiency virus (HIV), which causes AIDS, is concentrated mostly in blood and semen. The client should not share articles that may be contaminated with blood, such as razors and toothbrushes.

(2) HIV is not transmitted by sharing eating utensils.

(3) Someone with HIV does not need to limit time in public places.

(4) HIV is not transmitted by sharing food from serving dishes used by someone with AIDS.

5.   The answer is 4

The nurse prepares to administer a tuberculin (Mantoux) skin test to a client suspected of having tuberculosis (TB). The nurse knows that the tuberculin test will reveal which of these?

Category: Standard precautions/transmission-based precautions/surgical asepsis

(1)   The test cannot detect how long a person has been infected.

(2)   The test cannot detect whether the infection is latent (inactive) or active.

(3)   The test cannot detect whether the infection can be passed on to others.

(4)   CORRECT: A tuberculin skin test is performed to determine if a person has ever had TB or has been infected with the TB bacilli.

6. The answer is 1, 3, 4, 5, 6, 8, and 9

CORRECT OPTIONS: The nurse is concerned that the client's history of **untreated latent tuberculosis infection (LTBI)** and **HIV co-infection** are strong risk factors for progressing to tuberculosis (TB) disease. The nurse is concerned with abnormal clinical findings of **productive cough of four-month duration**, **night sweats**, **respiratory rate 24**, **heart rate 106 and irregular**, and **crackles in bilateral lung bases**.

INCORRECT OPTIONS: The nurse is not concerned with the client's 2+ radial pulses or pulse oximetry 95% on room air as these are normal adult assessments.

7. See explanation for answers

CORRECT OPTION: The nurse recognizes the client's clinical findings may indicate symptoms related to **primary tuberculosis (TB) disease**. Productive cough, night sweats, fever, weight loss, and abnormal lung sounds are present in clients who have active TB. INCORRECT OPTIONS: A pneumonia that develops after 48 hours of admission in a nonintubated client and not present at the time of admission is known as a hospital-acquired pneumonia. The client presented with respiratory symptoms at the time of admission. While hepatitis B and C virus can occur as co-infections with HIV, the client's clinical findings do not correlate with common manifestations of hepatitis (i.e., fatigue, hepatomegaly, jaundice, joint pain, and dark urine).

CORRECT OPTION: Immunosuppression from varying causes, cancer, and long-term corticosteroid use increases the risk for the development of TB. Clients living with **HIV** have a high risk for developing TB. INCORRECT OPTIONS: Inadequate hand hygiene does not promote the spread of TB, an infectious disease transmitted person to person through airborne droplets. Cigarette smoking is a risk factor for different lower respiratory disorders including lung cancer and obstructive pulmonary disease. Risk factors for TB include immunocompromised status, immigration from or recent travel to countries with a high prevalence of TB, institutionalization, and overcrowded living conditions.

CORRECT OPTION: Clients with **latent TB infection (LTBI)**, a condition when TB bacteria are inactive in the body, may develop TB disease if untreated. HIV infection is the strongest risk factor for progressing to TB disease among clients with LBTI. INCORRECT OPTIONS: A history of SUD does not increase the client's risk for the development of primary TB. Ingestion of contaminated water is a risk for other reemerging infections, but not a risk for the development of TB.

8. The answer is 4

CORRECT OPTION: **Airborne precautions** are used for diseases that are transmitted by smaller droplets and remain in the air for longer periods of time, such as TB, varicella virus, and rubeola virus.

INCORRECT OPTIONS: Contact precautions are used for clients who have illnesses acquired by direct contact with items in the client's environment. Examples of illnesses requiring contact precautions include *Clostridioides difficile* and methicillin-resistant *Staphylococcus aureus* (MRSA). Droplet precautions are used to protect against illnesses that are transmitted by larger droplets expelled at close contact such as influenza virus, pertussis, pneumonia, and meningitis. Protective environment precautions are focused on clients highly vulnerable to infection, such as clients who have received an organ transplant or hematopoietic stem cell transplant (HSCT).

9. See explanation for answers

CORRECT OPTIONS: The nurse plans goals to **reduce transmission of TB**, **improve pulmonary function**, and **promote TB therapy adherence**. Reducing transmission of TB is important in the acute care setting as it is an infectious disease usually spread from person to person by small airborne droplets expelled during talking or coughing that remain in the air over longer periods of time. Improving pulmonary function is a goal related to preventing further complication from TB such as scarring and residual cavitation in the lungs. Medication therapy is the cornerstone of TB treatment and fostering adherence is essential for effective treatment.

INCORRECT OPTIONS: The nurse does not include goals to decrease bleeding risk, teach dry powder inhaler use, or provide antifungal therapy. TB disease is not a risk factor for acute or chronic blood loss. Although HIV infection can alter platelet counts, there are no clinical signs or symptoms of thrombocytopenia in the client that indicate bleeding. Dry powder inhaler use is a method of medication delivery for clients with chronic obstructive diseases. Teaching its use is not indicated in the client who has TB. Antifungal therapy is used to treat fungal infections that can be opportunistic in immunocompromised clients; it is not indicated as a treatment for TB.

10. The answer is 2, 4, 6, and 7

CORRECT OPTIONS: The nurse appropriately implements airborne precautions by **placing the client in a single room with negative pressure airflow** or an airborne infection isolation room (AIIR). An infected client with TB expels smaller droplets that remain suspended in the air over longer distances that can be inhaled by another person. Air is filtered through a high efficiency particulate air filter so it is not returned to the inside ventilation system and instead exhausted to the outside. **A proper fitting HEPA mask, such as an N95 respirator, is worn by the nurse when entering the room** due to its highly effective protection from small droplets. **Closing the door to the room to control the direction of airflow** is an important isolation precaution for clients with TB to prevent transmission to health care workers. **Teaching the client proper cough etiquette**, such as covering the nose and mouth with paper tissues during coughing or sneezing, is a part of standard precautions in clients with symptoms of respiratory infection.

INCORRECT OPTIONS: In illnesses such as influenza, larger droplets are expelled into the air and spread at close contact. Droplet precautions require the nurse to wear a surgical mask when within 3 to 6 feet of the client in these circumstances. Shoe and hair coverings before entering the room are not required in airborne or standard precautions. A single room with positive pressure airflow creates a protective, contaminant free environment for clients who are highly vulnerable to infection, such as after hematopoietic stem cell or organ transplant.

11. See explanation for answers

Effective: Effective teaching includes the client statement about **medication adherence** and its importance in controlling the spread of infection. TB is communicable and taking medications is the best means to prevent transmission. While clients are infectious, exposure to close contacts should be minimized, **spending time outdoors is encouraged and reducing time in public areas is important**. The client's statement has indicated effective teaching about this information. Notifying the public health department is required and public health nurses provide follow up and assessment for adherence. **Sputum for AFB smear and culture is obtained at frequent intervals.**

Ineffective: **Close contacts of the client should be screened for TB**, and anyone testing positive for TB will need further evaluation. **Treatment failures occur when clients stop taking medication too soon or when taking it irregularly.**

12. The answer is 3

The nurse has just administered insulin to a client. Which is the appropriate action to dispose the insulin syringe and needle?

Category: Handling hazardous and infectious materials

(1) Needles should not be re-capped.

(2) Needles should not be re-capped and should be placed in puncture-resistant containers, not just any biohazard container.

(3) CORRECT: Needles and sharps should be placed in the nearest puncture-resistant container.

(4) Needles should not be broken.

13. The answer is 6, 3, 1, 2, 7, 4, 5

The nurse prepares to administer packed red blood cells (PRBCs) to a client. Arrange the following steps in the order the nurse should perform them. **All options must be used.**

Category: Error prevention

(1) The third step is to explain the procedure to the client.

(2) The fourth step is to obtain the client's vital signs.

(3) The second step is to assess that the client has a blood bank identification armband.

(4) The sixth step is to obtain the PRBCs from the blood bank according to hospital policy and perform a visual check of the blood.

(5) The last step is to perform a bedside identification and blood product verification by two licensed independent practitioners.

(6) The first step is to verify the physician order.

(7) The fifth step is to prime the transfusion tubing with a 0.9% sodium chloride solution.

14. The answer is 4

Two nurses prepare to lift a client up in bed. Which precaution should the nurses take to help avoid injuring their backs?

Category: Accident/injury prevention; Ergonomic principles

(1) When lifting or moving a client, nurses should maintain the natural curve of the spine and not bend at the waist.

(2) When lifting or moving a client, nurses should lift with the legs and not the back.

(3) When lifting or moving a client, place the bed in the Trendelenburg position if the client can tolerate it.

(4) CORRECT: The bed should be in a reasonably high position so the nurses do not have to lean.

15. The answer is 3

In the emergency department (ED), the nurse assesses a child suspected of having measles. Which infection control precaution should the nurse initiate?

Category: Standard precautions/transmission-based precautions/surgical asepsis

(1) Contact precautions are not used for measles.

(2) Droplet precautions are not used for measles.

(3) CORRECT: Airborne precautions are used to prevent the transmission of infectious agents that remain infectious over long distances when suspended in the air. Diseases requiring airborne precautions include, but are not limited to: measles, Severe Acute Respiratory Syndrome (SARS), varicella (chickenpox), and mycobacterium tuberculosis.

(4) Reverse isolation is not used for measles.

16. The answer is 3

A client presents to the emergency department reporting vaginal discharge, irritation of the vagina, and the need to urinate often. The nurse suspects a sexually transmitted infection (STI). The provider prescribes diagnostic testing of the vaginal discharge. Which STI should be reported to the local Department of Health?

Category: Standard precautions/transmission-based precautions/surgical asepsis

(1) Genital herpes is not a reportable disease.

(2) Human papillomavirus infection is not a reportable disease.

(3) CORRECT: Gonorrhea must be reported to the Department of Health. All US states have a reportable diseases list. It is the responsibility of the health care provider, not the client, to report cases of these diseases. Many diseases on the list must also be reported to the US Centers for Disease Control and Prevention (CDC). Examples of reportable infections include gonorrhea, chicken pox, and influenza.

(4) Trichomoniasis is not a reportable disease.

17. The answer is 1, 2, 5, and 6

A client who had a total hip replacement is disoriented to time, place, and person. The client is attempting to get out of bed and pull out the IV line that is infusing antibiotics. The client has bilateral soft wrist restraints and a vest restraint. Which intervention by the nurse are appropriate? **(Select all that apply.)**

Category: Use of restraints/safety devices

(1) CORRECT: Toileting and range-of-motion exercises should be provided every 2 hours while a client is in restraints.

(2) CORRECT: The client must be assessed frequently to ascertain when restraints can be removed, and this information must be documented.

(3) Restraints should never be tied to the side rails, because this can cause injury if the side rail is lowered without untying the restraint.

(4) A new health care provider prescription must be obtained every 24 hours if restraints are continued.

(5) CORRECT: The nurse should observe for correct placement of restraints.

(6) CORRECT: Restraints should be tied in knots that can be released quickly and easily.

18. See explanation for answers

Priority Concern	
Opportunistic infection.	✓

CORRECT OPTION: The nurse's priority concern is the client's risk for **opportunistic infection** and cancers that occur when the immune system is weakened. In this situation, organisms can cause severe illnesses that do not occur with functioning immune systems. When CD4 cells—cells that are needed to fight infection—decrease below 500 cells/mm^3, the immune system has difficulty fighting infections. HIV becomes more active when viral load increases and CD4 cells decrease. Candidiasis (thrush) is one of the more common infections that can occur along with symptoms of fever, night sweats, and diarrhea.

INCORRECT OPTIONS: Wasting syndrome attributed to HIV/AIDS is unintentional loss of 10% or more of ideal body mass along with weakness, fever, or diarrhea lasting more than 30 days. Peripheral neuropathy can commonly occur at any stage of HIV infection or as an adverse effect of antiretroviral (ART) medications. The client is not experiencing significant pain in the hands and feet. The client is not exhibiting common symptoms of venous thromboembolism (VTE), unilateral leg edema, pain, and tenderness. In addition, risk factors for VTE (e.g., venous stasis, blood hypercoagulability, endothelial damage) are not present.

Actions to Take	
Teach infection control including hand washing and total body hygiene.	✓
Provide referral for community-based support services.	✓

CORRECT OPTIONS: The client has immune deficiency due to HIV infection with significant implications for physiologic functioning as related to infection prevention. The nurse should **teach infection control including hand washing and total body hygiene**. Hand washing is an effective method to prevent the spread of organisms, and total body hygiene is important to decrease the risk for bacterial and fungal diseases. The nurse is an important resource to **provide referral for community-based support services**, which are critical for promoting adherence to antiretroviral (ART). The client may need assistance with housing, prescription medication coverage, food security, and social support.

INCORRECT OPTIONS: Post-exposure prophylaxis (PEP) is related to reducing the risk of acquiring HIV after a potential exposure. Effective PEP involves the use of prophylactic antiretroviral medications within 72 hours of exposure. Per the Centers for Disease Control and Prevention (CDC), standard precautions are used to reduce the risk of exposure to the HIV virus. The nurse does not educate about contact precautions, which are used as isolation precautions to prevent the transmission of infections spread by skin-to-skin contact or contact with other surfaces. Acyclovir is the medication of choice for herpes simplex virus and varicella-zoster virus; fluconazole is an effective treatment for candidiasis.

Parameters to Monitor	
CD4 + T-cell lymphocytes.	☑
Ability to eat and swallow.	☑

CORRECT OPTIONS: The nurse will monitor the client's **CD4+ T-cell lymphocytes**, as the primary marker of the client's immunocompetence. With progressive disease, CD4 cells decrease and problems related to immunosuppression can develop with less than 500 CD4 cells/mm^3, and severe problems when the CD4 cells are fewer than 200 cells/mm^3. The nurse should also monitor the client's **ability to eat and swallow.** For a client with a depressed immune system, oral candidiasis can progress into the client's esophagus, making swallowing extremely painful.

INCORRECT OPTIONS: The nurse does not monitor activated partial thromboplastin time (aPTT), urine ketones, or HIV antigen/antibody test. The aPTT is a measure of blood coagulation ability and is commonly used to evaluate the effectiveness of heparin therapy. Urine ketones are produced as a complication of diabetic ketoacidosis, when glucose utilization is impaired and fat is used for energy. The HIV antigen/antibody test is used to diagnose HIV infection. It tests for the virus, the antigen, and antibodies for HIV.

19. The answer is 3

Which action does the nurse implement **first** before administering medications to a client?

Category: Error prevention

(1) Scanning the medication label and the client's wristband might be correct if the institution has a bar coding system, but it is not the first thing you would do.

(2) Asking the client their name might be correct, but it is not the most complete answer.

(3) CORRECT: The 2024 National Patient Safety Goals require using at least two ways to identify clients. For example, use the client's name and date of birth. This is done to make sure that each client gets the correct medicine and treatment.

(4) The room number should never be used as a client identifier.

20. The answer is 1

The health care provider verbally prescribes a medication for a client during an emergency. Which steps should the nurse take next?

Category: Error prevention

(1) CORRECT: In an emergency, such as a "code," the prescription can be repeated back to the provider for confirmation before it is carried out. Closed-loop communication is a communication technique used to avoid misunderstandings. When the sender gives a message, the receiver repeats this back. The sender then confirms the message.

(2) The medication prescription should be confirmed with the provider first.

(3) The prescription should be repeated back to the provider for verification before it is administered.

(4) The nurse should confirm the prescription with the provider first.

21. The answer is 1, 2, and 5

The client has a prescription for the placement of a urinary catheter due to urinary retention. Which of these should the nurse do before starting the procedure? **(Select all that apply.)**

Category: Error prevention

(1) CORRECT: The nurse should confirm the client's identity, because a procedure requires proper identification.

(2) CORRECT: The nurse should confirm the client's medical record number via the wristband and prescription.

(3) The nurse must always properly identify clients for any and all treatments, not just for medication administration.

(4) A signed consent is not required before inserting a urinary catheter. The client has to verbally agree.

(5) CORRECT: The nurse should confirm the client's name via the wristband and prescription.

22. The answer is 4

Which action by the nurse is the **most effective means** of preventing infection?

Category: Standard precautions/transmission-based precautions/surgical asepsis

(1) The chemicals in Clorox wipes are caustic to the skin mucosa. The wipes are not intended to be applied directly to the skin. They are used for cleaning surfaces and equipment.

(2) Staff should decontaminate hands before having direct contact with clients, not just before reporting to work.

(3) Staff should perform hand hygiene before giving IV meds. The use of sterile gloves is not warranted in giving IV meds.

(4) CORRECT: If hands are not visibly soiled, the use of alcohol-based hand rub for routinely decontaminating hands is effective in preventing infection.

23. The answer is 2

The nurse cares for a client who is obese with pressure injuries. Treatment requires frequent turning and repositioning. The nursing unit has a special lift that allows for turning of clients and placement onto a bedpan without any lifting on the part of the staff. The client urgently requests the bedpan. Because the lift apparatus takes a few minutes to set up, which of action should the nurse take?

Category: Ergonomic principles

(1) Quickly assisting the client onto the bedpan is a tempting answer and might happen frequently in real life. However, it is not the best or safest option for the client or the nurse.

(2) CORRECT: Encourage the client to wait while the apparatus is set up. It is more important to prevent potential injury to the nurse. Nurses are commonly affected by ergonomic injuries related to lifting and moving clients.

(3) Lifting the client with the help of the unlicensed assistive personnel (UAP) is not the best or safest option for the client or the UAP.

(4) Encouraging the client to wear an incontinence brief is inappropriate.

24. The answer is 3

The nurse cares for client who has experienced multiple episodes of hyperglycemia not manageable by subcutaneous insulin injections. The client is prescribed an insulin drip for glycemic management which will be discontinued at bedtime, after which the client is NPO. The client's most recent blood glucose level, taken at 1500, was 60 mg/dL (3.3 mmol/L). Which action by the nurse is **best**?

Category: Error prevention

(1) The nurse has a duty to verify the prescription, given the change in circumstances. The blood glucose is now low, and continuing an insulin drip has the potential to drop it to a dangerous level.

(2) The nurse would recheck the client's blood glucose level only if there was reason to believe it might be in error.

(3) CORRECT: The best action is to contact the provider and discuss stopping the insulin infusion, based on the last blood glucose level.

(4) The nurse might ask a colleague for advice, but the best action is to discuss the situation with the provider.

25. The answer is 4

The adult children of a hospice home care client inquire about whether it is safe to hug their mother, because she has had a methicillin-resistant *Staphylococcus aureus* (MRSA) infection in the past. Which statement by the children would indicate a need for further teaching by the nurse?

Category: Standard precautions/transmission-based precautions/surgical asepsis

(1) A statement that "we should wash our hands frequently" is accurate.

(2) A statement that "we should use hand sanitizer" is accurate.

(3) A statement that "those of us with poor immune systems should be extra careful" is accurate.

(4) CORRECT: The family members do not have to wear gowns and gloves when interacting with their mother. The infection occurred in the past; even if it were still active, gowns and gloves would not be required. Staff wear PPE to prevent spreading these types of infections to other clients.

26. The answer is 1

The hospitalized client is receiving an intravenous infusion and the pump has malfunctioned. Which action by the nurse is **best** once the infusion is restarted with a functioning pump?

Category: Safe use of equipment

(1) CORRECT: The malfunctioning equipment should be labeled clearly and put in a separate area to be reviewed by the equipment department.

30. The answer is 2

The nurse discovers that a client received the wrong dose of intravenous antibiotic. Which is the most appropriate action by the nurse?

Category: Reporting of incident/event/irregular occurrence/variance

(1) Documenting the event in the client's medical record only is insufficient.

(2) CORRECT: The event should be recorded in both an incident report and in the client's medical record.

(3) Documenting in the client's medical record that an incident report was filed is incorrect. The incident report is for internal purposes of learning for the institution.

(4) Filing an incident report without documenting the event is incorrect; the incident is part of the patient's medical record.

CHAPTER 6

HEALTH PROMOTION AND MAINTENANCE

Health promotion and maintenance involves helping your clients achieve and continue to enjoy optimal health. You help people to identify that target state, discover their strengths and their needs, and then support their path to full health and wellness potential. Putting your enthusiasm into screening, education, and treatment efforts can make a significant difference in successful outcomes.

On the NCLEX-RN® exam, you can expect approximately 9 percent of the questions to relate to Health Promotion and Maintenance. This category focuses on the knowledge of expected growth and development principles, prevention and/or early detection of health problems, and strategies to achieve optimal health. Exam content related to Health Promotion and Maintenance includes, but is not limited to, the following areas:

- Aging process
- Ante/intra/postpartum and newborn care
- Developmental stages and transitions
- Health promotion/disease prevention
- Health screening
- High-risk behaviors
- Lifestyle choices
- Self-care
- Techniques of physical assessment

Let's now review the most important concepts covered by the Health Promotion and Maintenance category on the NCLEX-RN® exam.

Aging Process

The aging process unfolds gradually, starting with infancy (the first year of life). After that, school becomes the dividing marker. Thus preadolescent stages are divided into two: preschool (1 to 4 years) and school-age (5 to 12 years). Puberty marks the onset of the adolescent stage (13 to 18 years). Adulthood is divided into three parts: the working years (19 to 64 years), the retirement years (65 to 85 years), and the elderly years (over 85 years). As you review for the NCLEX-RN® exam, make sure you understand the special needs of each of these age groups so that you can provide the necessary care and education required.

Whichever stage your clients are in, you need to be able to assess their reactions to expected age-related changes. For example, an adolescent and an elderly person are going to react differently to a change in their residential location. A teenager will probably make that transition more easily than an elderly client who is coping with other physical and cognitive losses.

Ante/Intra/Postpartum and Newborn Care

To ensure the health of both mother and baby, pregnancies are now closely monitored from the moment a client knows she is expecting to several weeks after the baby is born.

Antepartum Care

Antepartum care is care given to the mother and baby before birth. It is also known as *prenatal care*. Antepartum care involves keeping track of the client's history and includes a number of important examinations.

Calculating Expected Delivery Date

Every mother wants to know her estimated date of delivery. A simple way to calculate this is to add 7 days and 9 months to the first day of the last menstrual period. Only 4 percent of births actually take place that day.

A pregnancy is considered *full term* between weeks 37 and 42. Birth occurring prior to week 37 is considered a *premature* birth, and later than week 42 is considered to be *overdue*.

Documenting the Mother's Current Health and Previous Health History

Documenting the mother's current health and previous health history is an important part of prenatal care. You should obtain data about blood pressure, weight, lifestyle, and family and genetic history; and ask about support systems, perception of pregnancy, and previous coping mechanisms. The absence of an in-place support system can be countered by putting the client in touch with a prenatal support group, for example. A referral is also appropriate if the client sees pregnancy as an illness, or if she has previously used denial or fantasy as coping mechanisms.

You also need to know which medications the client is using—prescribed, alternative, and over-the-counter. Category X medications have such a harmful effect on the developing fetus that they are contraindicated in pregnancy. These include:

- Birth control pills
- Accutane
- Some hyperlipidemia medications
- Warfarin (Coumadin)
- Ulcer drug (Cytotec)
- Vaccines for measles, mumps, and smallpox

You also need to test for the Rh factor, unless the mother is Rh-positive (has the factor) or both parents are Rh-negative (lack the factor). If the mother is Rh-negative and the father is Rh-positive, the mother needs to have Rho (D) immune globulin (RhoGAM) in the 28th week.

Ultrasounds are used to noninvasively confirm fetal viability, gestational age, fetal anatomy, and location of the placenta.

Sometimes an *amniocentesis*—withdrawing amniotic fluid for analysis—is done after the 14th week. The test is indicated for women over age 35 and those with a family history of genetic or metabolic problems.

Documenting Fetal Health

Fetal heart rate during routine prenatal exams should be 120 to 160 beats per minute.

Educating a New Mother-to-Be

Nutrition is an important part of prenatal care and education. An estimated 50 percent of pregnancies are unplanned, and the mother-to-be might not have been getting adequate nutrients. Pregnant teenagers need more protein, calcium, and phosphorus than pregnant adults, because their bones are still growing.

Weight gain should be limited to between 22 and 27 pounds—somewhat less if overweight, somewhat more if underweight. Substantial weight gain is deleterious to both mother and baby because it increases risk of preeclampsia. If the mother does not lose the extra pounds after childbirth, she increases her risk of diabetes and high blood pressure, which are linked to a greater risk of coronary artery disease, among other conditions.

You also need to be able to provide prenatal education about normal pregnancy events, such as *quickening* (the first perceptible fetal movement, typically at 17 to 19 weeks, but in some instances as early as 13 weeks or as late as 25 weeks). Some women might have some Braxton Hicks contractions after the 20th week.

It is equally important to educate about possible danger signals. Examples include:

- Vaginal bleeding
- Continuous headaches during the last three months
- Marked or sudden swelling of extremities during the last three months
- Dimness or blurring of vision during the last three months
- Severe, unrelenting abdominal pain
- Decreased fetal movement after 24 weeks

Recognizing Cultural Differences

Be aware of cultural differences in childbearing practices. Chinese Confucian women value modesty and self-control, so such women may remain stoic during pregnancy, asking few questions. For Mormon women, pregnancy is viewed as a time of personal and family growth, as it creates a connection with eternity. The Orthodox Jewish woman is considered ritually impure after her water breaks, so her Orthodox Jewish husband is unlikely to be in the delivery room. Instead, he prays in the waiting area.

Intrapartum Care and Education

Intrapartum care is defined as care that is given during labor and birth.

Identifying Onset of Labor

The three main factors that may cause labor to begin are the effect of hormones, the distension of the uterus, and the effect of oxytocin. Two recognizable signs of impending labor are the passage of a thick mucus plug from the cervix and rupture of the amniotic membranes. On average, the entire process from onset to birth lasts about 12 to 14 hours for a first baby. Subsequent labors tend to be shorter in length.

Care During Labor

Nursing care mirrors labor's four stages:

(1) **From 4 to 10 cm:** Assess cervical effacement and dilation, and need for analgesia.

(2) **From complete dilation to delivery of baby:** Assess newborn.

(3) **From delivery of baby to expulsion of placenta:** Usually within 5 to 20 minutes after birth; assess umbilical cord for two arteries and one vein.

(4) **Immediate recovery and observation:** Approximately 2 hours after birth; assess maternal vital signs, uterine fundal height, vaginal discharge, and bladder distention; assist breastfeeding efforts if indicated.

Postpartum Care and Education

The mother must be carefully observed after birth to identify serious complications, including the following:

- **Hemorrhage:** Report heavy clots or spurts of bleeding. Expect some blood in vaginal discharge for 3 to 6 weeks.

- **Infection or other illnesses:** Watch for a temperature over 100.4° F (38° C); sudden increase in perineal pain; unusually heavy or foul-smelling vaginal discharge; hot, tender, or red breast; dysuria; pain or swelling in the legs; and chest pain or cough.

Newborn Care and Education

One minute after birth, the physician rates five factors:

(1) Appearance (color)

(2) Pulse (heart rate)

(3) Grimace (reflex irritability)

(4) Activity (muscle tone)

(5) Respiration (respiratory effort)

This is known as the *APGAR score*. The value of each factor is 0 (not good), 1 (OK), or 2 (good). A total score of 10 is optimum.

Inform the mother of the warning signs of complications with her newborn, and explain when to call a doctor or take the baby to an emergency room. Those complications include:

- Has sunken or swollen soft spots on the head

- Has a fever higher than 100.4° F (38° C)

- Vomits more than once in 24 hours

- Is unable to keep down food or water
- Is not breathing easily

It is also important to assist the mother in performing newborn care. This is an ideal time to answer questions about parent-infant bonding. This is also the best time to provide contraception education, if needed. The client's menstrual cycle should begin in 6 to 8 weeks after giving birth, unless she is breastfeeding. Make sure your client knows about normal emotional stress (the *blues*) during her second or third postpartum week. Tell her to contact her physician if she experiences significant negative mood changes.

Developmental Stages and Transitions

The following sections provide an overview of life's milestones to review for the NCLEX-RN® exam.

Infants

Infants are newborn to 1 year old (0 to 12 months of age).

Expected Development

- **Physical:** May have swollen genitals and breasts, a misshapen head, milia (white spots) on face; exhibits sucking, grasping reflexes; able to focus; learns to grasp with thumb and finger
- **Cognitive and psychosocial:** Vocalizes sounds (coos); begins to respond selectively to words

Deviations

- Not rolling from tummy to side at 10 months
- Not transferring toys from hand to hand at 9 months

Special Needs

- Parent-infant bonding

Preschool-Age Children

Preschool-age children are 1 to 4 years old.

Expected Development

- **Physical:** Enjoys physical activities; has increasing bladder and bowel control; can manipulate small objects with hands; is able to dress and undress self; has refined coordination
- **Cognitive and psychosocial:** Becomes aware of limits; says "no" often; has a limited vocabulary of 500 to 3,000 words in very short sentences (3 to 4 words); believes that adults know everything; can use a pencil to draw shapes; is eager to learn; has a strong desire to please adults

Deviations

- Does not walk at 18 months
- Does not speak at least 15 words
- Does not imitate actions or words or follow simple instructions

- Talks excessively about violence or other mature topics
- Not interested in "pretend" play or other children

Special Needs

- Security and consistency of environment
- Protection from harmful situations caused by natural curiosity
- Some allowance for independence and playtime

School-Age Children

School-age children are 5 to 12 years old.

Expected Development

- **Physical:** Able to do a series of motions to perform activities, such as skipping or jumping rope
- **Cognitive and psychosocial:** Able to follow two-step directions; knows full name, age, and address; tends to identify with parent of the same gender

Deviations

- Bed-wetting late into childhood
- Verbal or outward expression of anxiety about school or home

Special Needs

- Developing scoliosis (sideways curvature of spine)
- Vision and hearing problems: important to discover at earliest stages

Adolescents

Adolescents are 13 to 18 years old.

Expected Development

- **Physical:** Shows increased interest in personal attractiveness; develops secondary sexual characteristics
- **Cognitive and psychosocial:** Struggles with sense of identity; forms strong peer allegiances; engages in risk-taking due to a sense of immortality

Deviations

- Persistent misbehavior, especially in school
- Aggression

Special Needs

- Understanding of puberty's effect on disposition and personality

Adults

Adults are 19 to 64 years old.

Expected Development

- **Physical:** Peak reached between 25 and 35 years old; might live for many years with a chronic condition
- **Cognitive and psychosocial:** From 19 to 34 years old—Erikson's stage of intimacy versus isolation; from 35 to 64 years old—Erikson's stage of generativity versus stagnation

Deviations

- Feeling that life is meaningless

Special Needs

- Learning lessons of workplace, long-term relationships, and parenting

Older Adults

Older adults are 65 to 85 years old.

Expected Development

- **Physical:** General slowing of physical functioning
- **Cognitive and psychosocial:** General slowing of cognitive functioning; Erikson's stage of ego integrity versus despair; interpersonal relationships continue despite changes and losses

Deviations

- Despair can arise from remorse for what might have been

Special Needs

- Learning lessons of successfully retiring from the workplace
- Keeping or losing long-term relationships

Very Old Adults

Very old adults are over 85 years old.

Expected Development

- **Physical:** Continued decline of physical functioning
- **Cognitive and psychosocial:** Continued decline of cognitive functioning; marked increase in changes and losses in relationships

Deviations

- Suicidal thoughts and behavior

Special Needs

- Acceptance of life's accomplishments and declines

Health Promotion/Disease Prevention

Traditionally, health has been defined as the absence of disease and disability. This philosophy, known as the medical model of health, has changed with the recognition that people can enjoy life even while experiencing challenges to medical health and variations to physical form. The World Health Organization now defines *health* as a state of physical, mental, and social well-being. Thus the phrase "health and wellness" expresses the goal of helping each client achieve optimal functioning regardless of current health status or disability.

During the continuum of life from infancy to old age, you need to be able to educate clients about their health and help them make changes to increase their wellness. Your approach is straightforward:

(1) Assess the client's perception of their own health status.

(2) Identify the client's health-oriented behaviors.

(3) At regular intervals, evaluate the client's understanding of health and wellness activities.

(4) Encourage client participation in behavior modification programs, as needed.

Health promotion concerns helping people to increase control over and to improve their health. Health promotion activities seek to empower individuals and their communities to organize, prioritize, and act on health issues. Disease prevention, on the other hand, involves efforts to stop the onset of a specific illness or condition, such a cancer.

You should be able to identify the important risk factors for disease/illness. The table lists the top three leading causes of death by age group, as identified by the Centers for Disease Control and Prevention.

CAUSE OF DEATH	UNDER 1	1–4	5–9	10–14	15–24	25–34	35–44	45–54	55–64	OVER 65
Birth defects	1	2	3							
Disorders related to premature birth	2									
Sudden infant death syndrome (SIDS)	3									
Unintentional injury		1	1	1	1	1	1	3	3	
Cancer			2	3			3	1	1	2
Suicide				2	3	2				
Homicide		3			2	3				
Heart disease							2	2	2	1
COVID-19										3

Adapted from the Centers for Disease Control and Prevention's "10 Leading Causes of Death, United States, 2022."

Health Promotion/Disease Prevention Programs

Health promotion/disease prevention programs include using community intervention techniques, such as holding health fairs or doing on-site education at elementary and high schools. Health promotion topics might include the following:

- **Healthy weight management:** The client's current weight should be assessed in comparison to a desirable weight. Know that a person with type 2 diabetes can improve glucose control by losing only 10 to 20 pounds.

- **Smoking cessation:** Factors associated with continued smoking include the strength of the nicotine addiction, continued exposure to smoking-associated stimuli (at work or in social settings), stress, depression, and habit. Continued smoking is more prevalent among those with low incomes, low levels of education, and psychosocial problems. Multiple factors often require multiple strategies.

- **Stress management:** Studies show a cause-and-effect relationship between stress and events including infectious diseases, traumatic injuries (such as motor vehicle crashes), and some chronic illnesses. Teaching stress reduction prevents other additional negative consequences.

- **Exercise:** Benefits include improved circulatory and respiratory systems; decreased cholesterol; lower body weight; delayed osteoporosis; and more flexibility, strength, and endurance.

- **Special diets:** Clients with hypertension should avoid foods high in sodium, such as processed, canned foods. Clients with high cholesterol should avoid saturated fatty acids (found in fatty meats) and trans fatty acids (found in deep-fried fast foods).

- **Complementary, alternative, or homeopathic therapies:** Examples include hypnosis, acupuncture, and massage. Some clients use over-the-counter remedies, vitamins, minerals, herbal medicines, or other approaches, such as a shaman.

- **Breast self-examination (BSE):** Beginning at puberty, females should develop breast self-awareness (i.e., familiarity with how breasts look and feel). Many clients do this through BSE undertaken monthly; should be done between day 5 and day 7 of their menstrual period. In menopause, BSE should continue monthly.

- **Testicular self-examination:** Testicular cancer is the most common cancer in males ages 15 to 35, and one of the most curable solid tumors. Teach clients that the best time to check is after bathing, when the scrotum is more relaxed. Any evidence of a lump or swelling should be reported to a physician.

- **Hormone replacement therapy (HRT):** HRT lowers the risk of osteoporosis-related bone fractures in postmenopausal women but increases the risk for coronary artery disease (CAD), breast cancer, deep vein thrombosis (DVT), and stroke.

- **Immunizations:** Hepatitis B vaccine is given to newborns. Infants get most immunizations from 2 to 12 months. Annual flu shots can start at 6 months. Meningococcal vaccine is recommended for previously unvaccinated college freshmen living in dormitories. Seniors over age 60 need vaccinations to prevent shingles (herpes zoster) and pneumonia.

- **Oral health:** Gum disease can allow bacteria to enter the body. Clients should schedule regular visits to dentists every 6 months beginning at age 2.

- **Mental health:** Teach ways to deal with stress and encourage seeking professional help during crises.

- **Stroke and heart disease prevention:** Clients should monitor blood pressure regularly, especially if they have a positive family history of hypertension.
- **Healthy joints:** Teach clients to do weight-bearing and stretching exercises regularly.
- **Bone health:** Diets need to include vitamin D and calcium to prevent osteoporosis.
- **Skin cancer prevention:** Teach clients to counteract the negative impacts of excessive sun exposure by using sunscreen, wearing protective clothing, or limiting time outdoors.

Health Screening

Health screening requires you to apply your knowledge of pathophysiology and risk factors linked to ethnicity and known population or community characteristics. Screening examples include:

- **Blood sugar check:** Levels more than 199 mg/dL without fasting or more than 125 mg/dL with fasting for 8 hours signal the need for a more complete workup.
- **Blood pressure check:** One-third of people whose blood pressures exceed 140/90 mmHg do not know it. Incidence of the *silent killer* is higher in the southeastern United States, especially among African Americans. Other risk factors are age over 60 years, inactive lifestyle, and hyperlipidemia.
- **Fasting lipid profile:** Adults should have a fasting lipid profile done at least once every 5 years. The total cholesterol value should be under 200 mg/dL, triglycerides (fatty acids) should be under 150 mg/dL, the low-density lipoprotein (LDL, the "bad" cholesterol that accelerates atherosclerosis) value should be under 100 mg/dL, and the high-density lipoprotein (HDL, the "good" cholesterol that removes cholesterol) value should be greater than 40 mg/dL for men and 50 mg/dL for women.
- **Colorectal screening:** Regular screening, beginning at age 50, is the key to preventing colorectal cancer. This screening can include fecal occult blood test (FOBT), sigmoidoscopy, colonoscopy, double-contrast barium enema (DCBE), or digital rectal exam (DRE).
- **Prostate screening:** Men should get a prostate-specific antigen (PSA) test beginning at age 50.
- **Mammograms:** Women should get a baseline mammogram between ages 40 and 50, after considering risk factors.

High-Risk Behaviors

High-risk behaviors are those lifestyle practices that increase the likelihood of illness, disease, or death. For example, in the case of HIV/AIDS, those activities include unprotected sex (anal, vaginal, or oral), using contaminated needles or sharing syringes, and coming in contact with bodily fluids (blood, semen, vaginal fluids, and saliva). Unprotected sex can also lead to other consequences, such as sexually transmitted diseases (STDs). Most safe sexual practices take some planning, such as having condoms available. An unplanned pregnancy can be avoided by taking birth control pills regularly.

Promote accident awareness to reduce deaths due to unintentional injuries. This includes using seat belts in automobiles, wearing helmets while biking, and using crosswalks.

Lifestyle Choices

Lifestyle is a characteristic set of behaviors and practices that range from habits and conventional ways of doing things to reasoned actions. Examples of lifestyle choices include being child-free; living in urban, rural, or suburban environments; educating children in public or private schools or home-schooling; and using alternative or homeopathic health care practices. Any of these choices might have an impact on your clients' health.

Self-Care

Self-care includes all activities that promote and maintain personal well-being without medical, professional, or other assistance or oversight. For developmentally delayed or elderly people, an inability to perform these tasks can curtail their ability to live independently. Your knowledge of in-home community resources might enable them to live in that environment longer. Your care plan might also need to involve clients (if able to give input), family members, friends, or paid staff inside or outside an institution.

Techniques of Physical Assessment

You should know the four methods or techniques of performing a physical assessment:

(1) **Inspection or purposeful observation:** Pay attention to outward details about the client, noting any deviations from expected age-related development. Note posture and stature, body movements, nutritional status by appearance, speech pattern, and vital signs. Individualize your approach. For example, with an obese young person, use an adult-size blood pressure cuff to get an accurate reading while assuring client comfort.

(2) **Palpation:** Use fingers and palms to apply a light touch or deeper pressure to gather data about the health of superficial blood vessels, lymph nodes, the thyroid, and the organs of the abdomen and pelvis.

(3) **Percussion:** Tap a part of the body and listen for the returned sound. This technique is often used on the chest and abdominal walls.

(4) **Auscultation:** Use a stethoscope to listen to sounds caused by movement of air or fluid within the client's body. This provides information about breath sounds, the spoken voice, bowel sounds, cardiac murmurs, and heart sounds. The stethoscope's bell (hollow cup) part of the endpiece can assess very-low-frequency sound, such as heart murmurs. The diaphragm (disc) part of the endpiece can assess high-frequency sounds from the heart and lungs.

Principles of Teaching/Learning

Principles of teaching and learning are techniques that allow you to share medical and health information with clients. You have been in school for some time, so it is second nature for you to absorb new information. For clients, you need to do the following:

(1) Use an organized approach to assess readiness and ability to learn.

   a. Consider age and developmental stage when teaching clients. For example, teaching adolescents might best be done by pointing them to trusted Internet sites, so that they can have a sense of autonomy in discovering health advice for themselves.

   b. Take into account clients' living situations. An example is an elderly person who is socially isolated due to decreasing sight and hearing or geographically isolated due to family and friends living far away.

   c. Encourage clients to establish their own goals and evaluate their own progress.

   d. Let clients demonstrate their understanding of information and practice their skills.

   e. After teaching, evaluate the results.

(2) Account for learning preference.

   a. Visual learners think in pictures, so use visual aids such as diagrams, videos, and handouts.

   b. Auditory learners best understand material through listening. Tell them about community lectures, discussions, and recordings.

   c. Tactile or kinesthetic learners prefer to learn via experience–moving, touching, and doing. Let the client hold a scale model of body organs to illustrate anatomy, for example.

(3) Identify barriers to client learning.

   a. Physical condition, such as decreased sight or hearing

   b. Financial considerations

   c. Lack of support systems

   d. Misconceptions about disease and treatment

   e. Low literacy and comprehension skills

   f. Cultural/ethnic background and language barriers

   g. Lack of motivation

   h. Environment

   i. Negative past experiences

   j. Denial of personal responsibility

This chapter reviewed aspects of childbirth to features of old age, and looked at health and wellness across the life span. Whatever your clinical setting, and whatever the reason clients seek medical help, you can rely on your grasp of basic health promotion and maintenance concepts. That knowledge will be evident when you successfully take the NCLEX-RN® exam.

Chapter Quiz

1. A client has just given birth. The baby looks healthy, with the exception of giving a grimace instead of a cry. Which of these would the nurse expect the obstetrician to say?

   1. "The APGAR score is 3."

   2. "The APGAR score is 6."

   3. "The APGAR score is 9."

   4. "The APGAR score is 12."

Refer to the Case Study to answer the next question.

The nurse in the pediatric clinic is caring for a 6-year-old client brought to the clinic by both parents.

History and Physical	Nurse's Notes

Well-child visit: The client has no history of medical issues or hospitalizations, and immunizations are up to date. The client is preparing to attend kindergarten next month. The client could have begun kindergarten last year, but the grandparent wanted to keep the client at home and the parents decided to wait until this year to send the child to school.

Physical: The client is a well-developed 6-year-old. Height 42 inches (106.68 cm), weight 50 lbs (22.67 kg). Body mass index (BMI) 19.9 (obese). Alert and answers questions appropriately. Eyes clear. No vision or hearing issues. Skin warm, dry. No visible rashes or bruising. Lungs clear, clear S1 S2 to auscultation. Abdomen soft and slightly protuberant with active bowel sounds. Parent denies any gastrointestinal issues. States client is a "picky eater" and will only eat cereal, macaroni and cheese, chocolate milk, and hot dogs. Consumes very few fruits or vegetables but does like apple juice. No genitourinary issues.

Psychosocial: The client is the youngest of three children. The siblings are ages 13 and 15. Both parents work full time, and a grandparent lives with the family and provides care when the parents are at work. Currently, the client spends all day with the grandparent and does not attend a preschool or other program. Client likes to work puzzles, draw, and play card games. Can "sound out" a few words when looking at a book and count to 100. The grandparent reads to the child frequently and has begun to teach the client to play the piano. The client expresses being excited to go to school "like my brother and sister do."

History and Physical	Nurse's Notes

Visit 1

Provided parent with information regarding balanced diet. Encouraged increased physical activity such as riding a bike, playing outside, going for walks. Parent reports the grandparent is unable to engage in much physical activity due to issues with arthritis. Parent states, "I think when my child starts school and meets other children there will be more opportunities for physical activities."

Visit (3 months later)

The 6-year-old child is at the clinic by appointment, accompanied by both parents. A parent states that a few weeks after school began, on school mornings, the client began to cry and throw temper tantrums and begged to stay home with the grandparent. For the past month, the child has begun to report headaches and stomachaches almost every morning; on a few mornings the client has vomited. As a result, the client has missed several days of school. These periods of illness do not occur on the weekends. The parents report the child stating "the other kids at school are mean to me."

Parents also report the child has been caught cheating when playing cards, and the child took some jewelry from the grandparent's room and hid it in a drawer. They are extremely concerned the child learned these bad habits from other children at school.

Current height: 42 inches (106.68 cm), weight 44 lbs (19.95 kg). BMI 17.5 (overweight). Vital signs stable, afebrile. Alert, talkative. Mucous membranes pink, moist. Eyes clear. Skin warm and dry, lungs clear, clear S1 S2. Abdomen soft with positive bowel sounds. Client denies pain at this time. Urinalysis negative for bacteria, ketones, protein.

2. The nurse reviews the child's history and assesses the child.

    Which **3** statements are correct for the nurse to provide the parents of this child?

    1. "You should set up a time to speak with your child's teacher as soon as possible."
    2. "It is perfectly normal for 5- and 6-year-olds to have these types of symptoms when they start school."
    3. "At least your child has lost some weight, which is a very positive thing."
    4. "Children this age need peer interaction, so returning to school is important."
    5. "It is not unusual for a 6-year-old to cheat in order to win, or to take and hide valuable or attractive objects."
    6. "At age 6, most children become more dependent on their parents or caregivers."
    7. "It sounds like your child's weight has been causing problems at school."
    8. "A 6-year-old is not acutely aware of body image, so issues with obesity are not typically a problem at this age."

3. A client with acne has been using isotretinoin. The client tells the nurse, "I recently learned I am pregnant." The client asks, "Will my pregnancy interfere with the medication's effectiveness?" Which is an appropriate response by the nurse?

   1. "The medication is contraindicated for pregnant women."
   2. "You will have to change the route of administration, because you are pregnant."
   3. "There is no reason you can't continue taking isotretinoin."
   4. "If the medication makes you look better, that will help you feel better about yourself."

4. The nurse is preparing for a women's health fair. Which is correct when teaching clients about the risks and benefits of hormone replacement therapy (HRT)?

   1. HRT is related to a decreased risk of deep vein thrombosis (DVT).
   2. HRT is related to an increased risk for coronary artery disease (CAD).
   3. HRT is related to an increased risk for osteoporosis-related bone fractures.
   4. HRT is related to a decreased risk of breast cancer.

5. The nurse provides education to a group of clients with type 2 diabetes mellitus. Which measure is **most** effective in attaining normal blood glucose levels for these clients?

   1. Decreasing sodium intake.
   2. Increasing potassium and calcium intake.
   3. Reaching recommended weight.
   4. Decreasing daily exercise.

6. A local high school is having a health fair. Which dietary choice does the nurse recommend as the most healthful for an adolescent whose serum cholesterol level is 300 mg/dL (7.8 mmol/L)?

   1. Medium rare cheeseburger.
   2. Vegetarian style pizza.
   3. Grilled chicken breast.
   4. Salad with extra dressing.

7. New parents are concerned about an unexpected characteristic of their newborn. Which finding would cause the nurse to contact the provider?

   1. Swollen genitalia.
   2. High-pitched crying.
   3. Misshapen head.
   4. Milia on the nose.

8. The nurse gives a primigravida client who is 35 years of age a Rh°(D) injection in the 28th week of pregnancy. Which client situation requires the nurse to take this action?

   1. Rh-positive mother and Rh-negative father.
   2. Rh-positive mother and Rh-positive father.
   3. Rh-negative mother and Rh-negative father.
   4. Rh-negative mother and Rh-positive father.

9. The nurse teaches a male client about testicular cancer. The nurse emphasizes that the client should be aware of which manifestation as an early sign of testicular cancer?

   1. Lumbar pain.
   2. Urinary frequency.
   3. Urinary urgency.
   4. Painless testicular enlargement.

10. An infant who is 3 months of age accompanies the parents to a seasonal flu clinic. Assuming that the child does not have a fever, can the nurse give the child the influenza vaccine?

   1. Yes, if regular immunizations are up to date.
   2. No, because the child does not meet criteria.
   3. Yes, because then the child won't get sick later.
   4. No, because it would interfere with regular immunizations.

11. A public health nurse visits a client at home three days after the client gave birth. Which finding should the nurse instruct the client to report to the health care provider?

    1. Vaginal drainage with streaks of bright red blood.
    2. Some discomfort at the site of the episiotomy.
    3. Feelings of fatigue late in the afternoon and evening.
    4. An elevated temperature without other symptoms.

12. The nurse provides discharge instructions to the parents of a newborn. In which situation would the nurse advise the parents to call the health care provider? **(Select all that apply.)**

    1. The newborn has a temperature higher than 100.4° F (38° C).
    2. The newborn vomits more than once in 24 hours.
    3. The newborn's respirations are even and unlabored.
    4. The newborn is unable to keep down food or water.
    5. The newborn has sunken or swollen soft spots on the head.

13. The client's first day of her last period was February 1. Which date should the nurse tell the client is the expected date of birth?

    1. November 8.
    2. October 8.
    3. December 1.
    4. November 20.

14. The client is 7 months pregnant with her first child. She is anxious because she feels some mild contractions at times. Which is the **best** response by the nurse?

    1. Inform the client to increase her bed rest to prevent the contractions.
    2. Inform the client the contractions are normal unless they increase in severity.
    3. Inform the client the contractions are a way of her body asking for more exercise.
    4. Inform the client she should avoid getting constipated and having gas as a result.

15. A client is 40 years of age and pregnant with her first child. The obstetrician asks the nurse to schedule the client for an amniocentesis. The client inquires why she needs amniocentesis. Which is the nurse's **best** response?

    1. "We routinely do an amniocentesis on all our clients to check the child's gender."
    2. "An amniocentesis is not invasive, so there is less risk than doing an ultrasound."
    3. "The standard for doing an amniocentesis is motherhood over the age 35."
    4. "If we know the baby's size, you can better count on having a vaginal birth."

16. The nurse educates a mother-to-be about possible danger signs during the last three months of pregnancy. Which finding would **not** be a cause for concern if experienced during pregnancy?

    1. Slight rectal bleeding.
    2. Continuous headaches.
    3. Marked swelling of hands.
    4. Blurred vision.

Refer to the Case Study to answer the next six questions.

The nurse is caring for a 17-year-old pregnant client admitted to a labor and delivery (L/D) unit.

Nurse's Notes

0800

Client is gravida 1 para 0 (G1P0) who is approximately 41 weeks gestation. Client presented to the Emergency Department (ED) at 0330 this morning after membranes ruptured spontaneously. Client was admitted to L/D at 0500. Since no spontaneous labor had begun, an IV oxytocin induction of labor has just been initiated. Cervix is 3 cm (1.18 inches) dilated and 50% effaced with the fetus in vertex presentation and at (−2) station. Fetal heart rate (FHR) baseline is 168 bpm with no decelerations noted. Moderate amount of green-tinged amniotic fluid noted on cervical exam.

1400

Cervix 6 cm dilated, 100% effaced, with the vertex at 0 station and continued leaking of green-tinged fluid. IV oxytocin continued at 12 milliunits/minute with contractions every 3–5 minutes lasting 45 seconds and palpably strong. FHR baseline 150 bpm with no decelerations and moderate variability observed. Client is becoming uncomfortable but declines offered analgesia.

1600

Client is currently tearful, restless, and anxious. Experiencing nausea and vomiting with contractions and reporting a feeling "like I need to have a bowel movement." States, "I can't do this! I want a C-section." Uterine contractions occurring every 2 minutes and lasting approximately 60 seconds. IV oxytocin infusing at 12 milliunits/minute. FHR 128 bpm with minimal variability.

17. Highlight tokenized information in the nurse's notes that is **most** concerning to the nurse. Tokenized options are enclosed in boxes.

0800: Client is gravida 1 para 0 (G1P0) who is approximately 41 weeks gestation. Client presented to the Emergency Department (ED) at 0330 this morning after membranes ruptured spontaneously. Client was admitted to L/D at 0500. Since no spontaneous labor had begun, an IV oxytocin induction of labor has been initiated. Cervix 3 cm (1.18 inches) dilated and 50% effaced with the fetus in vertex presentation and at (−2) station. Fetal heart rate (FHR) baseline 168 bpm with no decelerations noted. Moderate amount of green-tinged amniotic fluid noted on cervical exam.

1400: Cervix 6 cm dilated, 100% effaced, with the vertex at 0 station and leaking green-tinged fluid. IV oxytocin continued at 12 milliunits/minute with contractions every 3–5 minutes lasting 45 seconds and palpably strong. FHR baseline 150 bpm with no decelerations and moderate variability observed. Client is becoming uncomfortable but declines offered analgesia.

1600: Client is currently tearful, restless and anxious. Experiencing nausea and vomiting with contractions and reports a feeling "like I need to have a bowel movement." States, "I can't do this! I want a C-section." Uterine contractions occurring every 2 minutes and lasting approximately 60 seconds. IV oxytocin infusing at 12 milliunits/minute. FHR 128 bpm with minimal variability.

18. Which finding indicates the client is experiencing the transitional stage of labor? **(Select all that apply.)**

1. Nausea and vomiting.
2. Urge to push and bear down.
3. Fetal heart rate with minimal variability.
4. Anxiety and tearfulness.
5. Short contraction interval.
6. 100% effacement.
7. Green-tinged amniotic fluid.
8. Fetal heart rate < 160 bpm.

Nurse's Notes	Fetal Monitor Strip 1600

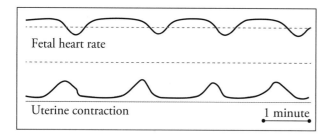

19. The nurse assesses the fetal monitor strip and notes the FHR and uterine contractions.

Complete the following sentence by choosing from the list of options.

The client is at risk for developing ⌈ Select from list 1 ⌉ due to ⌈ Select from list 2 ⌉ and ⌈ Select from list 3 ⌉.

(1)	(2)	(3)
meconium aspiration	late decelerations	post maturity
umbilical cord prolapse	variable decelerations	transitional stage of labor
fetal hypoxia and distress	early decelerations	spontaneous rupture of membranes

20. The nurse develops a plan of care for this client.

Which potential intervention is a priority for the nurse to implement when late decelerations are noted? **(Select all that apply.)**

1. Position the client on the left side.
2. Apply oxygen by mask at 5 L/min.
3. Explain the process of an emergency cesarean section.
4. Notify the provider.
5. Stop the IV oxytocin infusion.
6. Insert an indwelling catheter.
7. Give a bolus of primary IV fluids.
8. Encourage client to accept an IV analgesic.

| Nurse's Notes | Fetal Monitor Strip 1600 | Apgar Score |

Apgar Parameter	1 -Minute
Pulse	1
Respiratory Effort	0
Color	0
Reflexes	1
Muscle Tone	0

21. The client actively pushes for 90 minutes and vaginally delivers a viable infant weighing 10 lbs 4 ounces (4,694 grams). The nurse provides care for the newborn after reviewing the newborn's 1 minute Apgar score.

    For each 1-minute Apgar parameter below, specify the nursing interventions that are appropriate for the care of the client. **Each Apgar parameter may support more than 1 nursing intervention.**

Apgar Parameter	Nursing Intervention
Pulse 86 beats/minute	☐ Vigorously dry infant. ☐ Begin chest compressions. ☐ Administer epinephrine 1:1000 IV.
Respirations absent	☐ Clear oropharynx with bulb syringe. ☐ Provide positive pressure ventilation. ☐ Prepare to intubate newborn.
Color pale	☐ Encourage skin-to-skin bonding. ☐ Open supplies for an umbilical IV. ☐ Ensure the radiant heater is functional.
Facial grimace	☐ Check a rectal temperature. ☐ Stimulate Babinski reflex. ☐ Stimulate rooting reflex.
Muscle tone flaccid	☐ Briskly rub newborn's back. ☐ Stimulate Moro reflex. ☐ Mimic bicycle movement with newborn's legs.

22. The nurse reassesses the newborn at 5 minutes of age and documents the findings.

    For each assessment finding below, specify whether the finding indicates the newborn's condition has improved, not changed, or declined.

Assessment Finding	Improved	No Change	Declined
Pulse 112 beats/minute	○	○	○
Respirations 18, irregular	○	○	●
Acrocyanosis	○	○	○
Grimace	●	○	●
Arms and legs flexed with slight movement	○	○	○

23. The nurse teaches a group of mothers of toddlers how to prevent accidental poisoning from medications. The nurse teaches the mothers to store medications in which location?

    1. In a secure, locked place.

    2. In vials with childproof caps.

    3. On the highest shelf in the room.

    4. Disguised in different containers.

24. The nurse assesses an older adult couple, both 80 years of age, to determine if they can safely continue to live independently. The couple insist they are getting along fine but need help with grocery shopping and housekeeping. The nurse determines that they have difficulty in doing which of these?

    1. Activities of daily living (ADLs).

    2. Instrumental activities of daily living (IADLs).

    3. Daily living milestones (DLMs).

    4. Preventive health activities (PHAs).

25. The nurse gives a lecture at the senior center about preventative health activities for people over the age of 60 years. The nurse tells the clients that the Centers for Disease Control and Prevention (CDC) now recommends which vaccine for this age group?

    1. Shingles (herpes zoster).

    2. Diphtheria.

    3. Pertussis (whooping cough).

    4. Meningitis.

26. The nurse teaches about the challenges of smoking cessation. Clients attempting to quit smoking face which known challenges? **(Select all that apply.)**

    1. Stress and depression.

    2. Low level of income.

    3. High level of education.

    4. Psychosocial problems.

    5. Continued exposure to smoking-associated stimuli.

27. Stress reduction techniques include biofeedback and meditation. The nurse conducting classes on these methods knows that studies have shown a cause-and-effect relationship between stress and which of these? **(Select all that apply.)**

    1. Adverse medication effects.

    2. Infectious diseases.

    3. Motor vehicle accidents.

    4. Some chronic illnesses.

    5. Genetic diagnoses.

28. The nurse prepares for a community educational presentation. The topic is the leading cause of death for people from ages 1–44. What is the leading cause of death for this age group?

    1. Cancer.

    2. Heart disease.

    3. Unintentional injuries.

    4. Diabetes mellitus.

29. The nurse reviews the client's lipid profile to determine if education is needed to reduce the risk of heart disease. Match the appropriate part of the profile below on the left to the values on the right. **All options must be used.**

   1. Total cholesterol.

   2. HDL cholesterol for men.

   3. HDL cholesterol for women.

   4. LDL cholesterol.

   5. Triglycerides.

   A. More than 40 mg/dL.

   B. More than 50 mg/dL.

   C. Less than 100 mg/dL.

   D. Less than 150 mg/dL.

   E. Less than 200 mg/dL.

30. The nurse reviews the best approach to prepare three clients for surgery. Each has a different learning preference. Match the learning preference to the appropriate approach. **All options must be used.**

   1. Brochures about preparation activities.

   2. Models of the relevant anatomy.

   3. Discussions about the surgery.

   A. Auditory.

   B. Visual.

   C. Tactile.

Chapter Quiz Answers and Explanations

1. The answer is 3

A client has just given birth. The baby looks healthy, with the exception of giving a grimace instead of a cry. Which of these would the nurse expect the obstetrician to say?

Category: Ante/intra/postpartum and newborn care

(1) An APGAR score of 3 indicates a baby in poor health.

(2) An APGAR score of 6 indicates a less healthy baby.

(3) CORRECT: In 4 of the 5 categories of rating, the baby scored a 2. In the category of reflex irritability, the baby scored a 1, for a total APGAR score of 9.

(4) An APGAR score of 12 does not exist; the highest score is 10.

2. The answer is 1, 4, and 5

CORRECT OPTIONS: This 6-year-old child is exhibiting school phobia, or school refusal. A child experiencing school phobia has severe emotional distress about attending school. Behaviors may include anxiety, temper tantrums, or somatic symptoms. One of the first things the parent should do is **set up time to speak with the child's teacher(s)** to determine what may be occurring at school to trigger the behavior. **Six-year-old children need peer interaction**, and the situation must be explored and resolved so that the child can return to school. While the child's somatic symptoms and absence from school are cause for alarm, the **behaviors of cheating and stealing are not unusual for a child this age**. The child must be taught that these behaviors are not appropriate, but the actions alone are not cause for concern.

INCORRECT OPTIONS: While many children this age may have some nervousness about attending school, this child's symptoms are far more serious and must be investigated. The parents need to encourage the client to be more active and limit processed and high-calorie, low-nutrient foods; however, the loss of a few pounds while the client is stressed should not be viewed as a positive outcome. While children need their parents at age 6, they are becoming less dependent on them and more self-reliant and focused on peer interactions. The nurse cannot assume the child's weight is the cause of the issues the child is having; the situation needs to be explored further before any conclusions can be drawn. However, school-age children are very aware of body image and are concerned with anything which that set them apart from the "norm."

3. The answer is 1

A client with acne has been using isotretinoin. The client tells the nurse, "I recently learned I am pregnant." The client asks "Will my pregnancy interfere with the medication's effectiveness?" Which is an appropriate response by the nurse?

Category: Ante/intra/postpartum and newborn care

(1) CORRECT: Severe fetal abnormalities may occur if isotretinoin is used during pregnancy. The nurse should stress that the priority is the high risk of fetal abnormalities that the medication can cause rather than the effectiveness of the medication. Isotretinoin, is known to cause birth defects, including brain, heart, and face deformities, if women take it while pregnant.

(2) The nurse would not tell the client to continue taking this drug.

(3) The nurse would not tell the client to continue taking this drug.

(4) The nurse would not tell the client to continue taking this drug.

4. The answer is 2

The nurse is preparing for a women's health fair. Which is correct when teaching clients about the risks and benefits of hormone replacement therapy (HRT)?

Category: Health promotion/disease prevention

(1) HRT causes an increased risk of DVT.

(2) CORRECT: Current research counteracts earlier theories of a decreased risk of CAD.

(3) HRT causes a decreased risk of osteoporosis-related bone fractures.

(4) HRT causes an increased risk of breast cancer.

5. The answer is 3

The nurse provides education to a group of clients with type 2 diabetes mellitus. Which measure is **most** effective in attaining normal blood glucose levels for these clients?

Category: Health and wellness

(1) Decreasing sodium intake is not an effective way to attaining normal blood glucose levels in a client with type 2 diabetes mellitus.

(2) More potassium and calcium will not affect blood glucose.

(3) CORRECT: Losing only as much as 10–20 pounds improves blood glucose control.

(4) The client needs to increase, not decrease, daily exercise.

6. The answer is 3

A local high school is having a health fair. Which dietary choice does the nurse recommend as the most healthful for an adolescent whose serum cholesterol level is 300 mg/dL (7.8 mmol/L)?

Category: Health and wellness; Health promotion/ disease prevention

(1) The fat content of the main course (cheeseburger) needs to be lower due to the teenager's known elevated cholesterol level.

(2) The fat content of the main course (pizza) needs to be lower due to the teenager's known elevated cholesterol level.

(3) CORRECT: The fat content of a grilled chicken breast is the lowest of the choices.

(4) The fat content of the main course (salad with extra dressing) needs to be lower due to the teenager's known elevated cholesterol level.

7. The answer is 2

New parents are concerned about an unexpected characteristic of their newborn. Which finding would cause the nurse to contact the provider?

Category: Ante/intra/postpartum and newborn care

(1) Swollen genitals and breasts are normal due to maternal hormones.

(2) CORRECT: High-pitched crying is not normal and could be due to a neurological problem.

(3) A misshapen head is normal due to descent through the birth canal.

(4) Milia is normal due to blocked sebaceous glands.

8. The answer is 4

The nurse gives a primigravida client who is 35 years of age a Rh$_o$(D) injection in the 28th week of pregnancy. Which client situation requires the nurse to take this action?

Category: Ante/intra/postpartum and newborn care

(1) An Rh-positive mother does not need to worry about the Rh factor of the father.

(2) An Rh-positive mother does not need to worry about the Rh factor of the father.

(3) An Rh-negative mother does not need to worry about the Rh factor of the father, if it is the same as her status.

(4) CORRECT: An Rh-negative mother and Rh-positive father is the combined Rh status in which the mother could develop harmful antibodies.

9. The answer is 4

The nurse teaches a male client about testicular cancer. The nurse emphasizes that the client should be aware of which manifestation as an early sign of testicular cancer?

Category: Health promotion/disease prevention

(1) Among other serious causes, lumbar pain could be a sign of metastasis.

(2) Urinary frequency is not an early sign of testicular cancer.

(3) Urinary urgency is not an early sign of testicular cancer.

(4) CORRECT: Painless testicular enlargement is a common early sign of testicular cancer.

10. The answer is 2

An infant who is 3 months of age accompanies the parents to a seasonal flu clinic. Assuming that the child does not have a fever, can the nurse give the child the influenza vaccine?

Category: Health promotion/disease prevention

(1) The minimum age to receive a flu shot is 6 months; therefore the nurse cannot give the child the shot. CDC recommends that everyone 6 months of age and older get a seasonal flu vaccine.

(2) CORRECT: The minimum age to receive a flu shot is 6 months.

(3) The minimum age to receive a flu shot is 6 months; therefore the nurse cannot give the child the shot.

(4) The minimum age to receive a flu shot is 6 months; therefore the nurse cannot give the child the shot.

11. The answer is 4

A public health nurse visits a client at home three days after the client gave birth. Which finding should the nurse instruct the client to report to the health care provider?

Category: Ante/intra/postpartum and newborn care

(1) Vaginal drainage with streaks of bright red blood is normal for the first 3–6 weeks.

(2) The episiotomy area will continue to heal and is not a cause for concern, unless the discomfort rises to the level of persistent or increasing pain.

(3) Feelings of fatigue are normal after giving birth.

(4) CORRECT: A fever above 100.4° F (38° C) is reason to call the provider.

12. The answer is 1, 2, 4, and 5

The nurse provides discharge instructions to the parents of a newborn. In which situation would the nurse advise the parents to call the health care provider? (**Select all that apply.**)

Category: Ante/intra/postpartum and newborn care

(1) CORRECT: If a newborn has a fever higher than 100.4° F (38° C), the parents should call the provider.

(2) CORRECT: If a newborn vomits more than once in 24 hours, the parents should call the provider.

(3) There would be no need to call the health care provider in this instance.

(4) CORRECT: If a newborn is unable to keep down food or water, the parents should call the provider.

(5) CORRECT: A provider should evaluate the newborn immediately if the fontanels are either sunken or swollen.

13. The answer is 1

The client's first day of her last period was February 1. Which date should the nurse tell the client is the expected date of birth?

Category: Ante/intra/postpartum and newborn care

(1) CORRECT: November 8 is 9 months and 7 days later.

(2) October 8 is one month too early.

(3) By December 1, the baby would be overdue.

(4) By November 20, the baby would be overdue.

14. The answer is 2

The client is 7 months pregnant with her first child. She is anxious because she feels some mild contractions at times. Which is the **best** response by the nurse?

Category: Ante/intra/postpartum and newborn care

(1) Increasing bed rest is not necessary; Braxton Hicks contractions are normal at this stage in the pregnancy.

(2) CORRECT: Braxton Hicks contractions are normal at this stage in the pregnancy.

(3) More exercise is not necessary: Braxton Hicks contractions are normal at this stage in the pregnancy.

(4) Gas is not likely to be the cause of the contractions; Braxton Hicks contractions are normal at this stage in the pregnancy.

15. The answer is 3

A client is 40 years of age and pregnant with her first child. The obstetrician asks the nurse to schedule the client for an amniocentesis. The client inquires why she needs amniocentesis. Which is the nurse's **best** response?

Category: Ante/intra/postpartum and newborn care

(1) The most common reason for an amniocentesis is to check chromosomal abnormalities, not to check the child's gender.

(2) The ultrasound is not invasive; the amniocentesis is invasive.

(3) CORRECT: After age 35, the risk of infant chromosomal abnormality is greater than the risk associated with the procedure.

(4) The most common reason for an amniocentesis is to check chromosomal abnormalities, not to check the baby's size.

16. The answer is 1

The nurse educates a mother-to-be about possible danger signs during the last three months of pregnancy. Which finding would **not** be a cause for concern if experienced during pregnancy?

Category: Ante/intra/postpartum and newborn care

(1) CORRECT: Although hemorrhoids could cause rectal bleeding, it is vaginal bleeding that would concern the nurse.

(2) Continuous headaches is a symptom that would concern the nurse.

(3) Marked swelling of hands would concern the nurse.

(4) Blurred vision would concern the nurse.

17. See explanation for answers

0800: Client is gravida 1 para 0 (G1P0) who is approximately 41 weeks gestation. Client presented to the Emergency Department (ED) at 0330 this morning after membranes ruptured spontaneously. Client was admitted to L/D at 0500. Since no spontaneous labor had begun, an IV oxytocin induction of labor has been initiated. Cervix 3 cm (1.18 inches) dilated and 50% effaced with the fetus in vertex presentation and at (−2) station. Fetal heart rate (FHR) baseline 168 bpm with no decelerations noted. Moderate amount of green-tinged amniotic fluid noted on cervical exam.

1400: Cervix 6 cm dilated, 100% effaced, with the vertex at 0 station and leaking green-tinged fluid. IV oxytocin continued at 12 milliunits/minute with contractions every 3–5 minutes lasting 45 seconds and palpably strong. FHR baseline 150 bpm with no decelerations and moderate variability observed. Client is becoming uncomfortable but declines offered analgesia.

1600: Client is currently tearful, restless and anxious. Experiencing nausea and vomiting with contractions and reports a feeling "like I need to have a bowel movement." States, "I can't do this! I want a C-section." Uterine contractions occurring every 2 minutes and lasting approximately 60 seconds. IV oxytocin infusing at 12 milliunits/minute. FHR 128 bpm with minimal variability.

CORRECT OPTIONS: **Fetal post-maturity** is accompanied by an aging placenta, which can diminish sufficiency of gas exchange and increase the likelihood of intrauterine hypoxia. The presence of **green-tinged amniotic fluid** indicates that the fetus has endured some stress that stimulated the passage of some meconium prior to birth. Meconium, if present in the airway at birth and aspirated into the terminal airways with initial breaths, can lead to a chemical pneumonitis. Fetal heart rate variability is the interplay between sympathetic and parasympathetic nervous systems over a 10–minute period. Reduced variability is the single best predictor for determining fetal compromise. In this instance, the **heart rate baseline is within normal limits, but the minimal variability indicates concern for fetal well-being**.

INCORRECT OPTIONS: Spontaneous rupture of membranes alone is not concerning for fetal well-being until the duration of rupture exceeds 24 hours; at that time, risk for chorioamnionitis increases dramatically. Vertex presentation is expected and desired in active labor. Cervical evaluation at 1400 indicates sufficient progress in cervical change and fetal descent from the prior cervical assessment. Nausea, vomiting, and rectal pressure are all expected findings in labor as the second stage approaches.

18. The answer is 1, 2, 4, and 5

CORRECT OPTIONS: Maternal behavior suggesting the approaching second stage of labor may include episodic **vomiting**, an **urge to push** or feeling the need to have a bowel movement, and increased restlessness and **anxiety** as the fetus descends into the pelvis. **Contraction intervals** during this time are less than every 2 minutes with a shortened rest interval between contractions.

INCORRECT OPTIONS: Diminished fetal heart tone variability can be an indicator of decreased fetal tolerance of labor but is not exclusively related to the transitional phase of labor. Effacement of the cervix to 100% indicates the cervix has thinned as much as possible to allow advancement of dilatation;

effacement often occurs before the transitional phase of labor in a first pregnancy. Green-tinged amniotic fluid has been noted and is unchanged since admission, so its presence alone does not indicate the transitional phase of labor. Normal fetal heart range is 110–160 beats/minute; 128 beats/minute is within normal limits and not indicative of the transitional phase of labor.

19. See explanation for answers

CORRECT OPTIONS: **Late decelerations** are associated with uteroplacental compromise, which disrupts oxygen transfer to the fetus, leading to **fetal hypoxia and distress**. An aging placenta in a **post term pregnancy** can be the etiology behind the occurrence of late decelerations. Oxygen transport diminishes due to the intervillous hemorrhagic infarcts and thickened vessels that occur in the placenta as it ages. When oxygen supply is insufficient to meet the physiological needs of the fetus, nonreassuring fetal distress may occur.

INCORRECT OPTIONS: Meconium aspiration, if it occurs, would be apparent only through evaluation of the newborn after birth and upon visualization of the newborn's oropharynx. There is no indication in this question that umbilical cord prolapse has occurred. Variable decelerations are a visually abrupt descent to or ascent from the peak of a uterine contraction, and they indicate cord compression. Early decelerations are visually gradual, with the lowest point of the descent most often at the onset of the contraction and indicating fetal head compression in association with descent. While the fetus must negotiate the bony pelvis during the transitional or expulsive second stage of labor, the majority of fetuses without preceding compromise do not develop fetal distress strictly because they are navigating this phase of labor. Spontaneous rupture of membranes alone is not a distinct precipitator of fetal distress unless accompanied by umbilical cord prolapse.

20. The answer is 1, 2, 4, 5, and 7

CORRECT OPTIONS: **Positioning the client on the left side** enhances oxygenation and blood flow to the fetus by increasing maternal cardiac output. This is because the vena cava physically deviates to the right to empty into the right atrium. Enhancing oxygenation via O_2 **by mask** to the client provides extra oxygen to the baby through the mother; this intervention is indicated in the challenged fetal oxygenation state. Elevating the client's legs improves blood return to heart, which enhances maternal cardiac output and subsequent oxygenation to fetus. The nurse should **notify the provider** of the signs of uteroplacental compromise, which requires provider management. **Stopping the labor stimulant (i.e., oxytocin)** and **bolusing primary IV fluids** will diminish uterine contractility as a source of current fetal distress.

INCORRECT OPTIONS: Should the fetal status warrant a C-section, it is the role of the provider to explain the surgical procedure and gain client consent, not the nurse. If care progresses toward a C-section, insertion of an indwelling catheter would be performed; however, it is not a priority at this time for management of the late decelerations. Administration of an IV analgesic to the client at this time may further depress the fetal heart rate and may negatively impact fetal response to the distress indicated by the late decelerations.

21. See explanation for answers

Pulse 86 beats/minute: **Vigorously drying the infant** is an intervention that will warm and stimulate the infant. INCORRECT OPTIONS: Chest compressions and epinephrine are not indicated at this time, as the newborn's heart rate is not below 60 beats/minute.

Respirations absent: In the absence of spontaneous respirations in the newborn, **clearing the airway of any secretions**, followed by the implementation of **positive pressure ventilation** is the standard of care response in newborn resuscitation. INCORRECT OPTION: Tracheal intubation will be considered only if suctioning and positive pressure ventilation are ineffective.

Color pale: The pallor of the newborn can be associated with hypothermia as well as distress, so a **functional/consistent source of radiant heat** can be of assistance here. INCORRECT OPTIONS: Skin-to-skin bonding is important for physical, emotional, and social development but is delayed until the infant is physiologically stable. While an umbilical IV may ultimately be indicated in caring for this newborn, the priority during initial resuscitation efforts is providing warmth, clearing the airway, and stimulating breathing.

Facial grimace: **Checking a rectal temperature** may temporarily increase the heart rate and BP while also enhancing reflex irritability/response. INCORRECT OPTIONS: The Babinski reflex is the dorsi-flexion of the big toe and hyperextension of remaining toes in response to upward stroking of the plantar surface of the foot. The rooting reflex involves touching the newborn's mouth/cheek with the newborn response of turning toward the stimulus and opening the mouth. Evaluation of these reflexes is not a priority during resuscitation, nor will eliciting them enhance the infant's response to resuscitation efforts.

Muscle tone flaccid: **Rubbing the newborn's back** is another intervention designed to stimulate the infant. INCORRECT OPTIONS: The Moro (startle) reflex is an involuntary response to an external stimulus such as noise. As noted, evaluation of this reflex is not a priority during resuscitation. Mimicking bicycle movements of the newborn's legs helps with intestinal motion and can expel trapped gas but will not enhance resuscitation efforts for this newborn.

22. See explanation for answers

Improved: Overall Apgar score has improved for this infant; score is now 6 at 5 minutes of life. **Pulse is now > 100 beats/minute**, there is evidence of **respiratory effort**, skin shows improvement with pink color in all areas but hands and feet (i.e., **acrocyanosis**), and there is some **flexion of extremities**.

No Change: The reflex response of a **grimace** is unchanged after 5 minutes but likely will improve as supportive care continues.

23. The answer is 1

The nurse teaches a group of mothers of toddlers how to prevent accidental poisoning from medications. The nurse teaches the mothers to store medications in which location?

Category: Aging process; Developmental stages and transitions

(1) CORRECT: A secure, locked place is the only safe place to store medications that might be accidentally ingested by a toddler.

(2) Children have been known to pull childproof caps off, especially if the cap is not fully engaged.

(3) Children have been known to climb up on counters and other surfaces, so placing medications on a high shelf is not necessarily safe.

(4) The challenge is the toddler's natural curiosity, not whether the toddler recognizes the item as a medication vial. If containers are disguised, this might also cause a medication error.

24. The answer is 2

The nurse assesses an older adult couple, both 80 years of age, to determine if they can safely continue to live independently. The couple insist they are getting along fine but need help with grocery shopping and housekeeping. The nurse determines that they have difficulty in doing which of these?

Category: Aging process; Self-care

(1) ADLs are basic functions of self-care, such as feeding, dressing, and bathing. The Katz Index of Independence in Activities of Daily Living, commonly referred to as the Katz ADL, is a popular used to assess the client's functioning.

(2) CORRECT: Grocery shopping and housekeeping are two important IADL functions.

(3) Grocery shopping and housekeeping are not milestones.

(4) Grocery shopping and housekeeping are not prevention activities.

25. The answer is 1

The nurse gives a lecture at the senior center about preventative health activities for people over the age of 60 years. The nurse tells the clients that the Centers for Disease Control and Prevention (CDC) now recommends which vaccine for this age group?

Category: Health promotion/disease prevention

(1) CORRECT: The shingles vaccine reduces the risk of shingles by about half and the risk of postherpetic neuralgia by two-thirds.

(2) The diphtheria vaccine is given much earlier in life.

(3) The pertussis (whooping cough) vaccine is given much earlier in life.

(4) The CDC recommends that college freshmen living in dormitories get the meningitis vaccine, but this is unlikely to apply to those over age 60.

26. The answer is 1, 2, 4, and 5

The nurse teaches about the challenges of smoking cessation. Clients attempting to quit smoking face which known challenges? **(Select all that apply.)**

Category: Health promotion/disease prevention; High risk behaviors

(1) CORRECT: Stress and depression are known challenges to smoking cessation.

(2) CORRECT: Continued smoking is more prevalent among those with a low level of income.

(3) A low, not high, level of education has been found to be associated with continued smoking.

(4) CORRECT: Continued smoking is more prevalent among those with psychosocial problems.

(5) CORRECT: Continued exposure to smoking-associated stimuli is a known challenge to smoking cessation.

27. The answer is 2, 3, and 4

Stress reduction techniques include biofeedback and meditation. The nurse conducting classes on these methods knows that studies have shown a cause-and-effect relationship between stress and which of these? **(Select all that apply.)**

Category: Health promotion/disease prevention

(1) No association between stress and adverse medication effects is known at present.

(2) CORRECT: Research shows a relationship between stress and infectious diseases.

(3) CORRECT: Research shows a relationship between stress and traumatic injuries, such as motor vehicle accidents.

(4) CORRECT: Research shows a relationship between stress and some chronic illnesses.

(5) There is no relationship between stress and genetic disease processes.

28. The answer is 3

The nurse prepares for a community educational presentation. The topic is the leading cause of death for people from ages 1–44. What is the leading cause of death for this age group?

Category: Health promotion/disease prevention

(1) Cancer is not the leading cause of death for people from ages 1–44, according to the CDC.

(2) Heart disease is not the leading cause of death for people from ages 1–44, according to the CDC.

(3) CORRECT: Unintentional injuries are the leading cause of death for people ages 1–44, according to the CDC.

(4) Diabetes is not the leading cause of death for people from ages 1–44, according to the CDC.

29. The answer is 1 (E), 2 (A), 3 (B), 4 (C), 5 (D)

The nurse reviews the client's lipid profile to determine if education is needed to reduce the risk of heart disease. Match the appropriate part of the profile below on the left to the values on the right. **All options must be used.**

Category: Health promotion/disease prevention

(1) (E): Total cholesterol should be less than 200 mg/dL.

(2) (A): HDL cholesterol for men should be more than 40 mg/dL.

(3) (B): HDL cholesterol for women should be more than 50 mg/dL.

(4) (C): LDL cholesterol should be less than 100 mg/dL.

(5) (D): Triglycerides should be less than 150 mg/dL.

30. The answer is 1 (B), 2 (C), 3 (A)

The nurse reviews the best approach to prepare three clients for surgery. Each has a different learning preference. Match the learning preference to the appropriate approach. **All options must be used.**

Category: Principles of teaching/learning

(1) (B): Brochures about preparation activities are visual: the client needs to see words and pictures.

(2) (C): Models of the relevant anatomy are tactile: the client needs to touch the model.

(3) (A): Discussions about the surgery are auditory: the client needs to hear the words.

CHAPTER 7

PSYCHOSOCIAL INTEGRITY

Psychosocial integrity, along with physiological integrity, is a basic health need for all clients. It is the state of dynamic psychological and sociological homeostasis, which may be affected during periods of stress, illness, or crisis. Any threats to a person's emotional, mental, and social well-being can disrupt this homeostasis. Any change in adaptive and coping responses may result in counterproductive ways of thinking, communicating, feeling, and acting. When assisting clients with psychosocial needs, you must be able to anticipate, recognize, and analyze these types of responses.

On the NCLEX-RN® exam, you can expect approximately 9 percent of the questions to relate to Psychosocial Integrity. This category focuses on promoting and supporting the emotional, mental, and social well-being of clients experiencing stressful events, as well as clients with acute or chronic mental illness.

Exam content related to Psychosocial Integrity includes, but is not limited to, the following areas:

- Abuse/neglect
- Behavioral interventions
- Chemical and other dependencies/substance use disorder
- Coping mechanisms
- Crisis intervention
- Cultural awareness/cultural influences on health
- End of life care
- Family dynamics
- Grief and loss
- Mental health concepts
- Religious and spiritual influences on health
- Sensory/perceptual alterations
- Stress management
- Support systems
- Therapeutic communications
- Therapeutic environment

Now let's review the most important concepts covered by the Psychosocial Integrity category on the NCLEX-RN® exam.

Abuse/Neglect

Abuse includes physical abuse, physical neglect, sexual abuse, and emotional abuse and neglect. You should be familiar with your state's laws for reporting suspected or known abuse. In addition, you must be able to identify risk factors and recognize signs of possible abuse and neglect and their roles in follow-up care.

All suspected cases of child abuse *must* be reported to the appropriate agency or authority. It is not sufficient just to document the suspected abuse in the medical record. Risk factors for child abuse include:

- Past or present spousal abuse
- Perception of stress
- Life changes
- Age at birth of first child
- Education
- Little or no prenatal care
- Having an unlisted phone/not having a phone
- Low income
- Current unemployment
- Evidence of harsh discipline

Elder abuse can affect either sex, but usually the victims are women who are over 75 years of age, physically or mentally impaired, and dependent on the abuser for their care. Nurses can intervene by educating caregivers about the needs of older adults and making resources available to provide support. A legally competent adult, however, cannot be forced to leave the abusive situation.

Domestic/spousal abuse affects families at all socioeconomic levels. Risk factors for domestic abuse include:

- Planning to leave or having recently left an abusive relationship
- Having been in an abusive relationship in the past
- Poverty or poor living situation
- Unemployment
- Physical or mental disability
- Separation or divorce
- Abuse as a child
- Social isolation from family and friends
- Having witnessed domestic violence as a child
- Pregnancy, especially if unplanned
- Being younger than 30 years old
- Being stalked by a partner

In any abuse situation, you should communicate openly, encourage victims to share their problems, provide counseling and information about resources and coping strategies, provide support, and educate your clients. In addition, you should know how to plan interventions for victims and suspected victims, and help direct them to a safe environment. It is also important to evaluate a client's response to interventions.

Behavioral Interventions

Nurses can intervene, helping to restore a client's ability to evaluate reality correctly. Characteristics of altered mental processes that you should be familiar with include:

- Disorientation
- Altered behavioral patterns
- Altered mood states
- Impaired ability to perform self-maintenance activities
- Altered sleep patterns
- Altered perceptions of surroundings

The treatment plan should respond to the specific needs of the client for structure, safety, and symptom management. You should be able to evaluate the client's response to the treatment plan.

Nursing interventions that you should be familiar with include:

- Maintaining routine interactions, activities, and close observation
- Developing an open and honest relationship with respectful and clearly verbalized expectations
- Verbalizing acceptance of the client despite inappropriate behavior
- Providing role modeling through appropriate social and professional interactions with other clients and staff
- Encouraging the client to assume responsibility for their own behavior but verbalizing willingness to assist
- Providing positive reinforcement
- Orienting the client to reality
- Encouraging the client to attend group therapy sessions, if appropriate

You should also know how to help the client achieve and maintain behavioral self-control, including strategies that the client can use to decrease anxiety.

Chemical and Other Dependencies/Substance Use Disorders

Substance use disorders occur when the recurrent use of alcohol and/or drugs causes clinically and functionally significant impairment, such as health problems, disability, or failure to meet major responsibilities at work, school, or home. Substance use disorders are defined as mild, moderate, or severe; the level of severity is determined by the number of diagnostic criteria an individual meets.

These criteria include evidence of impaired control, social impairment, risky use, and pharmacological criteria.

Non-substance-related dependencies include gambling addiction, sexual addiction, and addiction to pornography, among others.

Nursing priorities when dealing with a client with chemical and other dependencies include:

- Maintaining the physiological stability of clients experiencing substance-related withdrawal or toxicity by providing symptom management. For example, benzodiazepines are often part of treating alcohol withdrawal, with its symptoms of tremors, diaphoresis, and elevated heart rate.
- Promoting client safety. This might include using restraining devices, even against a client's wishes, to ensure that the client does not get hurt.
- Educating the client about chemical and other dependency complications and dangers.
- Providing appropriate referral and follow-up.
- Encouraging and supporting involvement in an intervention process (counseling).
- Teaching friends and family members how to provide ongoing support, and encouraging their participation in support groups.
- Evaluating the client's response to the treatment plan.

Coping Mechanisms

How a client responds to life's stressors depends on the client's coping resources—for example, social support networks and problem-solving skills. Sociocultural and religious factors can also influence how a client handles problems. Some clients may not have the resources or skills to cope with stressors. You should be able to assess these client support systems, resources, and skills, as well as a client's response to illness and the emotional reaction of a family to a client's illness.

Characteristics of the inability to cope that you should be familiar with include:

- Verbalization of the inability to cope
- Inability to make decisions or ask for help
- Destructive behavior toward self or others
- Physical symptoms
- Emotional tensions
- General irritability

Factors related to the inability to cope include, but are not limited to:

- Diagnosis of a serious illness
- Change in health status
- Unsatisfactory support system
- Inadequate psychological resources
- Situational crises

You should also be familiar with the variety of different defense mechanisms your client may employ, and be able to evaluate whether uses of these mechanisms are constructive or not, such as:

- **Denial:** Completely rejecting a thought or feeling
- **Suppression:** Being vaguely aware of a thought or feeling but trying to hide it
- **Projection:** Thinking someone else has is the source of a negative thought or feeling
- **Acting out:** Performing an extreme behavior in order to express thoughts or feelings that feel impossible to express otherwise
- **Displacement:** Redirecting feelings toward one person or thing to another target
- **Isolation of affect:** "Thinking" a feeling but not really feeling it
- **Intellectualization:** Avoiding the emotion arising from an act or feeling by substituting a rational explanation
- **Regression:** Reverting to an old, usually immature behavior to give vent to feelings
- **Reaction formation:** Turning the feeling into its opposite
- **Rationalization:** Coming up with various explanations to justify a situation while denying personal feelings
- **Sublimation:** Directing a feeling into a socially productive activity
- **Dissociation:** Losing track of time and/or person, and instead finding another representation of self in order to continue in the moment

Additionally, you need to provide clients with opportunities to express their thoughts and feelings, help them set realistic goals, assist them in constructive problem solving, and provide teaching on methods, support systems, and available resources to cope with stress and tension.

Crisis Intervention

A crisis is an emotionally significant event or radical change of status in a person's life. It is an unstable and/or crucial time with the possibility of an undesirable outcome—a situation that has reached a critical stage. During a crisis, you should:

- Identify the client's history of the present problem.
- Identify the client's current feelings.
- Assess the client's support systems.
- Teach crisis intervention techniques to assist the client in coping.
- Assess the client's potential for self-harm or harm to others.

Goal planning is based on nursing assessment and diagnosis, and outcomes are compared to goals and the client's response.

Goals of crisis intervention include:

- Decreasing emotional stress and protecting the client from additional stress
- Assisting the client in organizing and mobilizing resources or support systems to meet the client's needs, and reaching a solution for that situation
- Returning the client to a pre-crisis level of functioning

Assessing the risk for suicide includes asking questions (from general to specific, as well as about plans and lethality), obtaining a history, assessing mental status, and assessing the signals given by the client that may indicate that they are at high risk for suicide. *The highest priority for patients at risk for suicide is safety. Thus, arrangements might have to be made to provide constant observation of the high risk client.*

Cultural Awareness/Cultural Influences on Health

Caring varies among different racial and ethnic groups in its expressions, processes, and patterns. Cultural competence requires you to understand the client's world views as well as your own, while avoiding stereotyping. You can obtain cultural information by asking questions, and then apply the knowledge to improve the quality of client care and outcomes. This requires flexibility on your part and respect for other viewpoints. To do so, you should:

- Listen carefully to the client.
- Learn about the client's beliefs regarding health and illness.
- Show respect, understanding, and tolerance of the client's cultural background and practices.
- Provide culturally appropriate care.
- Identify language needs and use appropriate interpreters, as necessary. Avoid bias and subjectivity by arranging for nonfamily translation assistance.
- Document how the client's language needs were met.

End of Life Care

A client has the right to make informed choices about their end of life care that reflect personal, cultural, and religious values.

Nurses provide support, education, and impartial interpretation of medical information in a way that clients and families can understand, which may include treatment options as well as the right to refuse treatment. This requires open, honest, sensitive communication and effective teamwork. You should encourage clients and families to express their goals and wishes, and then tailor the care plan to the needs of each client and family. As a nurse, you have an ethical and legal duty to respect the client's wishes, choices, and priorities.

You also need to prepare the client and family for what to expect during the final phase of a terminal illness, which includes the physical aspects of a deteriorating condition and the act of dying. As the client's death approaches, the family may become more anxious. It is important for you to teach the family about the signs and symptoms of impending death, as well as reassure the family that the health care providers are making the client as comfortable as possible. After the death, you acknowledge the loss, express sympathy, and provide the opportunity for the family to view the body, but only after asking if they wish to do so.

Family Dynamics

Family members ideally support each other by listening, empathizing, and reaching out to one another. When communication patterns are dysfunctional, the result can be gross misunderstanding, which may lead to hostility, anger, or silence.

You need to be able to assess a family's dynamics and ability to function constructively by closely observing how well family members communicate. You should also assess coping mechanisms that determine how families relate to stress, and evaluate resources and support systems available to the family.

Family units may be vulnerable to health problems based on various factors, such as heredity, developmental level, and lifestyle practices. You should plan interventions, such as encouraging participation in group/family therapy. That intervention can assist the family with realistic strategies that enhance family functioning, such as improving communication skills and identifying and utilizing support systems.

Grief and Loss

Grieving is a normal, subjective emotional response to loss and is essential for mental and physical health. How a client or family responds to loss, and how they express grief, varies widely. Factors that influence the process of grieving include age, stage of development, gender, culture, and personal reserves and strengths.

You should know the different stages of grieving and factors that influence how clients and families react to death to understand their responses and needs. You must also be knowledgeable about legal issues surrounding death, such as advance directives, autopsies, organ donation, and do-not-resuscitate (DNR) orders.

You also need to take the time to analyze your own feelings about death before you can effectively help others.

Additional nursing responsibilities include:

- Brainstorming ways to provide relief from loneliness, fear, and depression
- Helping clients maintain a sense of security
- Helping clients and families accept the loss
- Providing physical comfort measures
- Providing emotional support, structure, and continuity
- Allowing expression of thoughts and feelings

Mental Health Concepts

Mental health is a positive state in which one is responsible, displays self-awareness, is self-directive, is reasonably worry-free, and can cope with usual daily tensions. Mentally healthy individuals function well in society, are accepted within a group, and are generally satisfied with their lives.

Influences on mental health include inherited characteristics, nurturing during childhood, and life circumstances. Influences on maintaining mental health include interpersonal communication, the use of ego defense mechanisms, and the presence of support people.

Nurses focus on different aspects of care based on the identified needs or presenting problems of patients. You should also be able to apply your knowledge of client psychopathology to mental health concepts.

Religious and Spiritual Influences on Health

Religion and spirituality have a great influence on the health of clients and how they cope, and make a difference in physical and psychosocial outcomes. You should promote your clients' physical, emotional, and spiritual health, because this balance of well-being is essential to a client's overall health. You must strive to be an empathetic listener and attempt to identify your clients' spiritual needs. To accomplish this, the nurse should understand how spirituality influences clinical care.

Nurses should be knowledgeable about religious traditions and spiritual expressions other than their own. You should approach each client based on that client's distinct need, because people develop and nurture their own spirituality in different ways. Each client's spiritual beliefs or religious practice should influence how you care for that client. Clients have the right to receive care that respects their religious and spiritual values. At the same time, they have the right to refuse care on religious grounds.

Sensory/Perceptual Alterations

A disruption in a client's cognitive processes can lead to faulty interpretations of their surroundings.

Alterations in sensory perception, or altered thought processes, affect a client's ability to function within their environment, which may place the client at risk for harm. You should assist the client to function safely in health care settings.

Some factors that influence sensory function include developmental stage, culture, stress, medications, illness, lifestyle, and personality.

You need to identify clients at risk for sensory/perceptual alterations so you can initiate preventive measures. Examples of clients at risk include those who:

- Are confined in a nonstimulating environment
- Have impaired vision or hearing
- Have mobility restrictions
- Have emotional disorders
- Have limited social contact
- Are experiencing pain or discomfort
- Are acutely ill
- Are closely monitored (such as in the ICU)
- Have decreased cognitive ability (as in a head injury)

When dealing with such a client, you should organize nursing care to reduce unessential stimuli; orient the client to person, place, and time during every contact; and explain all nursing care.

Stress Management

Everyone experiences stress, which can result from both positive and negative experiences. A person's response to any change in homeostasis results in stress. Stress indicators can be physiologic (increased heart rate or respirations, muscle tension), psychological (anxiety, fear, anger), and/or cognitive (thinking responses). Consequences of stress may be physical, emotional, intellectual, social, spiritual, or any combination of these.

To minimize stress in a client, you should help the client to do the following:

- Determine situations that precipitate anxiety.
- Verbalize feelings, perceptions, and fears, as appropriate.
- Identify personal strengths.
- Recognize usual coping patterns.
- Identify new strategies.

You should also listen attentively, provide an atmosphere of warmth and trust, provide factual information as needed, encourage clients to participate in the plan of care, promote safety and security, and provide education. Responses to stress are called *coping mechanisms*.

Support Systems

A support system is a network of personal contacts that are available to clients for practical, emotional, or moral support when needed. Support systems are important to clients in that they enhance client learning, offer support, help the client perform required skills, and help the client maintain required lifestyle changes. Exploring the client's support system is a component of the initial assessment.

Caregivers might also need to be connected to outside resources. For example, community support groups are appropriate interventions for family members suffering from caregiver role strain.

Therapeutic Communication

You use therapeutic communication techniques to promote understanding and establish a constructive relationship with the client. Therapeutic communication is planned, and is client- and goal-directed. It means listening to and understanding the client while promoting clarification and insight. It enables the nurse to form a working relationship with the client and peers, using both verbal and nonverbal communication. Remember that *nonverbal communication* is the most accurate reflection of attitude.

You should be familiar with the foundations for a therapeutic relationship, which include:

- An understanding of the factors influencing communication
- Realization of the importance of nonverbal communication

- Development of effective communication skills
- Recognition of the causes of ineffective communication
- Ability to participate in a therapeutic communication process

You should also be familiar with the conditions essential for a therapeutic relationship, which include:

- Empathy
- Respect
- Genuineness
- Self-disclosure
- Concreteness and specificity
- Confrontation (limited to a well-established nurse/client relationship with an accepting, gentle manner)

It is important to understand the client's views and feelings before responding. You also need to recognize barriers to effective communication, such as:

- Failure to listen
- Improperly decoding the client's intended message
- Placing the nurse's needs above the client's needs
- Stereotyping, challenging, probing, and/or rejecting
- Being defensive
- Changing topics and subjects
- Passing judgment

Effective therapeutic responses include:

- **Using silence:** Allows the client time to think and reflect; conveys acceptance; allows the client to take the lead in the conversation
- **Using general leads or a broad opening:** Encourages the client to talk; indicates your interest in the client; allows the client to choose the subject
- **Clarification:** Encourages recall and details of a particular experience; encourages description of feelings; seeks explanation; pinpoints specifics
- **Reflecting:** Paraphrases what client says

Therapeutic Environment

Nurses provide care for clients who constantly interact with their environment. Clients may have unmet needs, be unable to care for themselves, or be unable to adapt to the environment due to health problems. You provide therapeutic care so clients can adapt to their environment.

The Nursing Process and Psychosocial Integrity

You utilize the nursing process (assess, diagnose, plan, implement, and evaluate) to promote a client's psychosocial integrity by conveying understanding, sensitivity, and compassion to a client who is experiencing stress, illness, or crisis. Promoting a client's psychosocial integrity is not just for the mental health client, but for *all* clients. The nursing process respects the client's autonomy, freedom to make decisions, and involvement in nursing care.

Although you need to identify emotional disorders and behaviors that indicate mental illness, a client does not need to be mentally ill for you to include psychosocial integrity in the care plan. You must possess sound knowledge and focused clinical experiences to be prepared to recognize and effectively intervene with *any* client whose state of dynamic psychological and sociological homeostasis is being threatened—whether or not the client has a mental illness.

Chapter Quiz

1. The nurse provides care for an older adult client who appears fully alert and oriented. As it gets later in the day, the nurse notices the client becoming increasingly confused and agitated. It would be **most** appropriate for the nurse to take which action?

   1. Reorient the client, and then turn on the lights and television to distract the client from their confusion.
   2. Encourage the client's alert roommate to talk with the client.
   3. Tell the client they are at home in their own bed to get the client to settle down and go to sleep.
   4. Reorient the client, pull the shades down, shut the lights and television off, and promote a quiet environment.

2. The nurse cares for a client who has expressed a desire to commit suicide. He has informed the nurse of plans to pursue this. The nurse requests a sitter to stay with the client around the clock, but the client says he does not want this. Which is the **most** appropriate response by the nurse?

   1. The nurse accepts the client's refusal, because clients have a right to refuse care.
   2. The nurse implements the intervention, because protecting the client's safety overrules the client's right to refuse care.
   3. The nurse checks on the client every hour to be sure he is safe and the sitter is fine.
   4. The nurse asks the unlicensed assistive personnel (UAP) to check on the client every 30 minutes to be sure he is safe.

3. A client scheduled to have surgery tells the nurse, "I'm very scared. I have never had surgery before and am afraid that I might not make it through." Which response by the nurse is **best**?

   1. "Why do you feel this way?"
   2. "Don't worry, you will be fine."
   3. "Why don't we take some time to fully explore why you feel this way?"
   4. "It's normal to be scared. You will be taken cared of. Tell me how you are feeling."

4. The nurse works on a busy locked psychiatric unit. The alarm is activated when someone tries to go through the locked doors without permission from the front desk. Which action does the nurse take after the alarm is activated?

   1. Reset the alarm from the front desk after verifying that everybody is safe and nobody has escaped from the unit.
   2. Reset the alarm from the location where the alarm was activated after verifying that everybody in the unit is safe.
   3. Reset the alarm from a client's room after doing a quick scan of the hallways and bathrooms.
   4. Reset the alarm from the front desk once the receptionist says everybody is accounted for.

5. The nurse cares for a client who is intoxicated, has signs of delirium, and attempts to get out of bed every few minutes. The client's gait is unsteady and the nurse is concerned that the client might fall. The provider prescribes wrist restraints. The client refuses the restraints. The nurse should take which action?

   1. Place the restraints in compliance with hospital policy.
   2. Refrain from placing restraints to honor the client's wishes, because the client has the right to refuse care.
   3. Call the provider for advice on how to proceed.
   4. Check on the client every hour to ensure the client's safety.

6. The clinic nurse cares for a client who appears intoxicated and drove to the appointment. The nurse is concerned about the client's ability to drive home. Which action should the nurse implement **first**?

   1. Call the police and confiscate the client's driver's license.
   2. Ask the client's permission to call a family member for a ride.
   3. Give the client a ride home to protect their privacy.
   4. Call clinic security to detain the client to protect their safety.

Refer to the Case Study to answer the next question.

The nurse is caring for an adult client who arrives at the outpatient mental health clinic.

| Nurse's Notes | Client History | Medications |

1330: Client arrives to clinic reporting extreme feelings of sadness and loneliness after the client's dog died in a tragic accident 6 weeks ago. Client states, "I can't stop crying and I haven't gone to work for the past week. I can hardly eat or sleep because I'm so upset." Client explains the dog was a trusted companion and provided much emotional support for the client. Client states, "I feel like I want to start cutting again and end my life. My mom encouraged me to come here and get help." Client appears well groomed, dressed appropriately, is tearful with flat affect, and makes little eye contact.

| Nurse's Notes | Client History | Medications |

Client reports living alone and working as a full time care giver for 2 young children. Client reports 3 inpatient behavioral health admissions in the past, with the most recent 9 months ago, when client demonstrated the inability to care for self and maintain safety. Client states, "I cut myself multiple times then, in an attempt to end my life. All the terrible events of my past just came crashing down on me." Client denies any medical issues.

| Client History | Nurse's Notes | Medications |

Medication	Dose	Route	Frequency
Fluoxetine	20 mg	PO	once daily
Olanzapine	5 mg	PO	once daily
Ethinyl estradiol-norethindrone acetate 30 mcg/1.5 mg tablets	1 tablet	PO	once daily
Multivitamin (MVI)	1 tablet	PO	once daily

7. The nurse is reviewing the client's assessment data and medication list to prepare the client's plan of care.

Complete the diagram by dragging from the choices below to specify what condition the client is most likely experiencing, 2 actions the nurse takes to address that condition, and 2 parameters the nurse monitors to assess the client's progress.

Action to Take		Condition Most Likely Experiencing		Parameter to Monitor
Action to Take				Parameter to Monitor

Actions to Take	Potential Conditions	Parameters to Monitor
Encourage the client to return to work within the next 2–3 days.	Obsessive compulsive disorder and homicidal thoughts.	Client's ability to agree to a safety plan.
Encourage the client to ventilate feelings.	Depression and suicidal thoughts.	Presence of persecutory delusions.
Determine if the client will get another dog.	Bipolar 2 disorder and suicidal thoughts.	Depression screening tool score.
Ask, "Are you thinking about ways to end your life?"	Schizoaffective disorder and generalized anxiety disorder.	Weight loss in the past 3 days.
Ask, "Were you a victim of sexual abuse as a child?"		Interest in hobbies.

8. The home care nurse makes a visit to the home of an older adult client who has episodic confusion but remains safe at home while occasionally alone. The nurse finds the client disheveled, confused, and agitated, and the home is messy. This degree of confusion is unusual for the client. The nurse takes the client's vital signs, which are BP 115/70 mmHg, HR 70 beats/minute, RR 16 breaths/minute, and temperature 98.7° F (37° C). Which action should the nurse implement **first**?

   1. Nothing, because the client's vital signs are stable.
   2. Plan to come back the following day to reevaluate the client.
   3. Sit down with the client and encourage client to verbalize feelings.
   4. Call the client's family to take the client to be evaluated by a provider.

9. The nurse provides care to a client, diagnosed with Alzheimer disease, who is agitated and pulling at things. Which action should the nurse implement when providing care to this client?

   1. Provide the client with therapeutic sensory devices.
   2. Cohort the client with another client who is agitated, because they will calm each other.
   3. Place the client in a room with several other clients.
   4. Leave the client alone for a set period of time to reduce environmental stimulation.

10. The nurse cares for a terminally ill client who has agreed to enter hospice care. Which statement by the spouse indicates a need for further teaching by the nurse?

   1. "You will help to make my spouse as comfortable as possible while in hospice care."
   2. "You will help my spouse get better so we can get back to our old life."
   3. "The goal is to make the end of my spouse's life as comfortable as possible."
   4. "You will provide me with much needed support during this difficult time."

11. The nurse cares for a client with a known past medical history for intravenous substance abuse. The client requests to go outside to smoke and promises to come right back. The client has a peripheral intravenous line in. Which action does the nurse implement based on the current scenario?

   1. Allow the client to go outside but set a time limit in which to return.
   2. Secure the intravenous line with occlusive dressing and call security to escort the client to an approved smoking area.
   3. Make a behavioral contract with the client that includes an agreement to have an unlicensed assistive personnel (UAP) accompany the client.
   4. Watch the client from the window to make sure the IV line stays open.

12. The nurse admits a non-English-speaking client who is accompanied by family members who speak English. The nurse needs to ask general admission questions. It is **most** appropriate for the nurse to take which action?

   1. Call the hospital's interpreter services to assist with asking the client questions.
   2. Ask family members the questions and document their responses.
   3. Ask family members to translate and ask the questions for the nurse.
   4. Document "Unable to obtain answers, client does not speak English."

Refer to the Case Study to answer the next six questions.

The hospice nurse is caring for an adult client with a diagnosis of advanced metastatic ovarian cancer.

History

The client was diagnosed with stage 3 ovarian cancer 2 years ago. At the time of diagnosis, the cancer had spread from the ovaries into the upper abdomen and lymph nodes. The client had exploratory surgery with total hysterectomy, bilateral oophorectomy, debulking of the tumor, and dissection of multiple lymph nodes. The client has also had several rounds of systemic treatment with chemotherapy.

Last week, the client began to experience abdominal pain, increasing fatigue, nausea, and shortness of breath (SOB). Magnetic resonance imaging (MRI) confirmed metastasis to the liver, mediastinal lymph nodes, and pleural space. The client developed a malignant pleural effusion on the left and underwent thoracentesis with placement of a left posterior chest tube for drainage. The client is on oxygen at 2L/min per nasal cannula (O_2 2L/min per NC) to maintain oxygen saturation > 90% and decrease dyspnea. The client has a subcutaneous venous access device (VAD) implanted in the right chest, which is currently accessed so the client can receive IV fluids and medications. The client is receiving oxycontin 40 mg PO every 12 hours. Pain has been well controlled.

The client is married and has 2 school-age children and a preschool aged child. The client has numerous siblings and both parents are living and are active in the client's care. The client's parents and siblings are adamant the client should continue chemotherapy and consider a clinical trial. The client and the client's spouse requested to speak with the palliative care team to discuss supportive care. Following a lengthy discussion, the client requested to be discharged home with hospice care to spend more time with family and be with the children. The client completed an advance directive. Client is requesting no resuscitation, no IV fluids, enteral feeding, or antibiotics. The client's spouse has been named the client's health care proxy.

13. The palliative care team requests that a nurse from a local hospice agency visits the client and family in the hospital to explain hospice care.

Complete the following sentences by choosing from the list of options.

It is very important for the client and family to understand that by electing home hospice care, the client [Select from list 1]. The focus of hospice care is to [Select from list 2]. Members of the hospice interdisciplinary team also assist the client with [Select from list 3]. It is very important for the hospice team to provide [Select from list 4]. The family should also understand that [Select from list 5].

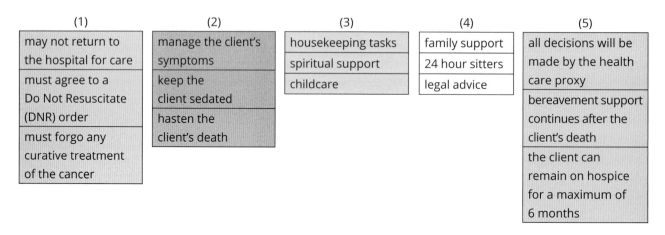

(1)	(2)	(3)	(4)	(5)
may not return to the hospital for care	manage the client's symptoms	housekeeping tasks	family support	all decisions will be made by the health care proxy
must agree to a Do Not Resuscitate (DNR) order	keep the client sedated	spiritual support	24 hour sitters	bereavement support continues after the client's death
must forgo any curative treatment of the cancer	hasten the client's death	childcare	legal advice	the client can remain on hospice for a maximum of 6 months

History	Nurse's Notes	Vital Signs

First visit to client's home since admission to hospice two days ago. Client's sibling, spouse, and parent are present. Client lying on right side with head of hospital bed elevated 60 degrees. Skin color and sclerae yellow; skin warm and dry. Client opens eyes to name and answers questions appropriately, but begins to cough and becomes very short of breath when attempting to speak. Absent lung sounds in left lower lobe; coarse rhonchi in upper lobe; right lung field clear, diminished in base. Left posterior chest tube dressing intact and dry. Bulge of right subclavian VAD is visible, but VAD is not accessed. Chest tube attached to disposable collection device draining cloudy serous drainage. Oxygen on at 2L/minute per nasal cannula.

Abdomen protuberant and firm with hypoactive bowel sounds throughout. Client's spouse states client has not had a stool since coming home. Client is diapered and voiding dark yellow urine. Lower extremities with 2+ edema and palpable pedal pulses. The client occasionally moans and grunts with movement. Client states, "I hurt so bad. It's worse when I cough." The spouse states, "We are trying to avoid giving that breakthrough medication. If we give too much, won't my spouse just stop breathing?"

Client's sibling states the client has refused to eat and is taking only occasional sips of water and cola. The sibling is very concerned about this and states, "The physician needs to put a feeding tube in or my sibling will starve to death!" The client's parent begins to cry and says, "We cannot do this at home. We need to go back to the hospital."

History	Nurse's Notes	Vital Signs

Vital Signs	Result
Temperature (axillary)	101.6° F (38.6° C)
BP	122/78
HR	98
RR	22
Pulse oximetry (O_2 2 L/min per NC)	91%

14. The client is discharged and admitted to home hospice care. Two days later, the hospice nurse makes a home visit, assesses the client, and obtains vital signs.

Drag the choices below to fill in each blank in the following sentence. Each choice will only be used once.

The nurse is **most** concerned about the client's _____ [Select from the list] and _____ [Select from the list].

lack of appetite
urine color
no stool since discharge
pain level
chest drainage
dyspnea
lower extremity edema
temperature

| History | Nurse's Notes | Vital Signs | Medications |

Medication	Dose	Route	Frequency
Oxycontin	40 mg	PO	Every 12 hours
Docusate sodium	100 mg	PO	Daily
Bisacodyl	5 mg	PO	Every 12 hours PRN constipation (no bowel movement × 3 days)
Acetaminophen suppositories	650 mg	Per rectum	Every 4 hours PRN mild pain or Temp > 101° F (38.3° C)
Ondansetron	4 mg	PO	Every 6 hours PRN nausea
Hydrocodone/ Acetaminophen	7.5 mg/325 mg	PO	Every 4 hours PRN breakthrough pain
Lorazepam	0.5 mg	PO	Every 6 hours PRN agitation

15. The nurse reviews the client's medications and talks with the family.

Which action does the nurse take **immediately**?

1. Call emergency medical services (EMS) to transport the client to the hospital.
2. Administer breakthrough pain medication.
3. Notify the physician of the sibling's request for a feeding tube.
4. Request the hospice chaplain to speak with the family.

16. At the hospice interdisciplinary meeting, the nurse discusses the client's increasing pain level and dyspnea with the hospice team. The nurse also expresses concerns about the family members' acceptance of the terminal diagnosis. The hospice team collaborates on an updated plan of care for the client.

For each nursing concern below, specify the potential nursing intervention that is appropriate for the care of the client at this time. **Each concern supports only 1 potential nursing intervention.**

Concern	Potential Nursing Interventions
Increasing pain	Select... ▾
	Increase the amount of oxycontin the client is receiving every 12 hours.
	Teach family members to medicate the client when pain reaches 7/10.
	Admit the client to the hospital for IV pain control.
Worsening dyspnea	Select... ▾
	Place the client on 100% non-rebreather face mask.
	Add liquid morphine as a PRN breakthrough medication.
	Encourage the family to suction the client's airway every hour.
Family's acceptance	Select... ▾
	Provide a pamphlet to the family about complicated grief.
	Encourage the caregiver and family to express fears and concerns.
	Tell the family members that death is an inevitable part of life.

17. The nurse provides education to the spouse and family about signs and symptoms of impending death.

Which statement is correct for the nurse to make? **(Select all that apply.)**

1. "If the client becomes incontinent, an indwelling urinary catheter will be required."
2. "As death approaches, the client's breathing becomes very peaceful and quiet until it ceases altogether."
3. "If you think the client has stopped breathing, call hospice right away and a nurse will come."
4. "It is not unusual for the client to become more responsive and animated soon before death."
5. "The client may lose the ability to swallow and the route of medications may need to be changed."
6. "If the urine becomes very dark then the client has developed an infection."
7. "When a client dies at home, the police must be notified."
8. "You can expect wide fluctuations in temperature before death."

18. Two nights later, the client's spouse notifies the hospice nurse on call that the client doesn't appear to be breathing. The nurse arrives at the home and assesses the client. The nurse pronounces the client's death and speaks with the spouse and family.

For each finding below, specify whether the findings are expected at the end of life or not expected.

Assessment Finding	Expected	Not Expected
The client was more alert and spent an hour with the children the previous day.	○	○
The client had very noisy breathing through the night with periods of gurgling.	○	○
The client was not responsive the last several hours.	○	○
The skin on the client's hands and legs became mottled.	○	○
The client spiked a high temperature a few hours ago.	○	○
The client had long periods of apnea before respirations ceased.	○	○
The client was extremely thirsty and requested IV fluids.	○	○
The client was incontinent of stool.	○	○

19. The nurse cares for a client diagnosed with alcohol abuse who reports having the last drink yesterday. The client exhibits tremors, diaphoresis, and tachycardia. Based on the current data, which action does the nurse implement **first**?

    1. Call the health care provider to report the symptoms and administer hydromorphone per the alcohol withdrawal pathway.
    2. Assess client every hour to monitor for worsening symptoms.
    3. Call the family and administer meperidine per the alcohol withdrawal pathway.
    4. Administer lorazepam per the alcohol withdrawal pathway.

20. A client with post-traumatic stress disorder (PTSD) appears to be experiencing a flashback. It is **most** appropriate for the nurse to perform which intervention?

    1. Encourage the client to tell the nurse how the client is feeling in that moment.
    2. Calmly reorient the client to the current situation.
    3. Assist the client in acting out the flashback event.
    4. Inform the client firmly that what the client is experiencing is not real.

21. An older adult client asks the nurse to kill the bugs that are crawling on the floor of the room. The nurse does not see any bugs and suspects the client is hallucinating. Which statement by the nurse to the client is **most** appropriate?

    1. "It may seem to you that there are bugs on the floor, but I do not see any bugs."
    2. "I see them too. They are crawling all over the floor. How should I kill them?"
    3. "Tell me how it make you feel to see these bugs."
    4. "Tell me, what do these bugs look like?"

22. The nurse provides care to a client who has experienced a depressed mood, decreased sleep, poor concentration, and poor appetite for the past 4 months. The nurse anticipates that the provider will prescribe which medication?

    1. Quetiapine.
    2. Haloperidol.
    3. Mirtazapine.
    4. Clonazepam.

23. The nurse provides care to a client who experiences a manic episode. It is **most** appropriate for the nurse to perform which intervention for this client?

    1. Give the client materials to make a collage.
    2. Encourage the client to use an exercise bike.
    3. Let the client attend a group about managing feelings.
    4. Ask the client to play a board game with other clients.

24. A client diagnosed with bipolar disorder makes a sexually inappropriate comment to the nurse. The nurse should take which action?

    1. Ignore the comment because the client has a mental health disorder and cannot help it.
    2. Report the comment to the nurse manager.
    3. Ignore the comment, but tell the incoming nurse to be aware of the client's inappropriate comments.
    4. Tell the client that it is inappropriate for clients to speak to any staff member that way.

25. The nurse cares for a hospice client who lives at home with an attentive spouse. The client's spouse quit work to care for the client. During the nurse's visit, the spouse expresses frustration and hostility toward the nurse. Which is an appropriate response by the nurse? **(Select all that apply.)**

   1. The nurse should encourage the spouse to verbalize feelings.
   2. The nurse should encourage the spouse to attend a caregiver support group.
   3. The nurse should encourage the spouse to go back to work part-time.
   4. The nurse should encourage the spouse not to verbalize negative feelings that may upset the client.
   5. The nurse should ignore the spouse's hostile behavior.

26. The nurse completes a health history for a client. The client has been taking lorazepam for 6 months. Which finding does the nurse anticipate when conducting the physical examination for this client?

   1. Excessive appetite.
   2. Physical dependence.
   3. Suicidal ideation.
   4. Seizure activity.

27. A client requires a blood transfusion. The client refuses based on religious beliefs. It is **most** appropriate for the nurse to take which action when providing care to this client?

   1. Confirm with the client that the client under-stands the potential risks of not having the blood transfusion.
   2. Tell the client that, regardless of personal beliefs, the client has to have the lifesaving transfusion.
   3. Call the legal department of the hospital immediately.
   4. Gently encourage the client to accept the transfusion.

28. The nurse works in a day program for clients with disabilities. The nurse notes that an adolescent client is frequently alone and often quiet. It is **most** appropriate for the nurse to take which action when providing care for this client?

   1. Allow the client alone time since the client prefer this.
   2. Make an effort to interact with the client periodically.
   3. Encourage the quiet client to join a youth group.
   4. Encourage others to interact more frequently with the client.

29. The nurse discovers a hospice client has expired. The family members are regrouping in the facility's waiting room. Which action by the nurse is **most** appropriate?

   1. Tell the family it would not be in their best interests to see their loved one.
   2. Encourage the family to view the body to help accept the situation.
   3. Provide condolences to the family and offer them viewing time.
   4. Tell the family "I will give you some time to spend with your loved one. Let me know if you need anything."

30. During the admission process, the nurse inquires about advance directives from the client. The client tells the nurse, "I do not want to make any medical decisions. I want my daughter to make these decisions for me." Which action does the nurse implement based on the current situation?

   1. Make sure that the written advance directives document the client's wishes.
   2. Tell the client that, being alert and oriented, the client should make their own medical decisions.
   3. Tell the client that due to confidentiality, the daughter will not be informed of details of the client's care.
   4. Encourage both the daughter and the client to work together on making medical decisions.

Chapter Quiz Answers and Explanations

1. The answer is 4

The nurse provides care for an older adult client who appears fully alert and oriented. As it gets later in the day, the nurse notices the client becoming increasingly confused and agitated. It would be **most** appropriate for the nurse to take which action?

Category: Therapeutic environment

(1) Although the nurse would reorient the client, the nurse would not turn on the lights and television in an attempt to distract. Clients with confusion can become increasingly more agitated with stimulation, such as lights and television.

(2) Encouraging the client's roommate to talk with the client is another inappropriate attempt at distraction.

(3) Reassuring clients is usually a good practice, but it is not appropriate unless the nurse is honest with the attempt to reorient to an accurate location, time, and place.

(4) CORRECT: Promoting a quiet environment decreases stimulation to prevent agitation. It also promotes the normal sleep-wake cycle, consistent with it being "later in the day."

2. The answer is 2

The nurse cares for a client who has expressed a desire to commit suicide. He has informed the nurse of plans to pursue this. The nurse requests a sitter to stay with the client around the clock, but the client says he does not want this. Which is the **most** appropriate response by the nurse?

Category: Crisis intervention

(1) Although clients do have the right to refuse care, in certain high risk-to-safety situations (e.g., suicide), nurses put measures in place to prevent harm.

(2) CORRECT: Protecting the client's safety trumps the client's right to refuse care.

(3) The nurse could check in on the client every hour in combination with other interventions. However, clients at high risk for suicide cannot be left alone for any time period.

(4) This answer is incorrect for the same reasons as answer choice (3): clients at high risk for suicide cannot be left alone for any time period, even for 30 minutes.

3. The answer is 4

A client scheduled to have surgery tells the nurse, "I'm very scared. I have never had surgery before and am afraid that I might not make it through." Which response by the nurse is **best**?

Category: Therapeutic communications

(1) Avoid asking "Why" questions because they imply disapproval with what the client is saying.

(2) Telling the client not to worry, and that the client will be fine, dismisses the client's feelings and provides false reassurance.

(3) The nurse must remain within the nursing scope of practice. The nurse is not a therapist, so asking the client to explore feelings with the nurse would not be appropriate.

(4) CORRECT: A response affirming that fear is normal, care will be provided, and feelings may be shared normalizes the client's experience, provides some reassurance, and allows the client to verbalize.

4. The answer is 2

The nurse works on a busy locked psychiatric unit. The alarm is activated when someone tries to go through the locked doors without permission from the front desk. Which action does the nurse take after the alarm is activated?

Category: Therapeutic environment

(1) Resetting the alarm from the front desk is not proper procedure.

(2) CORRECT: An alarm is a safety mechanism meant to alert staff to somebody at risk attempting to leave. When an alarm is activated, the nurse should first make sure that all clients are accounted for and safe, and then reset the alarm by going to the place where it was tripped.

(3) The nurse must be sure, based on firsthand knowledge, that all clients are safe. Resetting the alarm after a quick check of hallways and bathrooms would not be appropriate.

(4) The nurse must be sure, based on firsthand knowledge, that all clients are safe. Resetting the alarm based on the receptionist's report would not be appropriate.

5. The answer is 1

The nurse cares for a client who is intoxicated, has signs of delirium, and attempts to get out of bed every few minutes. The client's gait is unsteady and the nurse is concerned that the client might fall. The provider prescribes wrist restraints. The client refuses the restraints. The nurse should take which action?

Category: Chemical and other dependencies

(1) CORRECT: The nurse should place the restraints in compliance with hospital policy. This is a circumstance where the client's risk of harm and promotion of safety overrules the client's right to refuse.

(2) The client is at risk for fall due to intoxication and delirium; the nurse should place the restraints.

(3) The nurse, at some point, may call the provider for further assistance. The priority is the client's safety.

(4) The nurse could check on the client every hour, but only in addition to the needed ongoing safety measure of restraints or constant observation. A client could fall within minutes; an hour is too long to leave an at-risk client alone.

6. The answer is 2

The clinic nurse cares for a client who appears intoxicated and drove to the appointment. The nurse is concerned about the client's ability to drive home. Which action should the nurse implement **first**?

Category: Chemical and other dependencies

(1) The nurse's goal is to protect the client (and in this scenario, potentially the public as well), but calling the police immediately is not the best first option. The nurse may end up doing this but should first take the time to review other options.

(2) CORRECT: Asking the client's permission to call a family member is a better option because it includes the client in the choice. An intoxicated client may not make good choices, but the client may be amenable to good suggestions. Ideally, the nurse would find somebody (not the police) to get the client home safely. That would allow maintaining a trusting nurse-client relationship.

(3) The nurse should not overstep the boundaries and drive the client home.

(4) Calling clinic security to detain the client sounds less threatening than calling the police and might be done eventually, but the first option would be to enlist the client's family member.

7.   See explanation for answers

Condition Most Likely Experiencing	
Depression and suicidal thoughts.	☑

CORRECT OPTION: Feelings of sadness lasting at least 2 weeks, insomnia, loss of appetite, flat affect, and thoughts of suicide are consistent with a diagnosis of **depression and suicidal thoughts**. In addition, the client is prescribed fluoxetine, a serotonin selective reuptake inhibitor (SSRI), and olanzapine, an antipsychotic, which are commonly prescribed together to treat depression. Clients with a history of previous suicidal ideation or attempts are at a higher risk for future suicidality.

INCORRECT OPTIONS: Obsessive compulsive disorder (OCD) is characterized by persistent thoughts, images, or impulses accompanied by ritualistic behaviors in an attempt to reduce anxiety. Homicidal thoughts include the desire to kill another individual. Bipolar 2 disorder is characterized by depression alternating with periods of hypomania. Schizoaffective disorder contains elements of schizophrenia, including bizarre thoughts, feelings, emotions and behaviors, and a mood disorder, with periods of depression and/or mania. Generalized anxiety disorder is characterized by excessive worry, persisting for a period of time. The client's behaviors are not indicative of these conditions.

Actions to Take	
Encourage the client to ventilate feelings.	☑
Ask, "Are you thinking about ways to end your life?"	☑

CORRECT OPTIONS: **Encouraging the client to talk about feelings**, while conveying an attitude of acceptance, empathy, concern, and unconditional positive regard, may help relieve despair and hopelessness. Trust is enhanced and the client begins to believe self is a worthwhile person. Client's history of a suicide attempt and the statement "in an attempt to end my life" places this client at a greater risk for suicidal behavior. **Asking direct questions, and talking openly and in a matter-of-fact manner addresses the suicidal thoughts.** While this option is a closed-ended question, it is appropriate when the nurse is communicating with the client about suicide ideation. Active listening in a nonjudgmental manner provides some relief to the client. Further assessment, including the lethality of the suicidal thoughts, is a priority in the plan of care.

INCORRECT OPTIONS: When the client should return to work is decided by the client, not the nurse. Determining if the client will get another dog is not a priority at this time. The question regarding sexual abuse as a child is a closed-ended question, which is considered nontherapeutic.

Parameters to Monitor	
Client's ability to agree to a safety plan.	☑
Depression screening tool score.	☑

CORRECT OPTIONS: This client is at increased risk to follow through with the suicidal behavior based on the client's statement and history of previous suicide attempt. Completing a suicide attempt is more likely within 12 months of the previous attempt. **Formulating a short-term verbal or written contract** with a client, indicating the client will not harm self, gets the subject out in the open and some of the responsibility for safety is given to the client. While there are no guarantees, as the safety contract is not a legally binding document, it is a well-established means used for client safety. A standardized **depression screening tool**, such as the Beck Depression Inventory or the Hamilton Depression Scale, helps to determine the type and severity of depression. Using these tools at baseline and then periodically, helps the nurse understand the changes in depressive symptoms over time, and direct the plan of care.

INCORRECT OPTIONS: Persecutory delusions are behaviors exhibited in schizophrenia and psychosis, not depression. Monitoring weight loss in a client diagnosed with depression who reports decreased food intake is a priority, however, weight loss needs to be assessed over a period of at least one week. A safety plan and severity of depression are higher priorities than interest in hobbies.

8. The answer is 4

The home care nurse makes a visit to the home of an older adult client who has episodic confusion but remains safe at home while occasionally alone. The nurse finds the client disheveled, confused, and agitated, and the home is messy. This degree of confusion is unusual for the client. The nurse takes the client's vital signs, which are BP 115/70 mmHg, HR 70 beats/minute, RR 16 breaths/minute, and temperature 98.7° F (37° C). Which action should the nurse implement **first**?

Category: Crisis intervention

(1) Although the vital signs are within normal limits, the onset of worsening symptoms could be an indication of something more serious, so doing nothing would not be correct.

(2) The nurse may plan to come back the following day depending on what happens to the client in the next 24 hours, but as a first choice, this is not correct.

(3) Encouraging the client to verbalize feelings is not an appropriate intervention given the presenting symptoms.

(4) CORRECT: These are new symptoms, and the client does not appear safe to be alone. By contacting the family, the nurse is performing an intervention based on the assessment of the client. In the home care setting, assessing safety is prioritized, especially with new symptoms.

9. The answer is 1

The nurse provides care to a client, diagnosed with Alzheimer disease, who is agitated and pulling at things. Which action should the nurse implement when providing care to this client?

Category: Sensory/perceptual alterations

(1) CORRECT: Clients with Alzheimer disease often pick at items, such as buttons on clothing or medical devices, which poses a danger to them. Providing them with safely designed sensory devices serves the need of stimulating the senses as well as their urge to pick.

(2) Cohorting the client with another agitated client can worsen the problem due to increased stimulation.

(3) Placing the client in a room with several other clients can worsen the problem due to increased stimulation.

(4) Leaving the client alone could lead to injuries related to the agitation and picking.

10. The answer is 2

The nurse cares for a terminally ill client who has agreed to enter hospice care. Which statement by the spouse indicates a need for further teaching by the nurse?

Category: End of life care

(1) This is an accurate statement. The goal of hospice is to make clients as comfortable as possible during the remainder of their life.

(2) CORRECT: This is an inaccurate statement. The philosophy of hospice care is not to help a client recover, but to promote comfort and peace during the end of life. The presumption is that the client will not improve.

(3) This is an accurate statement. The goal of hospice is to make the end of life as comfortable as possible.

(4) This is an accurate statement. Hospice care involves the family as well as the client.

11. The answer is 3

The nurse cares for a client with a known past medical history for intravenous substance abuse. The client requests to go outside to smoke and promises to come right back. The client has a peripheral intravenous line in. Which action does the nurse implement based on the current scenario?

Category: Chemical and other dependencies

(1) Allowing the client to go outside for a set time could potentially be a part of an agreement with the client, but review the other choices first.

(2) The client has not shown any signs of eloping and has not threatened anyone. If the client tried to

elope, the nurse might then call security. At this point, the client has merely requested to go outside.

(3) CORRECT: Contracting with the client is the best choice. The nurse makes a compromise that the client can go outside but must be supervised while doing so. The client is a known abuser of intravenous substances, so sending the client outside alone could be a safety risk.

(4) Watching the client from the window is not an appropriate form of medical supervision.

12. The answer is 1

The nurse admits a non-English-speaking client who is accompanied by family members who speak English. The nurse needs to ask general admission questions. It is **most** appropriate for the nurse to take which action?

Category: Cultural awareness/cultural influences on health

(1) CORRECT: The only way to avoid bias and interjection by family members is by utilizing interpreter services at your hospital.

(2) Asking family members the questions and documenting their responses will result in obtaining answers to the questions and being able to create some documentation, but the responses should come straight from the client.

(3) Asking family members to translate and ask the questions is not appropriate. The responses should come straight from the client.

(4) Documenting "unable to obtain answers, client does not speak English" without trying another more appropriate method is a poor choice.

13. See explanation for answers

CORRECT OPTIONS: When a client elects hospice care, the client is agreeing to **forgo curative treatment of the admitting hospice diagnosis.** The client on hospice does not continue chemotherapy or other aggressive treatments. The **focus of hospice care is on management of symptoms, caregiver/family support, and quality of life.** Care includes physical, emotional, and **spiritual support.** When a client elects hospice, the hospice team continues contact with the client's family for **bereavement support for at least one year after the client's death.**

INCORRECT OPTIONS: A client who elects hospice may need to return to the hospital for symptom management if the symptoms cannot be managed in the home. The client also does not have to agree to a Do Not Resuscitate order to receive hospice care, although most clients will eventually request that they be allowed to die a natural death. When managing symptoms, the hospice team strives to relieve pain and other distressing symptoms without over-sedating the client if possible. The intent is not to hasten or postpone death, but to ensure quality of life remaining. The hospice team is comprised of nurses, physicians, chaplains, social workers, and unlicensed assistive personnel working together to meet the client's and family's needs. Hospice does not provide housekeeping services, childcare, 24 hour sitters, or legal advice. However, hospices do have many resources for such services they can share with clients and families.

It's important for the client and family to understand that the health care proxy will make decisions for the client when and if the client can no longer make wishes known. These wishes should be according to the preferences for care the client outlines in the advance directive. Once the client dies, the services of the health care proxy are complete. To elect hospice, the client's physician and medical director of hospice must agree that the client has a life expectancy of 6 months or less if the terminal illness continues its course. However, as long as the client continues to meet hospice criteria, the client may re-elect hospice services and remain on hospice.

14. See explanation for answers

CORRECT: Attention to symptom management is a priority for the client. Both **pain and dyspnea must be addressed immediately** to ensure the client's quality of life.

INCORRECT: It is not unusual for a terminally ill client to have a poor appetite or no appetite. The client's urine becomes dark amber or brown as fluid intake decreases. The client with hepatic involvement will also have very dark yellow or brown urine. The client may be becoming constipated from opioid use and poor intake of fluids. The client will also need to defecate less frequently with decreased oral intake. The client has prescribed medications that can be taken for constipation. The appearance of the chest drainage is expected, and the nurse would expect lower extremity edema with liver involvement and ascites. The client's temperature can be addressed, but is not a priority.

15. The answer is 2

CORRECT: The priority of care is **symptom management**. Pain that is not well-controlled is more difficult to treat and increases anxiety, agitation, and dyspnea. The client has orders for a **breakthrough pain medication**, which **should be administered immediately**. The nurse needs to address the spouse's misconceptions about the pain medication causing the client to stop breathing.

INCORRECT: Hospice care can be provided in the home. The client is not transported to the hospital unless symptoms cannot be adequately managed in the home and the hospice admits the client for treatment, or the client revokes hospice. The client specified no IV fluids and no enteral feedings in the advance directive. The sibling's concern and distress needs to be addressed by the nurse and possibly the social worker and chaplain. This is not the immediate concern.

16. See explanation for answers

Increasing pain: **Opiates are the medication of choice** for the control of pain and dyspnea, which are common symptoms in the dying process. **Proactive regimens** to prevent symptoms should be used. The client's **scheduled opiate dose should be increased**. Then, the client should receive breakthrough pain medication as needed for any pain exacerbations. If this regimen does not control pain, then a different medication, dosing schedule, or adjunctive medications should be tried. Nonpharmacologic pain management techniques should also be used. Mild pain is easier to control, therefore the client should receive medication before pain intensity becomes moderate to severe. Only if these measures did not control the client's pain should the client be moved back to the hospital for pain control. Beginning IV pain medication can occur in the home for this client with an implanted VAD.

Worsening dyspnea: **Liquid morphine sulfate is an excellent medication used for breakthrough pain and for dyspnea**. Administration of PO or sublingual liquid morphine sulfate provides relief of these symptoms within a few minutes. Administering high-flow oxygen will likely not improve the client's dyspnea, which is due to a combination of ascites and malignant pleural effusion. The client's dyspnea is not due to secretions occluding the airway; only occasional oral suction is used in hospice to clear the airway.

Family's acceptance: The client's family will **need a great deal of education and reassurance** to deal with the frightening symptoms, including education on how to provide care for the client in the home. Pamphlets and reading material can be helpful, but the nurse must first explore the family's concerns, fears, and questions. Telling the family that death is inevitable may be true, but does not address their concerns or ability to accept the client's prognosis.

17. The answer is 3, 4, 5, and 8

CORRECT: The family should be educated about hospice care and provided with contact information so that they can call with any questions or concerns. If the client dies or **appears to have died or had a change in condition, the family is encouraged to call hospice**. A **hospice registered nurse pronounces the client's death** in the the home and communicates with the medical director and funeral home. It is **not unusual for a client who has been minimally responsive to become more responsive and animated** for a short time as death approaches. **As swallowing function diminishes, medications are typically administered sublingually, transdermally, or via rectal suppository.**

Temperature can fluctuate prior to death. The client may spike an extremely high temperature and may also become very cold to touch as death approaches.

INCORRECT: Incontinence of urine and stool is expected as the client approaches death. The client can be diapered or the bed padded. The client does not have to be catheterized. Breathing may become very noisy and the client may even develop gurgling respirations, which can be very distressing for the family. Positioning the client to the side with the head of bed elevated can help. The client frequently has periods of apnea and gasping at the end of life. Dark urine is another expected finding and is due to the decreased oral intake, as well as the diminishing kidney function. It does not indicate infection has occurred. When a client under hospice care dies at home, neither the police nor emergency medical services (EMS) needs to be notified.

18. See explanation for answers

Expected: Periods of **increased alertness**, **gurgling respirations**, **decreased responsiveness immediately preceding death**, **mottling**, **fever**, **periods of apnea**, and incontinence are expected as death draws near.

Not Expected: The client is not expected to report **thirst** or hunger. Clients typically do not request **IV fluids**. Family members and caretakers are more likely to request aggressive treatment of symptoms because they are distressing to observe.

19. The answer is 4

The nurse cares for a client diagnosed with alcohol abuse who reports having the last drink yesterday. The client exhibits tremors, diaphoresis, and tachycardia. Based on the current data, which action does the nurse implement **first**?

Category: Chemical and other dependencies

(1) The nurse might call the health care provider at some point to report unmanageable symptoms, but hydromorphone is for pain and not for management of alcohol withdrawal.

(2) The nurse might assess the client every hour, but it is not the first thing the nurse would do. The nurse needs to intervene to prevent acute withdrawal.

(3) The nurse would not call the family unless the nurse had permission of the client, and would not give meperidine for withdrawal; it is for pain.

(4) CORRECT: Benzodiazepines such as lorazepam are often given as part of an alcohol withdrawal pathway; this client is clearly beginning to exhibit symptoms of withdrawal (tremors, diaphoresis, and an elevated heart rate).

20. The answer is 2

A client with post-traumatic stress disorder (PTSD) appears to be experiencing a flashback. It is **most** appropriate for the nurse to perform which intervention?

Category: Crisis intervention

(1) The client is in crisis mode. Encouraging the client to verbalize feelings is not going to bring the client back to reality.

(2) CORRECT: The nurse wants to calmly orient the client back to the reality of the moment, to the actual safe environment.

(3) Assisting the client in acting out the event is not an appropriate intervention. The nurse wants to encourage the client back to reality and not go further into the flashback.

(4) Although the nurse wants to orient the client to reality, this would not be done firmly. This could possibly cause more hostility or violence if the client feels a sense of heightened danger.

21. The answer is 1

An older adult client asks the nurse to kill the bugs that are crawling on the floor of the room. The nurse does not see any bugs and suspects the client is hallucinating. Which statement by the nurse to the client is **most** appropriate?

Category: Sensory/perceptual alterations

(1) CORRECT: This response validates what the client is seeing. To the client, a hallucination is real. However, the nurse must reorient the client to the appropriate reality and try to restore the client's feelings of safety.

(2) The nurse should not reinforce the hallucination.

(3) The nurse should not encourage verbalizing feelings during an active hallucination.

(4) It is not helpful to question or imply that the client is not seeing real bugs.

22. The answer is 3

The nurse provides care to a client who has experienced a depressed mood, decreased sleep, poor concentration, and poor appetite for the past 4 months. The nurse anticipates that the provider will prescribe which medication?

Category: Mental health concepts

(1) Quetiapine is not typically given for depression symptoms. It is usually given for bipolar disorder.

(2) Haloperidol is given for symptoms of schizophrenia, not depression.

(3) CORRECT: Mirtazapine is typically prescribed for depression.

(4) Clonazepam is more typically given for panic disorders.

23. The answer is 2

The nurse provides care to a client who experiences a manic episode. It is **most** appropriate for the nurse to perform which intervention for this client?

Category: Coping mechanisms

(1) Manic energy does not lend itself well to the patience and organization needed for a collage.

(2) CORRECT: The exercise bike would allow an outlet for the client's excessive energy.

(3) During the manic phase, clients do not have the patience to sit in a group and discuss feelings. This is not an appropriate intervention.

(4) During the manic phase, clients do not have the patience play a board game. This is not an appropriate intervention.

24. The answer is 4

A client diagnosed with bipolar disorder makes a sexually inappropriate comment to the nurse. The nurse should take which action?

Category: Mental health concepts; Behavioral interventions

(1) Clients have to be accountable for their own actions even if they have bipolar disorder. It is important to correct inappropriate behavior, and to encourage clients to interact socially in an acceptable way.

(2) The nurse's priority is to first communicate with the client; the nurse might want to report the incident to the nurse manager later.

(3) The nurse should not ignore the comment.

(4) CORRECT: The nurse should notify the client that this is inappropriate behavior and set up appropriate boundaries.

25. The answer is 1 and 2

The nurse cares for a hospice client who lives at home with an attentive spouse. The client's spouse quit work to care for the client. During the nurse's visit, the spouse expresses frustration and hostility toward the nurse. Which is an appropriate response by the nurse? **(Select all that apply.)**

Category: Support systems

(1) CORRECT: Verbalizing feelings is an appropriate intervention for family members suffering from caregiver role strain.

(2) CORRECT: Attending a support group is an appropriate intervention for family members suffering from caregiver role strain.

(3) It may not be possible or practical for the spouse to go back to work part time.

(4) Encouraging the spouse not to verbalize negative feelings interferes with natural expression and personal family conversations.

(5) Ignoring is not a therapeutic approach in communication.

26. The answer is 2

The nurse completes a health history for a client. The client has been taking lorazepam for 6 months. Which finding does the nurse anticipate when conducting the physical examination for this client?

Category: Chemical and other dependencies

(1) Excessive appetite is a possibility, but not the most likely.

(2) CORRECT: Clients can experience all types of side effects from benzodiazepines, but the most likely side effect from prolonged use is physical dependence.

(3) Suicidal ideation is a possibility, but not the most likely.

(4) Seizure activity is a withdrawal effect the nurse would monitor for if the client discontinued lorazepam abruptly.

27. The answer is 1

A client requires a blood transfusion. The client refuses based on religious beliefs. It is **most** appropriate for the nurse to take which action when providing care to this client?

Category: Religious and spiritual influences on health

(1) CORRECT: The nurse must be sure the client understands the potential risks of not receiving the transfusion.

(2) Clients do have the right to refuse care on religious grounds.

(3) Although the nurse may call the legal department at some future time, this would not be the first course of action in this situation.

(4) The nurse must be sure that the client comprehends the choice they are making, including risks and benefits. However, the nurse does not want to coerce the client into changing their mind.

28. The answer is 3

The nurse works in a day program for clients with disabilities. The nurse notes that an adolescent client is frequently alone and often quiet. It is **most** appropriate for the nurse to take which action when providing care for this client?

Category: Support systems

(1) It appears that the client has enough alone time, which could stunt the client's social growth. It could also defeat the purpose of a day program, which is to promote interaction among clients.

(2) Making an effort to interact with the client periodically does not lead to the client's personal growth. Therefore, it is not the best option.

(3) CORRECT: Participating in a youth group can help a teenage client with a disability develop social skills, use support systems, and feel more like a typical teenager.

(4) It would not be appropriate to talk about one client with other clients, for reasons of confidentiality and privacy.

29. The answer is 3

The nurse discovers a hospice client has expired. The family members are regrouping in the facility's waiting room. Which action by the nurse is **most** appropriate?

Category: Grief and loss

(1) It is not the nurse's decision whether a family wants to view a body or not. This is a paternalistic attitude to be avoided in this setting.

(2) The nurse should react to that particular family's needs or wishes, and not encourage or discourage in either direction.

(3) CORRECT: The nurse acknowledges the loss, expresses sympathy, and offers the viewing opportunity.

(4) This statement assumes the family wants to view the body without the nurse inquiring first.

30. The answer is 1

During the admission process, the nurse inquires about advance directives from the client. The client tells the nurse, "I do not want to make any medical decisions. I want my daughter to make these decisions for me." Which action does the nurse implement based on the current situation?

Category: Family dynamics

(1) CORRECT: As long as the client is not pressured into this decision and the nurse believes that it is being made of the client's free will, it is acceptable for the daughter to take over medical decision making for the ill parent.

(2) The client is entitled to have the daughter make the medical decisions for the client, if that is what the client wishes to do.

(3) The client is entitled to allow the daughter to be informed of the details of the client's care.

(4) The client is entitled to have the daughter make the medical decisions for the client, and the nurse should not encourage the client to do otherwise.

[CHAPTER 8]

PHYSIOLOGICAL INTEGRITY: BASIC CARE AND COMFORT

Providing basic care and comfort for your clients is one of your most important roles. Ensuring that your clients have adequate nutrition and hydration, personal hygiene, and rest and sleep, and that their elimination needs are being properly attended to, are important priorities. Being able to help your clients with nonpharmacological comfort interventions, mobility issues, and assistive devices is also part of providing them with basic care and comfort.

On the NCLEX-RN® exam, approximately 9 percent of the questions will relate to Basic Care and Comfort. Exam content related to this subcategory includes, but is not limited to, the following topics:

- Assistive devices
- Complementary therapies
- Elimination
- Mobility/immobility
- Nonpharmacological comfort interventions
- Nutrition and oral hydration
- Personal hygiene
- Rest and sleep

Let's now review the most important concepts covered by these subtopics on the NCLEX-RN® exam.

Assistive Devices

It is important to assess your clients for communication, speech, vision, and hearing issues, and help them learn how to compensate for deficits by using appropriate strengthening exercises, assistive devices, positioning, and/or other compensatory techniques. You will help clients select and learn how to use appropriate assistive devices, such as crutches, walkers, canes, hearing aids, and prosthetics, and evaluate whether the client is using them correctly.

Being able to communicate with clients who have visual and auditory deficits is also important. The following summarizes some techniques that you can employ.

Communicating with the Client with Visual Deficits

- Announce yourself and say your name when entering a client room.
- Stay in the client's field of vision, if possible.

- Use a warm, pleasant speaking voice; do not speak loudly.
- Explain procedures before starting them.
- Announce when you are leaving the room.

Communicating with the Client with Auditory Deficits

- Move where you can be seen by the client, or touch the client gently so the client knows where you are standing, before starting a conversation.
- Keep background noise to a minimum.
- Speak in a normal voice; do not shout.
- Look at the client when speaking so they can see your face/mouth for lip reading.
- Mime, write, or spell words, if needed.
- Pronounce words carefully.
- When changing the subject, slow down or use key words to indicate the change.

Complementary Therapies

Many Americans use health care approaches developed outside of conventional medicine. These approaches are referred to as "alternative" and/or "complementary" therapies. Although the two terms are often used interchangeably, they refer to different concepts. The National Center for Complementary and Integrative Health (NCCIH), a division of the National Institutes of Health (NIH), defines *complementary therapies* as nonmainstream practices used together with conventional medicine. *Alternative therapies* are defined as practices used in place of conventional medicine. True alternative medicine is uncommon. Most people who use nonmainstream approaches use them along with conventional treatments. The NCCIH uses the term *integrative health* to refer to the incorporation of complementary approaches into mainstream health care.

Researchers are currently exploring the potential benefits of integrative health in a variety of situations. Integrative health modalities have been shown to help patients manage their symptoms (from cancer, persistent pain, chronic fatigue, fibromyalgia, and many other conditions) and improve their quality of life.

Recent studies through the U.S. Centers for Disease Control and Prevention (CDC) suggest that as many as 38 percent of residents in the United States seek out complementary therapies. Examples of complementary therapies include but are not limited to acupuncture, aromatherapy, biofeedback, energy healing therapy (Reiki), special diets, and dietary supplements other than vitamins and minerals. The treatments promoted in integrative health are not substitutes for conventional medical care. They should be used in concert with conventional medicine. Certain therapies and products are not recommended at all or not recommended for certain conditions or people.

It is important that the nurse discuss with the patient any potential or ongoing use of complementary therapies to prevent adverse effects caused by interactions with mainstream therapies. For example, some supplements, such as ginkgo biloba, can increase the risk of bleeding or interact with traditional medications. Some patients who used dietary supplements as complementary therapies have reported hot flashes and/or gastric disturbances (nausea, constipation, etc.). In procedures in which the skin is pierced, such as acupuncture, infections may occur. More needs to be learned about the physiological effects, safety, and potential drug interactions of complementary therapies.

Elimination

Clients' elimination needs are important to their basic care and comfort, as well to as their health. You need to provide appropriate interventions for a client who has an alteration in elimination.

Urinary Issues

One of the most common urinary problems is a urinary tract infection (UTI).

Lower Urinary Tract Issues

- Urethritis, inflammation of urethra
- Cystitis, inflammation of the bladder
- Prostatitis, inflammation of the prostate

Upper Urinary Tract Issues

- Pyelonephritis, inflammation of the pelvis and parenchyma
- Incontinence
  - Stress
  - Reflex
  - Urge
  - Functional

Other Urinary Issues

- Urgency
- Pain or difficulty (dysuria)
- Frequency
- Hesitancy
- Polyuria (large volume at one time)
- Nocturia (excessive at night, interrupting sleep)
- Hematuria (red blood cells in urine)
- Retention

Be familiar with common urinary tests, including the bladder scan at the bedside. It is also important to teach clients how to maintain a healthy urinary tract—provide information and instruction about adequate hydration (1,500 to 2,000 mL/day), emptying the bladder completely, the impact of caffeine and alcohol, proper personal hygiene, and Kegel exercises. In addition, teach clients to recognize the signs of a UTI.

Foley catheters are used to drain urine. Catheters can cause infection, so it is highly important to use proper sterile techniques when inserting, maintaining, and removing them. You should also know how to perform irrigations of the bladder, eyes, and ears.

Bowel Issues

Be able to recognize potential bowel issues based on the age and health of a client. Common bowel problems include constipation (hard, dry stools that are difficult to pass), impaction (an accumulated mass of stool that cannot be passed), diarrhea (frequent passage of unformed/liquid stool), incontinence (inability to retain urine or stool), flatulence, and hemorrhoids. Bowel problems are diagnosed by abdominal x-ray, upper gastrointestinal (GI) barium test, barium enema, and upper (oral) and lower (rectal) endoscopy.

Treatments include the following:

- **Constipation:** Increase fluid intake, including hot liquids and fruit juices; advise a high-fiber diet.
- **Diarrhea:** Understand and treat underlying cause (which may be a virus, reaction to certain foods or medications, GI tract infection, etc.); typically, advise bland foods and a low-fiber diet, as well as to avoid spicy foods, alcohol, and caffeine while symptoms continue.
- **Flatulence:** Limit gum, carbonated beverages, cabbage, cauliflower, beans, and onions.

Care for ostomies (a surgically created opening in the abdominal wall through which feces can pass) is also an important part of basic care and comfort. Types and locations are as follows:

- **Ileostomy:** An opening into the distal end of the small intestine
- **Colostomy:** An opening into the colon

Ostomy care includes regularly assessing the condition of the stoma (the opening), making sure the skin around the stoma is clean and dry, and teaching the client how to care for the ostomy, including proper diet, fluid intake, and hygiene, and how to remove a food blockage.

It is also important to use proper skin care for clients who are incontinent, including the use of barrier creams and ointments. You should also be able to evaluate whether client elimination is restored to normal and whether it's maintained.

Mobility/Immobility

It is a nurse's responsibility to assess a client's mobility, gait, strength, motor skills, and use of assistive devices. You should be able to identify common causes of immobility, and complications associated with each. The main causes are:

- Pain
- Motor/nervous system impairment
- Functional problems
- Generalized weakness
- Psychological problems
- Side effect of medication

Complications of immobility can be physiological and/or psychological in nature. Physical complications can include:

- Atrophy, joint contracture
- Disuse osteoporosis

- Pressure ulcers
- Orthostatic hypotension
- Deep vein thrombosis
- Pneumonia and pulmonary embolisms
- Decreased peristalsis, constipation
- Kidney stones

Psychological complications can include body image issues, lack of social interaction, sensory deprivation, and depression.

Interventions should be implemented to counteract physiological and psychological complications. Active and passive range of motion exercises, positioning, and mobilization can be used to promote circulation. Turning, repositioning, and pressure-relieving support surfaces can be used to maintain skin integrity and prevent skin breakdown. Anti-embolic stockings and sequential compression devices can be used to promote venous return.

It is also important to know when orthopedic and assistive devices, such as crutches, walkers, canes, splints, traction, braces, or casts, are needed; you should be able to teach the client how to use them properly to maintain correct body alignment.

Nonpharmacological Comfort Interventions

It is important to be able to apply your knowledge of client pathophysiology to nonpharmacological interventions. Assess the client's need for pain management and implement comfort measures, as needed.

Therapies for comfort and treatment of inflammation/swelling can include heat, cold, or elevation of limbs. Use the pain scale and verbal reports to assess the effectiveness of the intervention.

Palliative Care

Nurses have an important role to play in palliative care, particularly in relation to pain and symptom management and the coordination of care. Assess a client's need for palliative care and provide counseling, as needed. Call in specialists from other disciplines, including doctors, psychologists, social workers, and clergy, as appropriate.

You should be able determine whether interventions are working and whether they are meeting the client's goals. The client's care may include pain management to improve comfort and quality of life, but may exclude painful treatments or heroic interventions.

You must respect a client's palliative care choices, and review those choices with the client periodically because they may change during the course of a client's disease. Assisting a client in receiving appropriate end-of-life symptom management, particularly as the client enters the active dying phase, is also important.

Nutrition and Oral Hydration

It is important to know the principles of nutrition, such as the basic food groups, their functions, and which foods fall within those groups. These include:

- **Carbohydrates:** Are converted to glucose, which the body uses for energy. Sources of carbohydrates include grain products (bread, pasta, and rice), fruits, milk, and products with high sugar content.

- **Proteins:** Are used to build and repair body tissue, such as muscles, and also for many essential body processes, such as nutrient transport and muscle contraction. Sources of protein include meat, poultry, fish, eggs, nuts, beans, peas, and lentils.

- **Fats:** Are used to insulate the body, provide energy, and store certain vitamins such as A, D, E, and K, which are soluble in fats and insoluble in water. Sources of fat include whole milk and milk products, oils, nuts, and certain meats.

Be familiar with general dietary guidelines, key nutritional concepts across a client's life span, and types of diets appropriate for specific conditions, for example, which foods would be appropriate for a client with heart disease (foods with low fat and low cholesterol) or inappropriate (foods with high fat and high cholesterol). You should also be able to apply your knowledge of mathematics to nutrition, such as by performing body mass index (BMI) calculations.

You can use the following to assess a client's ability to eat:

- Documented history
  - From patient
  - Nutritional screening initiatives (NSIs)

- Anthropomorphic measures
  - Height, weight, and body size
  - BMI
  - Basal metabolic rate (BMR)
  - Distribution of body fat (obesity)

- Lab/diagnostic measures
  - Albumin levels
  - Total lymphocyte count (TLC)
  - Hemoglobin levels

- Ability to chew and swallow

Assess clients for specific food/medication interactions, and consider client choices regarding nutritional requirements and dietary restrictions. Also monitor client hydration status. For example, be familiar with the signs and symptoms of both edema (excess fluid) and dehydration.

For clients unable to eat on their own, nutrition can be provided through continuous or intermittent tube feedings. This includes nasogastric, enterostomy (surgical), or percutaneous tubes. You should know how to maintain the tube insertion site, monitor it for infection and proper function, as well as ensure that the proper volume of formula is getting through. You should also recognize mechanical or metabolic problems and intervene, as needed. These include:

- Formula selection
- Formula adjustment
- Skin irritation
- Clogging
- Aspiration

Monitor the client's underlying condition to ensure the right dietary/feeding choices are made. Factors you must monitor include weight, protein measures, TLC, blood urea nitrogen (BUN), and creatinine levels, making adjustments as needed.

Personal Hygiene

It is important to assess your clients' personal hygiene and assist them in performance of both activities of daily living (ADLs) and instrumental activities of daily living (IADLs). Provide information on adaptations, such as shower chairs and hand rails.

Personal hygiene topics to know include care of skin, eyes, ears, nose, mouth, feet, nails, hair and scalp, perineal area, and prostheses. Care of the skin is particularly important. Know the measures to keep skin clean and moist, and how to prevent pressure points. Keeping skin clean can help prevent skin breakdowns and infections.

You should also know how to perform post-mortem care. After the patient is pronounced dead, nurses prepare the body for viewing by the family and transport to the morgue or funeral home. Family members should be given the option of seeing their loved one before or after post-mortem care is provided, or not at all, if that is their choice.

Rest and Sleep

It is important to know the physiology of sleep, the phases, normal sleep patterns, and how sleep differs at each developmental stage. Your knowledge of each client's pathophysiology will help you to provide the appropriate interventions, which could include the following:

- Keeping the environment conducive to quiet relaxation
- Promoting bedtime routines
- Promoting comfort
- Avoiding heavy meals before bedtime
- Promoting appropriate activity
- Providing pharmaceutical aids (sedatives or hypnotics) as needed

Chapter Quiz

1. The nurse performs dressing changes for a pediatric client with burns over 20% of the body. The client appears disoriented, has a fever of 101° F (38.3° C), and is crying in pain. Which nursing intervention would be the **most** appropriate in caring for this client?

   1. Gather equipment for the dressing change and explain the procedure to the child.
   2. Do a complete physical assessment and notify the provider of the findings.
   3. Administer appropriate analgesics and gather equipment for the dressing change.
   4. Offer the child an enticing distraction from pain, such as a video, music, or toy.

2. The nurse cares for a pediatric client a few hours after a tonsillectomy. Which nursing intervention is appropriate to promote adequate nutrition and oral hydration?

   1. Offer the child warm soup, watch for signs of bleeding, and suction vigorously to remove old blood.
   2. Offer ice chips; advance to cool, clear liquids; and suction gently to remove oral secretions as needed.
   3. Maintain the intravenous fluids appropriate for the child's weight for the next 24 hours and keep the child NPO.
   4. Offer soft, warm foods so the child will not be hungry; orange juice to provide vitamin C; and milk shakes for calories.

3. The nurse cares for a pediatric client who had an adenoidectomy and tonsillectomy 10 hours ago. The parents are in the room and prepare the child for bedtime. Which nursing intervention would be helpful to promote rest and sleep for this client?

   1. Provide a cool water rinse, adjust the head of the bed to a 30–45-degree angle, and offer an ice collar for discomfort.
   2. Encourage the parents to leave so the child can sleep.
   3. Suction the mouth vigorously before the child falls asleep.
   4. Offer an ice collar for discomfort, and assist the child in finding a position of comfort while promoting a patent airway.

4. The nurse cares for an adult client who is less than 24 hours post-op. In shift report, the nurse learns that the client rings the call light frequently, is anxious, and has been given pain medication as prescribed. Which intervention should the nurse include when caring for this client?

   1. Assure the client that anxiety is understandable, because the pain medication needs time to take effect.
   2. Assess other clients first, giving this client time to relax before evaluating the level of pain.
   3. Call the client's health care provider to increase the amount or frequency of pain medications prescribed.
   4. Provide a quiet environment, offer repositioning, straighten the bed linens, offer fluids, and assess the pain level.

5. The nurse cares for an adult client with bilateral leg fractures. The client has a long leg cast on the right lower extremity as well as traction applied to the left femur. Which is the main purpose served by the cast for this client?

1. Immobilizes the tibia and fibula and corrects deformities.
2. Keeps the client, who is in traction, more comfortable.
3. Immobilizes the pelvic bones for better healing.
4. Encircles the trunk and stabilizes the spine.

Refer to the Case Study to answer the next question.

The nurse in the orthopedic clinic is caring for an adult client following surgery to repair a fractured left ankle.

Client History	Nurse's Notes

Client is a well-developed, well-nourished adult who tripped while coming downstairs in the home. The client landed heavily on the left ankle and foot and experienced immediate pain and swelling. X-rays completed in the Emergency Department showed the client sustained a minimally displaced transverse fracture extending through the distal aspect of the left fibula with adjacent soft tissue swelling. The following morning, the client was taken to surgery for internal fixation of the joint.

The client was discharged home in a splint with instructions to be totally non-weight-bearing on the left foot. The client received a set of crutches and instructions from physical therapy prior to discharge. Return to orthopedic surgeon in 2 weeks for removal of sutures, x-rays, and casting of the left foot.

Client History	Nurse's Notes

Clinic Visit: 2 Weeks Postoperative

The client comes to the clinic today for suture removal and postoperative evaluation of left ankle. Client is accompanied by spouse. The client has been able to use the crutches to ambulate around the home and reports that pain has been well controlled with the pain medication. The client is wearing the splint on the left foot. The splint is clean and dry. The spouse states the client is elevating the foot and using ice when sitting down. Noted the client's crutch pads are placed directly against the axillae and the client leans on the crutches for balance when standing. The client is putting total body weight on the crutches in the axillae while ambulating from the waiting room to the examination room. Inspection reveals the client's axillae are reddened bilaterally.

Asked client if these are the crutches sent home at the time of discharge. The client states, "I have been using some crutches that belonged to my sibling. I didn't like using the ones that I brought home from the hospital. I like the hand grips on these better." The client asks how much longer the crutches will have to be used. The client reports, "They really hurt my armpits and make my hands tingle."

6. The nurse reviews the client's history and documents an assessment at the beginning of the visit.

Complete the diagram by choosing from the choices below to specify for which condition the client is at greatest risk, 2 instructions the nurse provides to address that condition, and 2 actions the nurse takes to verify the client understands the teaching provided.

Instruction to Provide		Action to Verify Understanding
Instruction to Provide	**Condition Most Likely Experiencing**	Action to Verify Understanding

Instructions to Provide	Potential Conditions	Actions to Verify Understanding
"The crutch pads should fit snugly into your axillae when you are standing with the crutches immediately to the side and in front of your feet."	Impaired wound healing.	Have the client demonstrate the proper way to use crutches to walk.
"Avoid leaning on your crutches to support your body weight and keep the affected foot off of the ground."	Radial nerve palsy.	Tell the spouse to frequently remind the client about the appropriate way to use the crutches.
"Use only the crutches which were measured for you by a therapist."	Fall with injury.	Ask the client, "Do you understand why you only use crutches fitted for you?"
"When using the crutches to ambulate, your arms should be perfectly straight."	Nonunion of fracture.	Instruct the client to avoid using crutches and purchase a standard walker.
"Your weight should be equally distributed in your hands and affected foot when using the crutches."		Check the distance between the crutch pads and axillae during the next visit.

7. The nurse cares for an client who has shortness of breath, cough, and pleural effusion. The provider asks the nurse to assist in the placement of a therapeutic and diagnostic thoracentesis. Which intervention should the nurse perform to assist this client?

   1. Make certain the consent is signed, witnessed, and filed in the electronic health record.
   2. Offer the client oral fluids as needed during the procedure.
   3. Help the client to lie flat with a pillow under the feet.
   4. Help the client to sit up and place arms over a bedside table, encouraging to remain still during the procedure.

8. The nurse cares for a newborn who is scheduled for circumcision. Which nonpharmacologic interventions should the nurse teach the parents to keep this client comfortable while the circumcision heals?

   1. Fasten the diaper tightly to avoid having it move around the wound.
   2. Apply petroleum jelly to gauze and place over the end of the penis.
   3. Offer feedings more often to soothe the newborn who is in pain.
   4. Wash the end of the penis vigorously to prevent infection.

9. The nurse cares for a quadriplegic client who is diagnosed with a C2-C3 fracture. Which measure does the nurse implement to keep the client comfortable, meet elimination needs, and prevent common causes of autonomic dysreflexia?

   1. Turn the client at least every 2 hours to prevent pressure injury on bony areas.
   2. Allow the client to sleep 8–10 hours without interruption each night to promote rest.
   3. Offer appetizing fluids every 2 hours during the day to promote hydration.
   4. Straight catheterize the client to prevent bladder distention and prevent bowel impaction.

10. The nurse cares for a pediatric client after an open reduction of the radius and ulna of the right arm. The client is now immobilized in a plaster cast splint reinforced with an Ace wrap. Which non-pharmacological nursing interventions will promote comfort for this client?

    1. Apply a heat pack to the approximate area of the surgical incision.
    2. Position the child so the cast is flat on the mattress for firm support.
    3. Elevate the cast on a pillow and apply an ice pack to the approximate area of the surgical incision.
    4. Do not move any part of the child's arm until the health care provider prescribes a specific position.

11. The nurse cares for an older client who is diagnosed with left-sided heart failure. Which nursing interventions reduce the workload of the heart and promote comfort and rest? **(Select all that apply).**

    1. Assist the client on short walks at least 2 times per shift to increase circulation.
    2. Raise the head of the bed to increase the reserve of the heart and to decrease the work of breathing.
    3. Offer the client stress-reduction strategies, such as mindfulness and meditation.
    4. Allow the client to lie flat to sleep and provide 2 liters oxygen via nasal cannula.
    5. Help the client walk to the bathroom rather than using a bedside commode.

12. The nurse teaches a client on the proper use of crutches. The client requires non-weight-bearing ambulation for 4–6 weeks. Which of these crutch gaits should the nurse teach this client for safe ambulation?

    1. The two-point gait.
    2. The three-point gait.
    3. The four-point gait.
    4. Swing-through gait.

13. The nurse finds a client in the bathroom reporting severe constipation. Which of these would be the appropriate order of nursing interventions to address the client's immediate elimination needs? **All options must be used.**

    1. Offer oral fluids to ease the constipation.

    2. Notify the provider.

    3. Offer PRN medications orally, if prescribed.

    4. Use a gloved hand with lubricant to manually assess for fecal impaction and to stimulate the rectal wall to loosen the fecal matter.

14. The nurse cares for a client who has recently had a vesicostomy. Which intervention should the nurse perform to assist this client with basic comfort and elimination?

    1. Apply an absorbent diaper or incontinence pads and dilate the opening once or twice a day as prescribed by the provider.

    2. Double-diapering the area is the only intervention needed.

    3. Apply a urine bag and change it daily.

    4. Double-diaper the area after applying a urine bag.

15. A client who has chronic pain asks the nurse about alternative therapies in conjunction with traditional treatment. Which form of alternative therapy could the nurse provide for this client?

    1. Music therapy or guided imagery.

    2. Acupuncture.

    3. Kegel exercises.

    4. None, nurses do not provide alternative treatments.

16. The nurse cares for an adult client with a fractured femur who must be maintained in traction for several days before surgical interventions can take place. The client has several abrasions, dirty hair, and healing wounds in the mouth. Which action should the nurse perform to address the personal hygiene needs of this client?

    1. Place everything within reach so the client can bathe unassisted.

    2. Assist with a bed bath, oral hygiene, and wash hair with a non-shampoo product for bed-bound clients.

    3. Allow a family member to bathe the client with the supervision of the nurse.

    4. Offer an oral rinse for hygiene, but postpone the bath until a later time due to the traction.

17. The nurse cares for an adult client with a long-bone fracture. The nurse encourages the client to move fingers and toes hourly, to change positions slightly every hour, and to eat high-iron foods as part of a balanced diet. Which of these foods or beverages should the nurse advise the client to avoid while on bed rest?

    1. Fresh-squeezed fruit juices.

    2. Large amounts of milk or milk products.

    3. Cranberry juice cocktail.

    4. No need to avoid any foods while on bed rest.

18. The nurse teaches personal hygiene to client with type 1 diabetes mellitus (DM). Which topics would be **most** appropriate for the nurse to teach this client?

    1. Dental care is not a top priority among clients with DM because it is not covered by insurance.
    2. Hair and nail care is the priority in the personal hygiene for clients with DM.
    3. Client with DM should keep skin clean and dry, especially the feet and in between toes.
    4. Personal hygiene is not included in diabetic teaching because it is an individual choice.

19. The nurse cares for a pediatric client in the ambulatory care clinic. The parents report a 24-hour period of gastrointestinal distress, including vomiting several times and 3 watery stools. Which action does the nurse perform to assist in maintaining nutrition for this client?

    1. Educate the parents on the signs of dehydration and the slow introduction of fluids to rehydrate the child.
    2. Offer no advice to the parents other than to suggest parents offer whatever foods the child feels like taking.
    3. Encourage the parents to offer the child milk products for the vitamins and rehydration.
    4. Encourage the parents to offer solid foods to improve the nutritional status quickly.

Refer to the Case Study to answer the next six questions.

The nurse is providing care in the home to an older adult client who has Parkinson disease (PD).

Nurse's Notes

The client is referred to home health services by a health care provider who evaluated progressive motor symptoms and mild changes in memory and thinking related to the client's PD. The spouse reports the client is encountering more difficulty with everyday activities, such as dressing and bathing, and is generally less active. The client is more limited in mobility and is having increased problems with coordination and balance. The client is sitting or lying for prolonged periods and forgets to move or cannot easily initiate a change in position. Additionally, the client is experiencing decreasing appetite with occasional episodes of dysphagia.

Assessment	Client Finding
General	Frail appearing.
	Face lacks expression.
	Slow monotone speech.
Neurological	Tremor at rest in right hand and forearm.
	Poor balance and gait coordination.
Integument	Skin, pink, warm, and dry.
	Right sacrum, 3 × 3 cm partial thickness skin loss with exposed dermis visible; pink, moist wound bed, without slough or granulation tissue.
	Right heel, intact skin with area of nonblanchable erythema.
Cardiovascular	Apical rate 72, regular, no murmurs.
	2+ radial pulses, equal.
	Capillary refill less than 2 seconds.
	No pedal edema.
Respiratory	Chest expansion equal.
	Lung sounds clear bilaterally.
Abdomen	Soft, rounded, nontender.
	Normoactive bowel sounds.
Musculoskeletal	Resistance to movement of arms and legs in passive range of motion (PROM).
	Stooped forward posture.
	Shuffling gait with short steps.
	Muscle strength, 3/5 bilaterally.

Vital Signs/ BMI/ Braden Scale	Results
BP	118/78 mmHg
Heart rate	72, regular
Respiratory rate	16, regular
Temperature (oral)	97.6° F (36.44° C)
Pulse oximetry	97% on room air
Body Mass Index (BMI)	18 kg/m² (underweight)
Braden Score	14 (moderate risk)

20. The nurse performs an assessment and documents nurse's notes.

    The nurse is concerned with which of these client findings? **(Select all that apply.)**

    1. Dysphagia.
    2. BMI 18 kg/m².
    3. Rounded abdomen.
    4. Sacrum with partial thickness skin loss and exposed dermis.
    5. Capillary refill less than 2 seconds.
    6. Shuffling gait with short steps.
    7. Prolonged periods of sitting or lying.
    8. Right heel, intact skin with area of non-blanchable erythema.

21. Complete the following sentences by choosing from the list of options.

    The nurse interprets the client's sacral wound as consistent with a [Select from list 1]. The nurse documents the area on the client's right heel as a [Select from list 2]. In addition to limited mobility, the nurse understands another risk factor for the client to develop pressure injuries includes [Select from list 3].

(1)	(2)	(3)
stage 1 pressure injury	stage 1 pressure injury	inadequate nutrition
stage 2 pressure injury	stage 2 pressure injury	poor skin perfusion
deep tissue injury	deep tissue injury	inadequate oxygenation

22. The nurse considers that the client's pressure injuries increase the risk for developing which of these complications?

    1. Anemia.
    2. Dehiscence.
    3. Infection.
    4. Evisceration.

23. Drag the choices below to fill in each blank in the following sentence. Each choice will only be used once.

When developing the plan of care, the nurse includes goals to _____ [Select from the list], _____ [Select from the list], and _____ [Select from the list].

| teach risk factors for stroke |
| promote adequate nutrition |
| reduce infection risk |
| educate about plasma exchange |
| heal pressure injuries |

24. The nurse implements client care twice weekly for the next four weeks. Care includes frequent skin and nutritional assessments.

For each goal below, specify the potential nursing interventions that are appropriate for the care of the client. Each nursing goal may support more than 1 potential nursing intervention.

Nursing Goal	Potential Nursing Interventions
Reduce infection risk	☐ Use principles of asepsis during skin care. ☐ Monitor for purulent drainage and odor. ☐ Report a decrease in the leukocyte count. ☐ Monitor for changes in temperature, pulse and respiration.
Heal pressure injuries	☐ Teach semi reclining positioning in bed or chair. ☐ Encourage individualized repositioning schedule. ☐ Use pressure redistribution devices, such as mattress overlays and chair cushions. ☐ After cleaning sacral injury, keep wound bed uncovered and dry.
Promote adequate nutrition	☐ Recommend diet intake high in calories, nutrients, and extra protein. ☐ Monitor prealbumin and albumin levels. ☐ Promote calcium supplements for collagen production. ☐ Encourage smaller, frequent meals with foods that are easy to chew and swallow.

25. The nurse evaluates the client after 4 weeks. Select **4** client findings which indicate the client has improved.

1. Consumes 90% of meals, twice daily protein drinks, and a vitamin C supplement.
2. Skin cool, pale, and frequently diaphoretic.
3. Right heel, intact skin with no areas of nonblanchable erythema.
4. Right sacrum, 1 × 2 cm partial thickness skin loss; pink moist wound bed.
5. Frequently semi reclines or slides down in bed or chair.
6. Client states the importance of performing passive range of motion exercises.

26. The nurse cares for a client diagnosed with pancreatic cancer. Which information does the nurse include when providing education to this client about nutrition and hydration?

    1. Drink clear water, progress diet rapidly as tolerated, and weigh daily.

    2. Puree foods, choose low-protein and low carbohydrates foods, and weigh weekly.

    3. Take herbal therapies, avoid vitamins supplements, and monitor weight weekly.

    4. Eat cool foods, and eat small but frequent high-protein and high-carbohydrate meals.

27. The nurse cares for a client who is on long-term enteral nutrition. The nurse reviews the infusion procedure with the client's daughter. The nurse states which of these as the rationale for infusing the formula through the gastrostomy tube at room temperature?

    1. "The formula tastes better when infused at room temperature."

    2. "Formula at room temperature is least likely to cause gastric discomfort."

    3. "There is no need to bring the formula to room temperature."

    4. "Room-temperature prepared formula reduces the risk of aspiration."

28. The nurse cares for a client recovering from a knee injury. Ambulation is still difficult for the client, and the physical therapist has suggested the client use a cane. Which statement **best** explains the use of a cane rather than a walker for this client?

    1. "The cane is just a reminder to use good posture."

    2. "The cane can be more dangerous than helpful, and another type of assistive device should be considered for this client."

    3. "The cane will help with fatigue while assisting the client with balance and support."

    4. "A cane does not offer any relief on weight-bearing joints."

29. The nurse reviews the forms of traction and the purposes for each before gathering equipment prior to the child's arrival. Match the type of traction on the left with the type of injury or indication on the right. **All options must be used.**

1. Bryant traction

2. Russell traction

3. 90-degree traction

4. Buck's traction

5. Cervical traction

A. Stabilizes a spinal fracture or muscle spasm

B. Used on the femur if skin traction is not suitable

C. Temporarily immobilizes a fractured leg

D. May reduce fractures of the hip or femur

E. Used in children younger than age 2 to reduce femur fractures or stabilize hips

30. The nurse assesses pain in an infant using the chart below. Which would the pain score be for an infant with a high-pitched cry, O_2 saturation of 96%, a grimace, and frequent periods of wakefulness?

	Score		
	0	1	2
Crying	No	High-pitched	Inconsolable
Requires O_2	No	< 30%	> 30%
Expression	None	Grimace	Grimace/grunt
Sleepless	No	Wakes frequently	Always awake

1. Score of 0.
2. Score of 2.
3. Score of 3.
4. Score of 4.

Chapter Quiz Answers and Explanations

1. The answer is 2

The nurse performs dressing changes for a pediatric client with burns over 20% of the body. The client appears disoriented, has a fever of 101° F (38.3° C), and is crying in pain. Which nursing intervention would be the **most** appropriate in caring for this client?

Category: Nonpharmacological comfort interventions

(1) The nurse would gather equipment, but not before addressing the crying child.

(2) CORRECT: The child may be suffering from an infection. The nurse recognizes that disorientation and fever are the first signs of sepsis in burn clients. It would be most appropriate to assess for the causes of fever and pain and notify the provider before proceeding.

(3) Analgesics may be appropriate but not before assessing the pain and source of fever and disorientation.

(4) Distractions may be offered after the assessment but they do not take priority over notifying the provider regarding the findings about the source of fever and pain.

2. The answer is 2

The nurse cares for a pediatric client a few hours after a tonsillectomy. Which nursing intervention is appropriate to promote adequate nutrition and oral hydration?

Category: Nutrition and oral hydration

(1) Warm liquids may increase bleeding and should be avoided the first few hours after surgery.

(2) CORRECT: The child may first take ice chips 1–2 hours after awakening, followed by cool, clear liquids without pulp or ice pops. Gentle suctioning may be necessary to remove secretions in the mouth and to keep the child from gagging. Suctioning should be kept to a minimum to avoid traumatizing the oropharynx.

(3) The health care provider may maintain an intravenous infusion postoperatively, but it is not necessary to keep the child NPO after the surgery. Ice chips or cool, clear liquids are soothing.

(4) Soft foods are not given in the first few hours after surgery to prevent emesis. Orange juice is acidic, and juices offered to a postoperative child should be alkaline. Milk products are controversial because they coat the throat and may cause the child to cough.

3. The answer is 4

The nurse cares for a pediatric client who had an adenoidectomy and tonsillectomy 10 hours ago. The parents are in the room and prepare the child for bedtime. Which nursing intervention would be helpful to promote rest and sleep for this client?

Category: Rest and sleep

(1) Semi-Fowler may not be a position comfortable for some children, so other positions may need to be considered.

(2) The parents should be encouraged to stay with the child and to participate in the care and comfort of the child, if possible.

(3) Suctioning should not be vigorous after an adenoidectomy or a tonsillectomy.

(4) CORRECT: Assist the child in finding a position of comfort. This may be prone, semi-prone, or semi-Fowler. An ice collar and a cool oral rinse will also aid in comfort.

4. The answer is 4

The nurse cares for an adult client who is less than 24 hours post-op. In shift report, the nurse learns that the client rings the call light frequently, is anxious, and has been given pain medication as prescribed. Which intervention should the nurse include when caring for this client?

Category: Nonpharmacological comfort interventions

(1) The client will probably be more reassured if physical comfort measures are taken, rather than just verbal assurances.

(2) Prioritizing is necessary, but avoiding an already anxious client may cause the nurse to overlook a serious symptom.

(3) The nurse may call the provider, if needed, after offering basic comfort measures and conducting an assessment.

(4) CORRECT: Changing the client's position, removing wrinkles in the bed linen, helping the client to take a drink, or limiting noise can help the client to rest and may reduce pain.

5. The answer is 1

The nurse cares for an adult client with bilateral leg fractures. The client has a long leg cast on the right lower extremity as well as traction applied to the left femur. Which is the main purpose served by the cast for this client?

Category: Mobility/immobility

(1) CORRECT: A long leg cast serves to immobilize the tibia and fibula by being placed above and below the knee and ankle joints.

(2) A long leg cast is not used for comfort for a client in traction.

(3) A long leg cast does not immobilize the pelvis.

(4) A body cast, not a long leg cast, encircles the trunk.

6. See explanation for answers

Condition Most Likely Experiencing	
Radial nerve palsy.	☑

CORRECT OPTION: Leaning on the underarm supports and pads of the crutches to support body weight can result in **injury to the axillae and compression of blood vessels and nerves**. The result can be numbness, pain, and tingling in the hands and numbness and pain in the axillae. Significant brachial plexus injury and radial nerve compression can also occur.

INCORRECT OPTIONS: The description of the client's visit indicates the client is keeping the affected foot off of the ground, and keeping the splint clean and dry. If the client was using crutches with worn or damaged tips, or using crutches inappropriately on stairs or wet surfaces, the client would be at higher risk for a fall with injury. The client is at less risk for impaired wound healing or nonunion of the fracture.

Instructions to Provide	
"Avoid leaning on your crutches to support your body weight and keep the affected foot off of the ground."	☑
"Use only the crutches which were measured for you by a therapist."	☑

CORRECT OPTIONS: The client should be instructed to balance with weight on the nonoperative leg using the crutches for support. The client **should not place the total body weight on the crutches for support**. The client's **affected or operative limb should not make contact with the ground** if the client is non-weight bearing. **The client should also use only the crutches which were provided at the time of discharge from the facility. Those crutches would have been measured and adjusted to fit the client by physical therapy.** Other crutches may be too tall or too short for the client, leading to injury or a fall.

INCORRECT OPTIONS: When the crutches are measured for the client, the crutch pads should be 2–3 fingerbreadths, or 1–2 inches, below the client's axillae when the client is standing with the crutches approximately 2 inches lateral and 4–6 inches anterior of the client's shoes. The client's elbow should be flexed approximately 15–30 degrees. The weight should be distributed equally in the client's hands when the client is propelling forward until the unaffected leg is back on the ground.

Actions to Verify Understanding	
Have the client demonstrate the proper way to use crutches to walk.	✓
Check the distance between the crutch pads and axillae during the next visit.	✓

CORRECT OPTIONS: The most effective way to determine if a client understands teaching which has been provided is to have the **client demonstrate** what has been learned. For this client, showing the nurse how the crutches are being used during ambulation will either verify the client has understood instructions or alert the nurse that the client needs further education. If the crutches are properly fitted to the client, and the **crutch pads are 1–2 inches from the axillae** at the next visit, the nurse can also determine that the client is following the teaching provided.

INCORRECT OPTIONS: Telling the spouse to remind the client is not an effective way to determine if the client understands the education provided. Asking the client a "yes/no" question is also not an effective way to determine understanding. There is no reason for the client to stop using crutches if they are used correctly. For a client who is non-weight-bearing, a standard walker would not be recommended.

7. The answer is 4

The nurse cares for an client who has shortness of breath, cough, and pleural effusion. The provider asks the nurse to assist in the placement of a therapeutic and diagnostic thoracentesis. Which intervention should the nurse perform to assist this client?

Category: Nonpharmacological comfort interventions

(1) The nurse should make certain the consent is signed before the start of a procedure, but that does not affect the client's comfort.

(2) Fluids should not be offered right before a procedure to avoid nausea and vomiting if pain is experienced.

(3) Lying flat with feet elevated is not the position of choice for a thoracentesis.

(4) CORRECT: Placing the client in a sitting position over a bedside table is the most comfortable and allows the best opportunity to remove fluid at the base of the chest

8. The answer is 2

The nurse cares for a newborn who is scheduled for circumcision. Which nonpharmacologic interventions should the nurse teach the parents to keep this client comfortable while the circumcision heals?

Category: Nonpharmacological comfort interventions

(1) Leaving the diaper slightly loose when fastening will be more comfortable.

(2) CORRECT: Petroleum jelly offers lubrication and helps stop the friction of the diaper over the raw area. The diaper should be left loosely fastened.

(3) Offering feedings more often than necessary may cause emesis and is not the best way to soothe a newborn.

(4) The end of the penis has a yellow exudate that is part of the healing process and should not be vigorously washed off. It will disappear with healing.

9. The answer is 4

The nurse cares for a quadriplegic client who is diagnosed with a C2-C3 fracture. Which measure does the nurse implement to keep the client comfortable, meet elimination needs, and prevent common causes of autonomic dysreflexia?

Category: Elimination

(1) Turning is necessary to prevent pressure injury and promote comfort, but it does not necessarily prevent an increase in blood pressure as seen with autonomic dysreflexia.

(2) Sleeping 8–10 hours is not related to autonomic dysreflexia.

(3) Offering fluids is a nursing measure but may not be related to autonomic dysreflexia because a client with a spinal cord injury may have a fluid restriction to help control blood pressure.

(4) CORRECT: Bladder distension and bowel impaction can result in autonomic dysreflexia, causing a critical increase in blood pressure.

10. The answer is 3

The nurse cares for a pediatric client after an open reduction of the radius and ulna of the right arm. The client is now immobilized in a plaster cast splint reinforced with an Ace wrap. Which nonpharmacological nursing interventions will promote comfort for this client?

Category: Nonpharmacological comfort interventions; Mobility/immobility

(1) Heat would not be appropriate, because it could cause, rather than reduce, swelling.

(2) The cast should be elevated for the first 24–48 hours and not be left flat on the mattress.

(3) CORRECT: Elevating the extremity and applying an ice pack will help to reduce swelling and may reduce pain. Repositioning is a comfort intervention.

(4) The child should not be totally immobile because it can lead to post-op respiratory complications.

11. The answer is 1, 2, and 3

The nurse cares for an older client who is diagnosed with left-sided heart failure. Which nursing interventions reduce the workload of the heart and promote comfort and rest? **(Select all that apply.)**

Category: Rest and sleep

(1) CORRECT: Taking short walks may provide distraction and increase mobility, circulation, and overall well-being if tolerated.

(2) CORRECT: Allowing the client to sit in an armchair makes it easier to breathe and is a safe alternative to an armless chair. It is also helpful to have the client raise the head of the bed when sleeping or napping. These are appropriate for a client with left-sided heart failure.

(3) CORRECT: Helping the client manage psychological stress will reduce the workload of the heart, because psychological stress can increase catecholamine production and increase heart rate and oxygen demand.

(4) A client in left-sided heart failure most likely will not tolerate lying flat, so this would not promote sleep and rest in this position.

(5) A bedside commode would reduce the work of getting to the bathroom and should be used.

12. The answer is 2

The nurse teaches a client on the proper use of crutches. The client requires non-weight-bearing ambulation for 4–6 weeks. Which of these crutch gaits should the nurse teach this client for safe ambulation?

Category: Assistive devices

(1) The two-point gait is an advanced four-point gait and allows for faster ambulation with minimal support.

(2) CORRECT: The three-point gait is the safest to use when one leg is injured. Both crutches and the injured leg move forward, followed by swinging the stronger lower extremity as the rest of the body weight is placed on the crutches.

(3) The four-point gait is used as a slow and stable gait for those who can bear weight on each leg.

(4) Swing-through gait is used for clients with lower extremities that are paralyzed and/or in braces.

13. The answer is 4, 3, 2, 1

The nurse finds the client in the bathroom reporting severe constipation. Which of these would be the appropriate order of nursing interventions to address the client's immediate elimination needs? **All options must be used.**

Category: Elimination

(1) This is last in the appropriate order of nursing interventions. Oral fluids should be increased but will not impact the immediate pain and constipation.

(2) Relief of the immediate pain is the priority. After an attempt to manually remove the impaction, and offering a PRN medication, the provider should be notified.

(3) PRN medications do not offer immediate relief and may not be effective if the impaction is solid. After a manual exam assessment, and an attempt to remove the stool, it would be appropriate to offer a PRN medication orally, if ordered, to prevent a repeat incident.

(4) The first nursing intervention should be manual assessment and removal of the fecal impaction. This will offer immediate relief while helping to assess what needs to be relayed to the provider.

14. The answer is 1

The nurse cares for a patient client who has recently had a vesicostomy. Which intervention should the nurse perform to assist this client with basic comfort and elimination?

Category: Elimination

(1) CORRECT: A vesicostomy is performed when chronic neurogenic bladder and frequent urinary tract infections become problematic. Hydration, cleansing and drying of the area, absorbent diapers, and daily dilation of the opening are all

appropriate care to prevent infection and to provide comfort. A cutaneous vesicostomy is a form of urinary diversion characterized by a small opening in the anterior bladder wall that is brought through the lower abdominal wall near the midpoint between the pubic bone and the umbilicus.

(2) Double diapers alone are not enough to keep the child comfortable and free from infection.

(3) It is not customary to apply a urine bag over the opening of a vesicostomy.

(4) The addition of a urine bag to double diapers will not keep the child comfortable and free from infection.

15. The answer is 1

A client who has chronic pain asks the nurse about alternative therapies in conjunction with traditional treatment. Which form of alternative therapy could the nurse provide for this client?

Category: Alternative therapy; Nonpharmacological comfort interventions

(1) CORRECT: Music therapy and guided imagery have been proven to increase a client's ability to perform activities of daily living by helping to focus on something other than pain.

(2) Acupuncture must be performed by a skilled practitioner and is not typically done by a staff nurse.

(3) Kegel exercises are done independently by the client to tighten the muscles of the pelvic floor. They do not provide pain relief.

(4) Nurses may participate in many forms of alternative therapies as nursing interventions when trained properly.

16. The answer is 2

The nurse cares for an adult client with a fractured femur who must be maintained in traction for several days before surgical interventions can take place. The client has several abrasions, dirty hair, and has healing wounds in the mouth. Which action should the

nurse perform to address the personal hygiene needs of this client?

Category: Personal hygiene

(1) The client may be able to do some of his bath, but it would not be possible for him to cleanse his own back and other areas while maintaining traction.

(2) CORRECT: Assisting with the bath allows inspection of the skin for any pressure areas; gentle teeth brushing and hair cleansing are nursing measures and promote comfort while maintaining the traction.

(3) A family member should not be responsible for inspecting the skin and maintaining the traction. These are nursing responsibilities.

(4) Oral care is important but the bath should not be postponed and can easily be done with the client in traction. It will promote comfort and healing.

17. The answer is 2

The nurse cares for an adult client with a long-bone fracture. The nurse encourages the client to move fingers and toes hourly, to change positions slightly every hour, and to eat high-iron foods as part of a balanced diet. Which of these foods or beverages should the nurse advise the client to avoid while on bed rest?

Category: Nutrition and oral hydration; Mobility/immobility

(1) Fruit juices can be taken while on bed rest.

(2) CORRECT: Too much milk increases the demand on the kidneys to excrete calcium and can lead to kidney stones.

(3) Cranberry juice can be taken while on bed rest and also aids in prevention of urinary tract infections.

(4) Some foods should be avoided or limited while on bed rest. For instance, milk and milk products should be avoided or limited while on bed rest to avoid kidney stone formation.

18. The answer is 3

The nurse teaches personal hygiene to client with type 1 diabetes mellitus (DM). Which topics would be **most** appropriate for the nurse to teach this client?

Category: Personal hygiene

(1) Oral care is an important part of diabetic hygiene to prevent cavities and infections.

(2) Hair care and nail care is not the most important part of personal hygiene, although it is important for self-esteem.

(3) CORRECT: Skin care is essential to prevent infection and skin breakdown. This is especially true for the feet, where a client may not see or may have reduced sensation.

(4) Personal hygiene is definitely a part of self-care teaching for an insulin-dependent client.

19. The answer is 1

The nurse cares for a pediatric client in the ambulatory care clinic. The parents report a 24-hour period of gastrointestinal distress, including vomiting several times and 3 watery stools. Which action does the nurse perform to assist in maintaining nutrition for this client?

Category: Nutrition and oral hydration

(1) CORRECT: Signs of dehydration would be part of parental teaching, and a slow introduction of clear liquids advancing to other liquids is appropriate.

(2) It would not be appropriate for the nurse to suggest that the parents offer whatever foods the child feels like taking, without first educating the parents about the signs of dehydration.

(3) Milk products would not be the first type of fluids offered for a child who has been vomiting. Milk is harder to digest and may exacerbate vomiting or diarrhea.

(4) Solid foods are introduced later, after liquids are offered over several hours, once vomiting has stopped.

20. The answer is 1, 2, 4, 6, 7, and 8

CORRECT OPTIONS: The nurse is concerned with abnormal clinical findings of **dysphagia, BMI 18 kg/m^2, sacrum with partial thickness skin loss and exposed dermis**, and **intact skin with area of non-blanchable erythema on right heel**. In clients with PD, a **shuffling gait with shorter steps** is a fall concern to the nurse. The nurse is also concerned with **prolonged periods of sitting or lying** as a risk for potential impaired skin integrity.

INCORRECT OPTIONS: The nurse is not concerned with the client's rounded abdomen and capillary refill less than 2 seconds as these are normal assessment findings.

21. See explanation for answers

CORRECT OPTIONS: The nurse interprets the client's abnormal skin findings according to the National Pressure Injury Advisory Panel (NPIAP) stages. The client's **sacrum injury is consistent with a stage 2 pressure injury**, which is identified as partial thickness skin loss with exposed dermis and pink, moist wound bed. The **right heel injury is consistent with a stage 1 pressure injury**, characterized as a localized area of intact skin with nonblanchable erythema. Including limited mobility, the nurse recognizes the client's risk factors to develop pressure injuries include **inadequate nutrition**. The client is underweight, evidenced by a BMI of 18, and is experiencing appetite loss with periods of dysphagia. Calorie, protein, and vitamin intake must be maintained to prevent and heal pressure injuries.

INCORRECT OPTIONS: A deep tissue injury is an area of either nonintact or intact skin with nonblanchable deep red or maroon discoloration; the client's injured skin areas are not relatable with this description. The client has capillary refill, less than 2 seconds, pink, warm, dry skin, and 2+ pedal pulses. These are indicators of arterial flow to the extremities and do not indicate reduced circulation to the skin and subcutaneous tissue, a risk factor for the development of pressure injuries. The client has adequate oxygenation status, evidenced by heart rate and respiratory rate within an acceptable adult range, pulse oximetry of 97% on room air, and clear lung sounds.

22. The answer is 3

CORRECT OPTION: The skin's primary function is to protect and provide a barrier against the external environment, including invading pathogens. Skin pressure that is not relieved can lead to destroyed cutaneous tissue; progressive inflammatory damage can result in chronic **infection** and sepsis.

INCORRECT OPTIONS: Anemia is not a complication from pressure injuries. Anemia is a risk factor for the development of pressure injuries, and wound healing may be delayed because less oxygen is delivered to the tissues. Dehiscence and evisceration are not complications of pressure injuries. Dehiscence is a complication of wound healing that occurs as disruption of previously joined wound edges, usually when a primary healing site has opened. Evisceration occurs with an abdominal wound when intestines protrude through separated wounds edges.

23. See explanation for answers

CORRECT OPTIONS: The nurse plans goals of **promoting adequate nutrition, reducing infection risk**, and **healing pressure injuries**. Promoting adequate nutrition is important especially in clients who are nutritionally deficit as pressure injuries are prone to develop and are resistant to healing. Reducing infection risk is a goal because a stage 2 pressure injury may be considered colonized with bacteria that potentially can cause infection. Healing pressure injuries is a goal related to impaired skin and tissue integrity, which if not treated, can progress to infection, sepsis, and potentially death.

INCORRECT OPTIONS: PD is associated with degeneration of dopamine storage cells and is a chronic neurodegenerative condition with an unknown etiology that may be associated with various environmental and genetic factors. Teaching about stroke risk factors is not a goal for clients with PD. Stroke risk is associated with multiple risk factors; prevention focuses on modifiable risk factors such as obesity, smoking, and hypertension. Educating about plasma exchange, that is removal of plasma and plasma components to reduce circulating antibodies, is not a goal for PD. Plasma exchange may be used as treatment for various autoimmune disorders, e.g. myasthenia gravis.

24. See explanation for answers

Reduce infection risk: The nurse implements **principles of asepsis during skin care**, including hand hygiene before and after care, as an essential action in reducing wound infection. The nurse **monitors for purulent drainage and odor** that may indicate the presence of infection. The nurse is alert for signs of inflammation and infection, indicated by a **rise in temperature, pulse, and respirations**. INCORRECT OPTION: The nurse should report an *increase* in leukocytes, a sign that may indicate infection; the nurse does not report a decrease in leukocytes.

Heal pressure injuries: The nurse recognizes that removing pressure, friction, and shear, and increasing mobility are needed for a pressure injury to heal. In clients with mobility problems, the nurse should teach methods of repositioning that reduce pressure, friction, and shear. **Frequency of repositioning should be individualized** to client risk factors and overall condition. Some clients need repositioning every 30 minutes and others every 2 hours. **Devices that redistribute weight, such as mattress overlays and wheelchair cushions**, are indicated for relieving pressure, especially in clients who have limited mobility. INCORRECT OPTIONS: Semi reclining in a chair or bed, raising the head of the bed, or sliding down in bed increase the shearing force on the sacrum and should be avoided. After cleaning a stage 2 injury with a non-cytotoxic agent, such as saline, it is important for the nurse to *cover* the injury with a dressing that keeps the wound bed slightly moist, not dry. A moist environment allows re-epithelialization to occur more rapidly.

Promote adequate nutrition: The nurse recognizes that nutritional status is important for wound healing. A **diet high in protein, calories, and nutrients** can decrease nutritional deficiencies and is essential for tissue repair. An increase in metabolic rate requires protein to reverse negative nitrogen balance. Without adequate carbohydrates for energy, the body utilizes protein for energy. Monitoring **prealbumin and albumin levels** provides information about nutritional effectiveness of therapies. Nutrients associated with tissue healing are vitamin C, A, copper, and zinc. Good nutrition and maintaining weight are necessary in clients with PD who have dysphagia and bradykinesia. **Smaller, frequent meals with foods that are easy to chew and swallow** may help prevent malnutrition. INCORRECT OPTION: Calcium provides various functions in the body, but it does not promote skin healing.

25. The answer is 1, 3, 4, and 6

CORRECT OPTIONS: The nurse evaluates the client's appetite and nutritional status as improved as evidenced by the client consuming **90% of meals, twice daily protein drinks, and a vitamin C supplement**. Improved appetite, protein, and vitamin C consumption are nutritional elements needed for wound healing. **The right heel, intact skin with _no_ areas of nonblanchable erythema** is an improvement from the prior assessment of right heel _with_ an area of nonblanchable erythema. **Right sacrum, 1 × 2 cm partial thickness skin loss, pink; moist wound bed,** indicates improvement and healing as the size of the pressure injury has decreased. The **client statement of the importance of performing passive range of motion exercises** indicates understanding of the role of mobility and exercise in preventing skin breakdown.

INCORRECT OPTIONS: Skin that is cool, pale, and frequently diaphoretic is at risk for injury. Excessive moisture increases maceration, softening of the skin, that increases vulnerability to breakdown. Shearing force on the sacrum is increased when the head of the bed is raised; the semi reclining position should be avoided.

26. The answer is 4

The nurse cares for a client diagnosed with pancreatic cancer. Which information does the nurse include when providing education to this client about nutrition and hydration?

Category: Nutrition and oral hydration

(1) It is more appropriate to progress the diet slowly to avoid nausea and vomiting.

(2) Pureed foods may cause nausea and gagging, low-protein foods do not offer enough nutrients, and daily weights are the norm.

(3) Herbal therapies have not been researched enough to be certain that they would not interfere or compromise cancer treatments when ingested. Topical herbal treatments may be of use for comfort.

(4) CORRECT: Foods high in both protein and carbo-hydrates will help to increase calorie intake. Both cool foods (which have less odor) and small, frequent meals help ward off nausea.

27. The answer is 2

The nurse cares for a client who is on long-term enteral nutrition. The nurse reviews the infusion procedure with the client's daughter. The nurse states which of these as the rationale for infusing the formula through the gastrostomy tube at room temperature?

Category: Nutrition and oral hydration

(1) There would not be a taste to formula given through the G-tube.

(2) CORRECT: Cold formula through the G-tube can cause discomfort and cramping.

(3) It is most appropriate for the comfort of the client to bring the formula to room temperature before administering.

(4) Temperature has nothing to do with the risk of aspiration.

28. The answer is 3

The nurse cares for a client recovering from a knee injury. Ambulation is still difficult for the client, and the physical therapist has suggested the client use a cane. Which statement **best** explains the use of a cane rather than a walker for this client?

Category: Assistive devices

(1) A cane is not used as a reminder for good posture; it is used for comfort and support.

(2) A cane is safe when used properly.

(3) CORRECT: A cane offers support and can give the client relief of joint pain and fatigue, and promote a safe way to ambulate when a lower extremity is injured.

(4) A cane does offer relief on weight-bearing joints when used properly.

29. The answer is 1 (E), 2 (D), 3 (B), 4 (C), 5 (A)

The nurse reviews the forms of traction and the purposes for each before gathering equipment prior to the child's arrival. Match the type of traction on the left with the type of injury or indication on the right. **All options must be used.**

Category: Mobility/immobility

(1) (E): Bryant's traction is used in children younger than age 2 to reduce femur fractures or stabilize hips.

(2) (D): Russell's traction may reduce fractures of the hip or femur.

(3) (B): 90-degree traction is used on the femur if skin traction isn't suitable.

(4) (C): Buck's traction is used to temporarily immo-bilize a fractured leg.

(5) (A): Cervical traction is used to stabilize a spinal fracture or muscle spasm.

30. The answer is 3

The nurse assesses pain in an infant using the chart below. Which would the pain score be for an infant with a high-pitched cry, O_2 saturation of 96%, a grimace, and frequent periods of wakefulness?

Score

	0	1	2
Crying	No	High-pitched	Inconsolable
Requires O_2	No	< 30%	> 30%
Expression	None	Grimace	Grimace/grunt
Sleepless	No	Wakes frequently	Always awake

Category: Rest and sleep

(1) A score of 0 is incorrect, because the infant has a grimace (1), periods of wakefulness (1), and a high-pitched cry (1).

(2) A score of 2 is incorrect, because the infant has a grimace (1), periods of wakefulness (1), and a high-pitched cry (1).

(3) CORRECT: A pain score of 3 is the closest evaluation with the information given. The infant has a high-pitched cry (1), an adequate O_2 saturation (0), a grimace (1), and periods of wakefulness (1).

(4) A pain score of 3 is the closest evaluation with the information given. The infant has a high-pitched cry (1), an adequate O_2 saturation (0), a grimace (1), and periods of wakefulness (1).

CHAPTER 9

PHYSIOLOGICAL INTEGRITY: PHARMACOLOGICAL AND PARENTERAL THERAPIES

Pharmacological and parenteral therapies involve the provision of care related to the administration of all forms of medication as well as parenteral/IV therapy. Generic names of medications are used in a fairly consistent manner, while the brand/trade name may vary. Therefore, you should expect to see the use of generic medication names only on the NCLEX-RN® exam. Some test items may also refer more broadly to general classifications of medications.

On the NCLEX-RN® exam, you can expect 16 percent of the questions to relate to the Pharmacological and Parenteral Therapies subcategory. Exam content includes, but is not limited to, the following areas:

- Adverse effects/contraindications/side effects/interactions
- Blood and blood products
- Central venous access devices
- Dosage calculation
- Expected actions/outcomes
- Medication administration
- Medication handling and maintenance
- Parenteral/intravenous therapies
- Pharmacological pain management
- Total parenteral nutrition

Now let's review some of the most important concepts related to these subtopics.

Adverse Effects/Contraindications/Side Effects/Interactions

It is important to assess clients for actual and potential side effects and adverse effects of medications, including prescription, over-the-counter, and herbal medications. This requires knowledge of all medications a client is taking, and information on preexisting conditions.

Provide clients with information on common side effects and how to manage them. This includes letting clients know when to call or notify their primary health care provider regarding side effects. Also know when to contact the client's primary health care provider regarding side effects of medication or parenteral therapy for clients who are hospitalized.

Be able to identify signs and symptoms of an allergic reaction, which include the following:

- **Skin:** Redness, itching, swelling, blistering, weeping, crusting, rash, eruptions, or hives (itchy bumps or welts)
- **Lungs:** Wheezing, tightness, cough, or shortness of breath
- **Head:** Swelling of the face, eyelids, lips, tongue, or throat; headache
- **Nose:** Stuffy nose, runny nose (clear, thin discharge), or sneezing
- **Eyes:** Red (bloodshot), itchy, swollen, or watery
- **Stomach:** Pain, nausea, vomiting, diarrhea, or bloody diarrhea

In addition, you must know which procedures are appropriate for counteracting adverse effects due to medication or parenteral therapy, and how to implement them. And of course, document client response to actions taken to counteract adverse effects.

Blood and Blood Products

One of the most important aspects of dealing with blood products is the correct identification of clients to ensure the right products are used. Identify the client according to facility/agency policy prior to administration of red blood cells/blood products. The steps involved include reviewing the prescription for administration, ensuring the blood is the correct type, ensuring the identity of the client, checking that crossmatching is complete, and ensuring client consent.

Before administering any blood products, check the client for appropriate venous access for product administration, select the correct needle gauge, and check the integrity of the access site. Understand when it is appropriate for a client to be an autologous donor (i.e., use the client's own blood), and the procedures for autologous blood donation:

- Four to six weeks prior to surgery
- Every three days if hemoglobin levels are satisfactory
- Good for rare blood types, transfusion reactions, prevention of blood-borne disease transmission
- Not good if client has an acute infection, a low hemoglobin count, or cardiovascular disease

Know the different blood types (ABO and Rh blood group systems) and compatibilities based on blood type, Rh factors, antibody screening, and crossmatching. Be familiar with the procedures employed after blood is drawn for typing, including the use of special client identification bracelets, and how to match the bracelets with the unique blood donor number on a sample or identification tag on any unit of blood the client receives.

It is also important to know the various blood components and what they are used for:

- **Whole blood:** Not normally used; mainly situations of major hemorrhage
- **Red blood cells (RBCs):** Anemia, blood loss
- **Fresh frozen plasma (FFP):** Coagulation deficiency
- **Platelets:** Thrombocytopenia
- **Albumin:** Shock, blood loss, low protein levels due to surgery or liver failure
- **Cryoprecipitate:** Blood loss or immediately prior to an invasive procedure in clients with significant hypofibrinogenemia

To administer blood products safely, and evaluate client response to administered products, follow the procedure detailed below:

(1) Verify client consent.

(2) Check client's baseline vital signs.

(3) Check physician's order.

(4) Identify a stable vein, and then choose a needle with the proper gauge.

(5) Set up equipment and start IV.

(6) Obtain correct component from blood bank.

(7) Verify client identification and related information (use second nurse to double-check).

(8) Hang blood.

(9) Begin transfusion at a slow rate (2 mL per minute).

(10) Monitor client vital signs after the first 15 minutes and thereafter in accordance with facility policy.

(11) After 15 minutes, increase rate of infusion.

(12) Monitor client vital signs and lung sounds for one hour after transfusion is complete.

(13) Document all activities in the client's medical record.

It is important to know how to respond to common complications from blood transfusions, including transfusion reactions (allergic, febrile, or hemolytic), circulatory overload, blood-borne infections, electrolyte imbalance, and iron overload. If complications occur, they must be documented in the client's medical record.

Central Venous Access Devices

Provide information to clients regarding reasons for and care of central venous access devices (CVADs). Types of CVADs include the following:

- **Tunneled catheter:** A tunneled catheter is placed in a central vein, tunneled under the skin, and then brought out through the skin. Examples include Hickman and Broviac.
- **Implanted port:** A port is inserted under subcutaneous tissue and attached to a catheter, which is threaded into the superior vena cava. Examples include Mediport and Port-a-Cath.

- **Peripherally inserted central catheter (PICC):** PICCs are inserted into a basilic or cephalic vein just above or below the antecubital space of the client's right arm by a doctor or specially trained IV therapy nurse. The catheter terminates in the superior vena cava. PICCs often remain in place for long periods of time.

Know how to access an implanted CVAD to provide medication and/or nutrition for a client, as well as how to care for a client with a CVAD. This includes:

- Maintaining strict sterile procedures to minimize risk of infection
- Flushing line periodically with normal saline solution
- Checking port placement
- Changing dressing

Dosage Calculation

Medications are prescribed in specific amounts or weights per volume for liquids. You should be able to perform the calculations needed for proper medication administration. The common formulas for calculating dosages include the following:

- Ratio and proportion
- "Desired over have"
- Dimensional analysis

Be aware of rounding rules when calculating dosages, as well.

Dosages are calculated using body weight in kilograms, so you convert between pounds and kilograms. Most often, you multiply the body weight by the dosage order per kilogram. You can also calculate volume using standard pharmaceutical math calculations. To calculate single dosages, divide the total daily dose by the number of doses per day. You can also use a nomogram (a type of graph) to calculate dosages based on body surface area.

In addition to dosage calculation for medications for adults, it is important to know the differences between adult and pediatric dosages and how to calculate pediatric dosages. It's also important to know how to help children swallow pills and how to give medications to infants.

Oral Medications

When tablets are scored, they may be broken and given as partial doses. Do not break or crush extended release tablets. Abbreviations to know include the following:

- **CR:** Controlled release
- **CRT:** Controlled release tablet
- **LA:** Long acting
- **SA:** Sustained action
- **SR:** Sustained release

- **TR:** Timed release
- **XL:** Extended length
- **XR:** Extended release

Enteral Medications

Enteral medications are administered through a tube. Know the correct tube placement for the following types of tubes:

- Nasogastric (through the nose and into the stomach)
- Nasointestinal (through the nose, past the stomach, and into the small intestine)
- Percutaneous (through the skin directly into the stomach)

It is important to know how to care for a client receiving enteral medication. Flush the tube with 30 mL water before administering the medication. Use a solution/elixir form of medication, when available.

Injectable Medications

The following steps comprise the procedure for injecting medications:

- Choose a needle based on volume and type of medication, destination site, client size, and viscosity of medication.
- Maintain sterility when assembling the syringe and needle.
- Withdraw medication from the vial/ampule.
- Use anatomical landmarks (intramuscular, intravenous, and/or subcutaneous).
- Wash hands and put on gloves.
- Cleanse area with alcohol swabs and wait for it to dry.
- Inject medication.
- Discard the syringe and needle into a sharps container.
- Remove gloves.
- Wash hands.

Topical Medications

Understand how to administer the following types of topical medications:

- Skin
- Nasal
- Optical
- Otic (ear)
- Vaginal
- Rectal

Inhaled Medications

You should be able to explain how to use a metered-dose inhaler (MDI) medication to your clients. A spacer is a device that attaches to the MDI to help deliver the medicine to the lungs instead of the mouth.

Expected Actions/Outcomes

You are expected to obtain information on prescribed medications for clients by reviewing the formulary and consulting the pharmacist, as needed. You must also understand the likely effects and outcomes for any oral, intradermal, subcutaneous, intramuscular, or topical medications prescribed for your client.

Evaluate and document a client's use of medications over time, including prescriptions, over-the-counter medications, and home remedies. This includes explaining effects and outcomes to clients and families.

Medication Administration

It is important to understand the general principles of medication administration, including how medications are named (generic versus brand name or trade name). The nurse must verify several facts before administering medication to a client. Here are "rights" to use when administering client medications:

(1) **Right client:** Identify the client in two ways, such as checking the client's armband and asking the client to state their name, if able. Do not use the room number as a method to identify the client.

(2) **Right medication:** Know both the generic name and its brand equivalent; also double-check the medication prescription.

(3) **Right time:** Verify that the medication is being given at the proper time (with meal, a.m./ p.m., etc.)

(4) **Right dose:** Make sure the dose that is administered is a safe amount.

(5) **Right route:** Check the medication order to verify the route of administration, such as oral, IV, or suppository.

(6) **Right site:** Verify that the medication can be applied to a particular site on the body and that sites are rotated with each application.

(7) **Right documentation:** Document details immediately after the medication is administered.

Review pertinent data prior to administration of medication. This includes vital signs, lab results, allergies, potential medication interactions, medical history, and current diagnosis.

Know the drug name, dosage, route, frequency, and special parameters for withholding doses or administering additional doses. Check each medical order for accuracy: ensure that it includes the date, time, and client's last name, and that it is signed by the prescribing physician. This is important because you are responsible if you administer a drug based on an incorrect order.

It is important to understand the basic concepts of pharmacology, including:

- **Pharmacokinetics:** How the body absorbs, distributes, and metabolizes medications
- **Absorption routes:** GI tract, respiratory tract, and skin
- **Distribution:** How a drug moves through the body from absorption site to action site
- **Metabolism:** Conversion of a drug by enzymes into a less-active, excretable substance
- **Excretion:** Elimination of drug and metabolites from the body

The basic principles of medication administration are:

- Make sure the medication order is accurate.
- Check for client allergies.
- Assess the client to be sure the medication makes sense.
- Check all other medications the client is taking.
- Calculate the proper dosage.
- Check the expiration date of the medication.
- Label all medications.

You are responsible not only for preparing and administering but also for documenting medications given by common routes (oral or topical), as well as by parenteral routes (IV, IM, or subcutaneous). This may include mixing medications from two vials when necessary, such as when administering a mixed dose of insulin.

You are expected to be able to adjust/titrate dosages of medication based on the assessment of physiologic parameters of each client. This includes giving insulin according to blood glucose levels and titrating medication to maintain a specific blood pressure.

Nurses must properly dispose of unused medications according to facility/agency policy. In addition, it is your responsibility to educate clients about medications, including their potential side effects, how to take them, and how to handle side effects and/or allergic reactions.

Medication Handling and Maintenance

In addition to observing the "rights" of medication administration, nurses must ensure the safe handling, storage, and disposal of medications.

Medication carts increase the portability of medications. The nurse is responsible for maintaining a controlled environment for medication storage in this mobile setting. There are many types of medicine carts, but most have individual drawers to hold medications for each patient. Unless all drawers are locked, the cart should never be left unattended in an unsecured area such as a hallway. When not in use, the medication cart should be stored in the designated area behind a locked door.

Controlled substances require additional security measures; they should not be placed in regular medicine drawers, which are not adequately secure. When controlled substances are included in the medication cart, it must be a cart equipped with double-locking drawers. These more secure medication drawers are made specifically to hold controlled substances.

Many hospitals use an automated drug dispensing system with computerized access. These systems require usernames, passwords, and sometimes barcodes for access and keep records automatically, providing enhanced security. Some automated systems provide an individual drawer for each patient, while others have an individual drawer for each medication, like a mini-pharmacy.

When a client is discharged from a health care facility or no longer needs a specific medication, unused medication may remain. Agencies vary in terms of how they dispose of unused medications. Refer to your facility's policies and procedures relating to the disposal of unused medications.

Parenteral/Intravenous Therapies

It is important to know the basics of intravenous therapy, including the indicators, types of fluids used (isotonic solutions, hypertonic solutions, and hypotonic solutions), and equipment (catheters and needles, infusion pumps, electronic delivery devices, regulators, controllers, mechanical infusion devices, and tubing). There are four types of infusion therapy: peripheral, central, continuous, and intermittent. Know when each should be used.

As with medication dosages, apply mathematic concepts when administering intravenous and parenteral therapy. To calculate an IV drip rate, use the following formula to calculate drops per minute:

(Total number of milliliters ÷ total number of minutes) × drip factor = gtt/minute

You will be provided with the drip factor in the question stem on the NCLEX-RN® exam.

Know which veins to access for various therapies; you should be able to prepare clients for intravenous catheter insertion, insert and remove a peripheral intravenous line, and monitor the use of an infusion pump, whether it's intravenous or patient controlled analgesia (PCA). You should also be able to maintain an epidural infusion.

If a client needs intermittent parenteral fluid therapy for nutritional purposes, educate the client and evaluate the client's response. You should also be able to monitor and maintain infusion sites and track the rates of infusion to ensure they are correct.

Pharmacological Pain Management

To determine client need for administration of a PRN pain medication, question the client about their level of pain using a pain rating scale from 1 to 10, or a visual scale using images of faces with different expressions. Be aware of nonverbal indicators, such as facial expressions or sounds.

Know how to provide pain management appropriate for client age and different diagnoses (pregnant clients, children, and older adults).

Document pain mediation administration according to facility/agency policy, and comply with regulations governing controlled substances (such as counting narcotics and wasting narcotics), and evaluate and document client use and response to pain medications.

Total Parenteral Nutrition

Total parenteral nutrition (TPN) is nutrition provided intravenously for clients who are unable to tolerate oral or enteral feedings. It may be used in both home and hospital environments.

Know how to administer, maintain, and discontinue TPN. This includes knowing the ingredients of the solution: amino acids, dextrose for carbohydrates, vitamins and minerals, trace elements, electrolytes, and water, and sometimes lipids, insulin, and heparin. You should also know the components of different solutions that need to be used depending on the client's nutritional needs and disease state. Clients who may need TPN are those with GI tract issues, who are recovering from GI surgery, or who have experienced trauma. Clients with high nutritional needs may also require TPN.

Access sites for TPN include peripheral lines through veins (for supplements only, not when a client needs nutrition replacement; these should only be used for 2 weeks or less) and central lines, which are more typical (often a PICC line).

Be aware of the following as you manage a client receiving TPN:

- There is a risk of pneumothorax during catheter insertion for a PICC line.
- Examine the IV insertion site during each shift for signs of infection.
- Do not use the IV line for anything other than TPN.
- Inspect the bag of solution for particles prior to hanging.
- Monitor the client's blood glucose level.
- Measure daily weight to determine/adjust fluid balance.
- Monitor other lab results, such as electrolytes, protein, prealbumin/albumin, creatinine, lymphocytic count, and liver function.

Know the rates of administration of TPN, how to monitor clients for adverse effects, and how to taper down use of TPN. (Do not discontinue TPN abruptly.) Possible complications include fluid overload, air embolism, infection/sepsis, hyperglycemia, and hypoglycemia.

Finally, you should be able to evaluate outcomes of TPN, including satisfactory weight gain and fluids, and electrolytes within normal limits.

Chapter Quiz

1. The nurse conducts a home visit with a client who has a history of angina. Which client statement demonstrates to the nurse that further teaching about nitroglycerin therapy is required?

   1. "I take a tablet about 10 minutes before I walk up the stairs."
   2. "I take no more than 3 doses in a 15-minute period of time."
   3. "I keep the tablets in a glass dish by the bedroom window so they are readily available."
   4. "I will call my provider immediately if I experience blurred vision, nausea, and vomiting."

2. The nurse assesses the peripheral IV site of a client receiving a doxorubicin infusion who has suspected extravasation. After stopping the infusion and disconnecting the IV tubing, which action does the nurse do **next**?

   1. Apply a hot compress to the IV site.
   2. Apply a cold compress to the IV site.
   3. Elevate the affected extremity.
   4. Attempt to aspirate the residual drug.

3. The nurse prepares to discharge a client on warfarin therapy. The nurse's discharge teaching should include which instruction?

   1. Increase intake of green and leafy vegetables.
   2. Take herbal remedies to manage cold symptoms.
   3. Avoid consumption of alcoholic beverages.
   4. Take the medication only on an empty stomach.

Refer to the Case Study to answer the next six questions.

| History and Physical | Laboratory Results |

Client is a 28-year-old involved in a 2-vehicle MVA last night. The client was transported to the emergency department (ED), and was extremely hypotensive and dyspneic upon arrival at 2330. The client was diagnosed with several rib fractures on the left chest, a hemopneumothorax, and ruptured spleen. In the ED, a 28 French chest tube was placed in the client's left posterior chest and immediately drained 500 mL blood. The client was transported to the operating room and underwent a splenectomy and exploratory laparotomy. Estimated blood loss (EBL) during surgery was 1,300 mL. The physician ordered stat laboratory tests in the Post Anesthesia Care Unit (PACU). The client was transported to the ICU in stable condition at 0400.

The client's parents and spouse are present and provided past medical history. The client's weight is approximately 180 lbs (81.64 kg) and height is 74 inches (188 cm). The client has no illnesses, takes no medications, is active, and exercises regularly. The client has an allergy to shellfish, but no medication allergies. Past surgical history includes an appendectomy at age 8, and an intermedullary nailing of a fractured femur at age 16. The parents state the client received blood at the time of the orthopedic procedure.

| History and Physical | Laboratory Results |

Laboratory Test	Result 0315	Interpretation
Blood type	A positive	Type A Rh positive
White Blood Cell (WBC) Count	11,500/mm^3 (11.5 $\times$ 10^9/L)	high
Red Blood Cell (RBC) Count	4.2 million/mm^3 (4.2 $\times$ 10^{12}/L)	low
Hemoglobin (Hgb)	7 g/dL (70 g/L)	low
Hematocrit (Hct)	26% (0.26)	low
Platelet Count	280,000/mm^3 (280 $\times$ 10^9/L)	normal

4. The nurse reviews the client's history and physical and lab results, and prepares to admit the client to the intensive care unit.

    Which **3** findings indicate the client may need a blood transfusion?

    1. Client was dyspneic on arrival to ED.
    2. Estimated blood loss before and during surgery.
    3. Allergy to shellfish.
    4. Hemoglobin 7 g/dL (70 g/L).
    5. Hematocrit 26% (0.26).
    6. Platelets 280,000/mm^3 (280 $\times$ 10^9/L).
    7. WBC count 11,500/mm^3 (11.5 $\times$ 10^9/L).
    8. History of previous blood transfusion.

5. Which information from the client's history alerts the nurse that the client has an **increased** risk for a blood transfusion reaction?

    1. The client had previous blood transfusions.
    2. The client has an allergy to shellfish.
    3. The client has no spleen.
    4. The client has no appendix.

History and Physical	Laboratory Results	Orders

Physician's Orders 0400

- Admit to intensive care unit (ICU).

- Allergies: Shellfish.

- Vital signs every 1 hour $\times$ 4, then every 4 hours.

- NPO except for ice chips, oral medications.

- Chest tube setting -20 mmHg continuous wall suction.

- Oxygen 2 L/min per nasal cannula to keep SpO$_2$ > 92%.

- Encourage incentive spirometer every hour while awake.

- IV dextrose 5% in 0.9% normal saline (D$_5$NS) at 125 mL/hour.

- Transfuse blood on arrival to ICU.

- Indwelling urinary catheter to bedside drainage.

- Portable AP and lateral chest x-rays in the morning.

- Physical therapy (PT) to get client up in chair and ambulate in room in a.m.

- Hydromorphone 2 mg IV every 3 hours for severe pain (pain 7–10/10).

- Hydrocodone/acetaminophen 10 mg/325 mg 1 tablet PO every 4 hours PRN moderate pain (pain 4–6/10).

- Acetaminophen 500 mg PO every 4 hours PRN mild pain or temperature > 100.8° F (38.22° C).

- Ondansetron 4 mg IV every 6 hours PRN nausea.

- Piperacillin/tazobactam 3.375 g IV every 6 hours.

6. The nurse reviews the physician's orders.

Drag the choices below to fill in each blank in the following sentence. Each choice will only be used once.

In order to transfuse blood, the nurse must **first** clarify the physician's order to specify the

_____ [Select from the list], _____ [Select from the list], and

_____ [Select from the list].

| type of blood product |
| donor number |
| type of tubing to be used |
| size of IV catheter |
| Rh factor |
| volume to be given |
| frequency of vital signs |
| rate of infusion |

| History and Physical | Laboratory Results | Orders | Nurse's Notes |

0600: Client is resting quietly with eyes closed. Rouses to name and is oriented × 4. Moves all extremities spontaneously and to command. Client has some scratches and bruises on left cheek and shoulder. Skin warm, dry. Lung sounds clear in upper lobes, diminished in left lower lobe. Chest tube intact to −20 mmHg wall suction with scant amount sanguineous drainage in tubing. Chest tube dressing dry and intact. Abdomen soft, hypoactive bowel sounds left upper quadrant. Dressing dry and intact to left abdomen. Indwelling urinary catheter draining clear yellow urine to bedside bag. Pedal pulses 2+ bilaterally.

Client states pain 3/10 in left chest with coughing and movement. Client was medicated for pain with hydromorphone 2 mg IV 10 minutes ago. IV D_5NS infusing at 125 mL/hr per pump to 18 gauge IV catheter in right forearm. Site intact without redness or swelling. Client has an 18 gauge IV catheter to saline lock in the left hand. Site with poor blood return and does not flush easily. Left hand swollen. IV catheter removed. Vital signs: T (oral) 98.8° F (37.1° C), HR 82, RR 14, BP 128/70.

7. The nurse documents a client assessment and plans to administer the first unit of PRBCs.

   For each timeframe below, specify the potential nursing interventions that are appropriate for the care of the client. Each timeframe may support more than 1 potential nursing intervention.

Time Frame	Potential Nursing Interventions
Before starting the transfusion	☐ Ensure the consent is signed. ☐ Obtain and record baseline vital signs. ☐ Insert a 22 gauge IV catheter and start an infusion of Dextrose 5% in Water (D_5W). ☐ Verify the client by name and number and check blood compatibility with an LPN/LVN or RN.
During the infusion	☐ Infuse the unit of blood in less than 4 hours. ☐ Assign an unlicensed assistive personnel (UAP) to remain with the client for the first 15 minutes. ☐ Hold IV medications until the blood transfusion is completed. ☐ Administer the blood using filtered tubing.
After the infusion	☐ Auscultate lungs and obtain vital signs. ☐ Discard the blood bag and tubing in the client's trash. ☐ Send a urine specimen for culture and sensitivity. ☐ Document the volume infused and time of infusion.

8. 0700: One hour after the first transfusion is initiated, the client reports a headache, having chills, and feeling "anxious." The vital signs are temperature (oral) 100.4° F (38° C), RR 18, HR 92, BP 136/78. The client's skin is warm, flushed, and dry. The lungs are clear; client denies dyspnea.

Complete the following sentences by choosing from the list of options.

The nurse will **immediately** [Select from list 1]. It is a **priority** for the nurse to [Select from list 2]. When this action is complete, the nurse will [Select from list 3]. The nurse will contact the physician and prepares to administer [Select from list 4].

(1)	(2)	(3)	(4)
place the client in high Fowler position	remove the blood tubing down to the catheter hub	keep the IV line open with new IV tubing primed with 0.9% normal saline	a diuretic
stop the blood transfusion	flush the client's blood tubing with 0.9% normal saline	start an IV below the infusion site and place to saline lock	epinephrine
encourage the client to deep breathe and cough	remove the IV catheter and culture the tip	prepare the client for central venous access device placement	an antipyretic

9. The nurse assesses the client 30 minutes later.

Which assessment finding indicates the client will require further interventions?
(Select all that apply.)

1. Blood pressure 92/62.
2. Respirations 16/min.
3. Temperature 100° F (37.7° C).
4. Audible wheezing.
5. Urticaria and pruritus.
6. Client drowsy and disoriented.
7. Hemoglobinuria.
8. Client reports chest pain 2/10.

10. A client takes amitriptyline hydrochloride to manage neuropathic pain. The client reports severe xerostomia. Which action does the nurse ask the client to implement to help relieve the xerostomia?

    1. Increase caffeine intake.
    2. Decrease fluid intake.
    3. Increase dietary sodium.
    4. Chew sugar-free gum.

11. Prior to administering digoxin 0.125 mg PO to a client diagnosed with chronic heart failure, the nurse notes that the apical pulse is 56 beats/minute. Which action should the nurse implement **next**?

    1. Administer the drug and recheck the pulse in one hour.
    2. Withhold the drug and notify the provider.
    3. Obtain a 12-lead electrocardiogram (ECG).
    4. Send a blood sample to the laboratory for a serum drug level.

12. The nurse reviews routes of medication administration with the client who is diagnosed with metastatic cancer. The nurse knows that the rectal route of administration is contraindicated when which manifestation is present?

    1. Nausea and vomiting.
    2. Difficulty swallowing.
    3. Neutropenia.
    4. Fever.

13. A client is admitted for gastrointestinal bleeding. The client has a platelet count of 15,000/mm^3 (15 × 10^9/L). A platelet transfusion is prescribed by the health care provider. Which is required for platelet transfusions? **(Select all that apply.)**

    1. ABO compatibility.
    2. Rh compatibility.
    3. Crossmatching.
    4. A specialized platelet filter.
    5. Verification of two patient identifiers.

14. A client's red blood cell transfusion is discontinued due to an acute hemolytic transfusion reaction. Which strategy **best** minimizes the client's risk of such a reaction?

    1. The nurse ensures the client's temperature does not increase more than 1.8° F during the transfusion.
    2. The nurse verifies all client-identifying information according to protocol before transfusing blood.
    3. The nurse administers meperidine for severe rigors.
    4. The nurse administers acetaminophen prior to the transfusion.

15. A client is receiving a blood transfusion. The nurse observes that the client is experiencing diarrhea, abdominal pain, and chills. Which action should the nurse take **first**?

    1. Assist the client to the bathroom.
    2. Stop the blood infusion.
    3. Administer meperidine.
    4. Get a warming blanket.

16. The nurse aspirates a central venous catheter prior to drug administration but is not able to verify blood return. The nurse does not feel resistance when flushing or see any fluid leakage, swelling, or redness around the catheter site. Which next steps are appropriate? **(Select all that apply.)**

    1. Flush the catheter with saline, using a 10-mL syringe and a push-pull technique.
    2. Request that the client cough and reattempt aspiration.
    3. Administer IV medication and observe for signs and symptoms of catheter malfunction.
    4. Place the client in Trendelenburg position and while attempting to aspirate blood.
    5. Follow institutional protocol to initiate a declotting protocol.

17. A client with known heparin-induced thrombocytopenia (HIT) is undergoing chemotherapy and is having a central venous access device placed. Which type of central venous access device **best** minimizes the risk of HIT-related complication?

    1. Hickman.
    2. Broviac.
    3. Groshong.
    4. Port.

18. A client has been instructed by the provider to increase warfarin sodium dose from 5 mg to 7.5 mg. The client only has 5-mg tablets available. How many tablets should the nurse instruct the client to take?

    1. 0.5.
    2. 1.
    3. 1.5.
    4. 2.

19. The nurse prepares to set up an intravenous infusion of normal saline (NS) 1,000 mL over a 6-hour period. The tubing drop factor is 10 gtt/mL. How many gtt/minute should the nurse infuse the NS?

    1. 12 gtt/minute.
    2. 28 gtt/minute.
    3. 33 gtt/minute.
    4. 36 gtt/minute.

20. The nurse prepares a dopamine hydrochloride infusion to start at 5 mcg/kg/minute for a client who weighs 165 lb (75 kg). The dopamine is available as 400 mg in 250 mL of D_5W. How many mL/hour does the nurse set the infusion pump to administer the dopamine?

    1. 14 mL/hour.
    2. 16 mL/hour.
    3. 22.5 mL/hour.
    4. 37.5 mL/hour.

21. A client is prescribed doxorubicin 60 mg/m^2 as part of cancer therapy. The client is 5 ft 6 in tall, weighs 145 lb, and has a body surface area of 1.75 m^2. What is the correct dose that the nurse should administer the doxorubicin? Round your answer to the nearest whole number.

    _____ mg

22. A client is admitted with sickle cell anemia and expresses concerns about becoming addicted to pain medicine. The nurse explains the difference between physical dependence, tolerance, and addiction. Which finding is associated with addiction?

    1. Withdrawal symptoms when the drug is abruptly stopped.
    2. Withdrawal symptoms when the drug dose is reduced.
    3. Habitual and compulsive use of a drug.
    4. A state of adaptation.

23. A client has been prescribed amphetamine and dextroamphetamine for attention-deficit/hyperactivity disorder (ADHD). The nurse explains that the client should be alert for which adverse reaction?

    1. Weight gain.
    2. Depression.
    3. Somnolence.
    4. Bradycardia.

24. The nurse administers a medication intramuscularly by Z-track method. Place the following steps in the appropriate order. **All options must be used.**

    1. Withdraw the needle.
    2. Administer the drug intramuscularly (IM) in the dorsogluteal site.
    3. Release the skin.
    4. Displace the skin lateral to the injection site.

25. A client admitted with chronic heart failure takes furosemide. Which statement, if made by the client, **best** demonstrates understanding of the side effects associated with furosemide?

   1. "My blood pressure might be abnormally high."
   2. "I should eat more foods such as bananas and apricots."
   3. "I should take the drug before I go to bed."
   4. "I should not take the medication with food."

26. The nurse administers vancomycin 1 g every 12 hours. Which statement indicates that the client may be experiencing an ototoxic adverse reaction?

   1. "I hear ringing in my ear."
   2. "The IV is burning."
   3. "My skin is very itchy."
   4. "I have a bad taste in my mouth."

27. A client is prescribed lisinopril. Which instruction should the nurse give the client to minimize a potential adverse reaction of lisinopril?

   1. Eat fruits and vegetables high in iron.
   2. Rise slowly from a lying to a sitting position.
   3. Increase fluid intake.
   4. Avoid aspirin-containing drugs.

Refer to the Case Study to answer the next question.

The home health nurse is responding to a call from the spouse of an older adult client.

| History | Admission Notes | Visit Notes | Flow Sheets |

Client has diagnoses of heart failure (HF), chronic kidney disease (CKD), osteoarthritis, and hypertension. The client lives with the spouse in an independent living facility. The client was admitted to the hospital for worsening lower extremity edema and dyspnea. The client received IV diuretics while in the hospital, and lower extremity edema and dyspnea improved. After a three-day hospital stay, the client was discharged home with adjustments to the home medications. Home health skilled nursing was ordered for disease management and medication teaching.

| History | Admission Notes | Visit Notes | Flow Sheets |

Day of Home Health Admission

Client was discharged from the hospital yesterday. Client is awake and alert, oriented × 4. Vital signs stable, recorded on flow sheet in client's home folder. No weight gain since discharge from hospital. Skin warm, dry. Mucous membranes moist. Lungs clear bilaterally, clear S1 S2. Abdomen soft with bowel sounds present × 4 quadrants. Client states voiding clear yellow urine. Trace edema in bilateral ankles. 2+ pedal pulses. Reviewed client's home medications. The client reports, "I typically need to take ibuprofen 2 to 3 times per day for my arthritis." Client and spouse verbalize understanding of medication changes and a low-sodium diet. Client records weight, blood pressure, and pulse each morning at 0800. Client scheduled to be seen next week.

Medication Reconciliation			
Current Medication	**Dose/Route**	**Frequency**	**New/Changed**
Losartan	50 mg PO	Daily	No change
Metoprolol	25 mg PO	Twice daily	No change
Furosemide	40 mg PO	Twice daily	Changed: Increased from 20 mg PO twice daily
Amlodipine	5 mg PO	Daily	No change
Ibuprofen	400 mg PO	Every 6 hours	PRN arthritis pain

| History | Admission Notes | Visit Notes | Flow Sheets |

Home Health Day 5

Responding to call from spouse this morning. Spouse reports the client has not felt well for the past couple of days. This morning the client feels "too weak to get out of bed."

Assessment: Client is lying in bed. Wakens to name. Oriented to person, but did not remember coming home and thought this was the hospital. Reorients easily. Skin pale and cool. Mucous membranes dry, lips cracked and dry. Tenting present on clavicle. Lungs clear. Clear S1 S2. Abdomen soft with faint hypoactive bowel sounds × 4 quadrants. Faint pedal pulses bilaterally. No ankle edema bilaterally. Client reports headache. States, "I just feel too dizzy when I try to sit up. I have to lie back down." The client has reported nausea, but no vomiting. Spouse reports client has only been able to drink a few sips of water and broth this morning. The client's spouse also states that the client has been voiding large amounts of light yellow urine, but this morning, voided only a small amount of dark amber urine. The client has continued to take medications as prescribed.

| History | Admission Notes | Visit Notes | Flow Sheets |

Home Health Flow Sheet			
Data	Day of Discharge	Home Health (HH) Admission	Visit 1 (HH Day 5)
Temperature (oral)	98.2° F (36.8° C)	98.8° F (37.1° C)	97.4° F (36.3° C)
BP	142/78	138/78	102/66
HR	82	78	88
RR	16	16	22
Pulse oximetry (room air)	95%	96%	94%
Daily weight	182 lb (82.5 kg)	182 lb (82.5 kg)	176 lb (79.8kg)

28. The home health nurse reviews the client's history and admission notes, then assesses the client and records information on the flow sheets.

Complete the following sentence by choosing from the list of options.

The client is at high risk for developing [Select from list 1] due to [Select from list 2] and [Select from list 3].

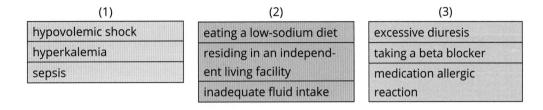

(1)	(2)	(3)
hypovolemic shock	eating a low-sodium diet	excessive diuresis
hyperkalemia	residing in an independent living facility	taking a beta blocker
sepsis	inadequate fluid intake	medication allergic reaction

---

29. The nurse administers doxorubicin IV push to a client with breast cancer. Which effect should the nurse explain is to be expected during therapy with doxorubicin?

1. Burning at the IV site during administration.
2. Red-colored urine.
3. Permanent alopecia.
4. Teeth discoloration.

30. The nurse prepares to infuse total parenteral nutrition (TPN) to a client. Which actions are appropriate for the nurse to perform in TPN administration? **(Select all that apply.)**

1. Follow aseptic technique.
2. Use a designated IV filter.
3. Apply a surgical mask to the client.
4. Label the tubing with date and time.
5. Check TPN bag expiration.

Chapter Quiz Answers and Explanations

1. The answer is 3

The nurse conducts a home visit with a client who has a history of angina. Which client statement demonstrates to the nurse that further teaching about nitroglycerin therapy is required?

Category: Adverse effects/contraindications/side effects/interactions

(1) Taking a nitroglycerin tablet prior to exertion is an appropriate way to help prevent angina-related symptoms induced by activity.

(2) Taking no more than 3 doses in a 15-minute period of time is appropriate nitroglycerin dosing instructions.

(3) CORRECT: Nitroglycerin tablets may lose effectiveness if not protected from light. Therefore, they should be stored in dark containers such as a brown glass bottle.

(4) Blurred vision is a significant side effect of nitroglycerin therapy that should be immediately reported to the provider. Nausea and vomiting could signify low blood pressure due to the nitroglycerin.

2. The answer is 4

The nurse assesses the peripheral IV site of a client receiving a doxorubicin infusion who has suspected extravasation. After stopping the infusion and disconnecting the IV tubing, which action does the nurse do **next**?

Category: Adverse effects/contraindications/side effects/interactions

(1) Hot compresses should not be applied in an doxorubicin-associated extravasation.

(2) Although a cold compress is recommended in an doxorubicin-associated extravasation, it should not be applied until residual drug removal has been attempted.

(3) Although elevating the arm for 48 hours is recommended, this should not be done until after the residual drug has been removed.

(4) CORRECT: The first step the nurse should take is to attempt to remove any residual drug using a 1–3 mL syringe.

3. The answer is 3

The nurse prepares to discharge a client on warfarin therapy. The nurse's discharge teaching should include which instruction?

Category: Adverse effects/contraindications/side effects/interactions

(1) The intake of foods containing vitamin K should not be altered from baseline.

(2) Herbal medications may interfere with the effectiveness of warfarin.

(3) CORRECT: Alcohol can increase the anticoagulant effect of warfarin and should be avoided.

(4) Warfarin can be taken without regard to food intake, although gastrointestinal upset may be diminished if taken with food.

4. The answer is 2, 4, and 5

CORRECT OPTIONS: The client's **estimated blood loss** of at least 1,800 mL is very significant and represents about 35% of the client's blood volume. Significant loss of blood will likely require a blood transfusion. Indications for a blood transfusion include a **hemoglobin** of < 6 g/dL (60 g/L) or 6−10 g/dL (60−100 g/L) depending on the client's symptoms. The client's **hematocrit** alone is not the best determinant of a need for a blood transfusion, but in the context of a low hemoglobin and known blood loss, is another indication of a need for a blood transfusion.

INCORRECT OPTIONS: The client's dyspnea in the ED can be attributed to the hemopneumothorax, and would not be an indication of a need for a transfusion. An allergy to shellfish does not indicate a need for blood. The client's platelets are within normal limits. An elevated WBC count indicates infection, not anemia or blood loss. A history of previous transfusion does not impact the client's need for blood at this time, but could impact the client's ability to be a blood recipient.

5. The answer is 1

CORRECT OPTION: A client who has had **previous blood transfusions** may have developed antibodies which could cause a transfusion reaction when the client subsequently receives another blood product. The nurse should also ask the parents if the client had any type of reaction to the previous transfusion.

INCORRECT OPTIONS: The risk of an allergic reaction to blood products, based upon passive transfer of food allergen from donor to client, is extremely low. Neither being without a spleen nor having an appendectomy places the client at increased risk for transfusion reaction.

6. The answer is 1, 6, and 8

CORRECT OPTIONS: There must be a valid physician's order to transfuse blood products. A type and cross match order is not an order to transfuse. The order should include the **type of blood product** to be given, such as packed red blood cells (PRBC), platelets, fresh frozen plasma (FFP), or washed red blood cells. The order should also include the **volume to be given**. This may be "1 unit," etc. The exact volume may vary from unit to unit. A unit of PRBC usually ranges from 200−250 mL. Finally, the physician should specify the **rate of infusion**. The physician might prescribe "give each unit over 2 hours," or "administer over 3 hours." The physician can also specify any special conditions, such as the use of a diuretic between units of PRBCs, or placing the blood on a warmer.

INCORRECT OPTIONS: The donor number is not known until the blood product is retrieved from the blood bank. It is verified by the nurse prior to administration. The Rh factor is determined by the type and crossmatch and is also verified by the nurse when checking the blood. The type of tubing, frequency of vital signs, and size of the IV catheter needed are part of standard nursing practice and facility policy and procedure. They are not specified by a physician order.

7. See explanation for answers

Before starting the transfusion: The nurse must **ensure the consent is signed** and the procedure has been explained to the client. The nurse will **obtain and record baseline vital signs**, usually on a blood transfusion record or document. Two nurses must **verify the client's identity and check the blood compatibility information** prior to giving blood products. This may be two RNs or an RN and an LPN/LVN. INCORRECT OPTION: The adult client must have an IV catheter of at least 20−18 gauge to infuse blood, and 0.9% normal saline is the only fluid which should be given with blood. Lactated ringer (LR) and D_5W may cause hemolysis of the blood cells.

During the infusion: **PRBCs should not hang for more than 4 hours**, so the nurse must ensure the infusion is completed before that time limit. **PRBCs should always be administered using filtered tubing**. INCORRECT OPTIONS: The RN, not the LPN/LVN or a UAP, must stay with the client for the first 15−30 minutes of a transfusion, as this timeframe is when transfusion reactions are most likely to occur. IV medications and fluids are not held during a blood transfusion and are not piggybacked in or injected into transfusion tubing. The nurse will need to plan care so that the client continues to have vascular access, which may mean inserting another IV catheter in order to infuse the blood and maintain the other infusing fluids and medications.

After the infusion: The nurse should perform an assessment and carefully **listen to the lungs** for evidence of fluid volume overload or airway restriction that could occur with an allergic reaction. The nurse will also **obtain a final set of vital signs** and **document the volume of blood infused and the time the infusion ended**. INCORRECT OPTIONS: Blood tubing and the blood bag should either be disposed of in a bag designated for hazardous waste, or, in some facilities, returned to the blood bank or laboratory. A urine specimen is not routinely collected and sent after a blood transfusion. However, a urine specimen would be collected in the event of a hemolytic transfusion reaction.

8. See explanation for answers

CORRECT OPTION: The client's symptoms indicate the client is having a febrile, nonhemolytic reaction, which is the most common blood transfusion reaction. For any transfusion reaction, the nurse must **stop the blood transfusion immediately**. INCORRECT OPTIONS: The client's temperature is elevated, but the client is not hypotensive, does not have a rash or urticaria, and is exhibiting no respiratory distress. Therefore, placing the client in an upright position and encouraging the client to cough and deep breathe is unnecessary.

CORRECT OPTION: It is a priority for the nurse to **remove the blood tubing down to the catheter hub**. INCORRECT OPTIONS: When a client is having a transfusion reaction, all effort should be made to keep the client from receiving any more of the blood in the tubing. Flushing the blood tubing with 0.9% normal saline is unsafe and would introduce more blood from the tubing into the client and could make the situation worse. Removing the catheter and culturing the tip is important if an infection at the site is suspected.

CORRECT OPTION: It is also important to **replace the blood tubing with tubing that is primed with 0.9% NS** and maintain vascular access with that fluid while treating the client. INCORRECT OPTIONS: The IV catheter does not need to be removed. Therefore, it would not be appropriate to place an IV below the infusion site, and the client does not require a central venous access device.

CORRECT OPTION: For a febrile, nonhemolytic reaction, the client will need to receive an **anti-pyretic** and be monitored closely. The reaction should be carefully documented and the client would need to receive washed PRBCs for future transfusions. INCORRECT OPTIONS: A diuretic is given when a client has transfusion-associated circulatory overload (TACO), and epinephrine is given for anaphylactic reactions.

9. The answer is 1, 4, 5, 6, and 7

CORRECT OPTIONS: If the client's condition declines, the nurse must take further action. Indications of a deterioration in condition include **hypotension**, **wheezing**, **urticaria** and **itching**, a **change in the level of consciousness**, and the **presence of blood or hemoglobin in the urine**.

INCORRECT OPTIONS: A respiratory rate of 16 is normal and requires no intervention. The temperature and pain level have both decreased, indicating improvement.

10. The answer is 4

A client takes amitriptyline hydrochloride to manage neuropathic pain. The client reports severe xerostomia. Which action does the nurse ask the client to implement to help relieve the xerostomia?

Category: Adverse effects/contraindications/side effects/interactions

(1) Increasing caffeine intake will not relieve xerostomia.

(2) Decreasing fluid intake will not relieve xerostomia.

(3) Increasing dietary sodium will not relieve xerostomia.

(4) CORRECT: Strategies to reduce xerostomia (dry mouth) include increasing fluid intake and chewing sugar-free gum.

11. The answer is 2

Prior to administering digoxin 0.125 mg PO to a client diagnosed with chronic heart failure, the nurse notes that the apical pulse is 56 beats/minute. Which action should the nurse implement **next**?

Category: Adverse effects/contraindications/side effects/interactions

(1) Unless the provider's prescription specifies otherwise, when the client's apical pulse drops below 60 beats/minute, the nurse should hold the dose (not give) and notify the provider.

(2) CORRECT: Unless the provider's prescription specifies otherwise, when the client's apical pulse drops below 60 beats/minute, the nurse should hold the dose (not give) and notify the provider.

(3) Although an ECG may be indicated, it is not generally the first course of action.

(4) Although obtaining a serum digoxin level may be indicated, it is not generally the first course of action.

12. The answer is 3

The nurse reviews routes of medication administration with the client who is diagnosed with metastatic cancer. The nurse knows that the rectal route of administration is contraindicated when which manifestation is present?

Category: Adverse effects/contraindications/side effects/interactions

(1) The rectal route of administration may be preferred when a client has nausea and vomiting.

(2) The rectal route of administration may be preferred when a client has difficulty swallowing.

(3) CORRECT: The rectal route of administration should NOT be used in clients who have anal or rectal lesions, mucositis, thrombocytopenia, or neutropenia.

(4) The rectal route of administration may also be appropriate for a client who has a fever.

13. The answer is 1, 2, 4, and 5

A client is admitted for gastrointestinal bleeding. The client has a platelet count of 15,000/mm^3 (15 × 10^9/L). A platelet transfusion is prescribed by the health care provider. Which is required for platelet transfusions? **(Select all that apply.)**

Category: Blood and blood products

(1) CORRECT: The donor and recipient should be ABO-compatible.

(2) CORRECT: The donor and recipient should be Rh-compatible.

(3) Crossmatching is not typically required for platelet and plasma product transfusions because these blood products contain no red blood cells.

(4) CORRECT: Platelets are administered using specialized platelet filters. Platelets must be infused through a filter, which can be found in either a platelet or standard component administration set, which contains a 170−260 micron filter.

(5) CORRECT: Safety standards require the use of two patient identifiers such as full name and date of birth.

14. The answer is 2

A client's red blood cell transfusion is discontinued due to an acute hemolytic transfusion reaction. Which strategy **best** minimizes the client's risk of such a reaction?

Category: Blood and blood products

(1) Monitoring the client's temperature may help to promptly alert the nurse to a reaction but does not prevent it from occurring.

(2) CORRECT: The most common cause of an acute hemolytic transfusion reaction is the administration of ABO-incompatible blood. By verifying client-identifying information according to hospital policy, the nurse can minimize the risk of a client being transfused with ABO-incompatible blood.

(3) Administering meperidine may alleviate symptoms associated with a reaction but does not prevent it from developing.

(4) Administering acetaminophen may be indicated to prevent hypersensitivity reactions, but this action will not minimize the risk of an acute hemolytic transfusion reaction from taking place.

15. The answer is 2

A client is receiving a blood transfusion. The nurse observes that the client is experiencing diarrhea, abdominal pain, and chills. Which action should the nurse take **first**?

Category: Blood and blood products

(1) Assisting the client to the bathroom may be an appropriate comfort measure, but it is not the priority action.

(2) CORRECT: Signs and symptoms of a transfusion reaction may include chills, diarrhea, fever, hives, pruritus, flushing, and abdominal or back pain. The nurse's first action should be to stop the transfusion.

(3) Meperidine may alleviate rigors, which the client was not experiencing.

(4) Getting a warming blanket may be an appropriate comfort measure, but it is not the priority action.

16. The answer is 1, 2, and 5

The nurse aspirates a central venous catheter prior to drug administration but is not able to verify blood return. The nurse does not feel resistance when flushing or see any fluid leakage, swelling, or redness around the catheter site. Which of these are appropriate next steps? **(Select all that apply.)**

Category: Central venous access devices

(1) CORRECT: Flushing the catheter with saline using a 10-mL syringe and a push-pull technique are appropriate steps to try to verify blood return in a central venous catheter.

(2) CORRECT: Instructing the client to cough before reattempting aspiration is an appropriate step to try to verify blood return in a central venous catheter.

(3) Administering IV medication (particularly cytotoxic medications) and fluids should not be performed until other steps are taken to verify proper placement of the catheter by assessing for patency and blood return.

(4) Putting the client in Trendeleburg position to aspirate blood return is not an evidence-based practice.

(5) CORRECT: Initiating a declotting protocol per policy is an appropriate step to try to verify blood return in a central venous catheter.

17. The answer is 3

A client with known heparin-induced thrombocytopenia (HIT) is undergoing chemotherapy and is having a central venous access device placed. Which type of central venous access device **best** minimizes the risk of HIT-related complication?

Category: Central venous access devices

(1) A Hickman does not contain valves and is routinely flushed with heparin.

(2) A Broviac does not contain valves and is routinely flushed with heparin.

(3) CORRECT: A Groshong is a valved catheter that does not require heparin flushing.

(4) A port does not contain valves and is routinely flushed with heparin.

18. The answer is 3

A client has been instructed by the provider to increase warfarin sodium dose from 5 mg to 7.5 mg. The client only has 5-mg tablets available. How many tablets should the nurse instruct the client to take?

Category: Dose calculation

(1) Taking half a tablet would only provide 2.5 mg of warfarin sodium.

(2) Taking one tablet would only provide 5 mg of warfarin sodium.

(3) CORRECT: Taking one and a half tablets containing 5 mg of warfarin sodium each will achieve a total dose of 7.5 mg.

(4) Taking two tablets would provide 10 mg of warfarin sodium.

19. The answer is 2

The nurse prepares to set up an intravenous infusion of normal saline (NS) 1,000 mL over a 6-hour period. The tubing drop factor is 10 gtt/mL. How many gtt/minute should the nurse infuse the NS?

Category: Dose calculation

(1) 12 gtt/minute is not the correct rate of infusion.

(2) CORRECT: 28 gtt/minute is the correct rate of infusion, calculated as follows: 1,000 mL/6 hours × 10 gtt/mL/60 minute/hour = 27.8 or 28 gtt/minute.

(3) 33 gtt/minute is not the correct rate of infusion.

(4) 36 gtt/minute is not the correct rate of infusion.

20. The answer is 1

The nurse prepares a dopamine hydrochloride infusion to start at 5 mcg/kg/minute for a client who weighs 165 lb (75 kg). The dopamine is available as 400 mg in 250 mL of D_5W. How many mL/hour does the nurse set the infusion pump to administer the dopamine?

Category: Dosage calculation

(1) CORRECT: The correct rate of infusion is 14 mL/hour, arrived at as follows: Convert 400 mg/250 mL to mcg/mL by dividing 400 mg/250 mL and multiplying the result (1.6 mg/mL) by 1,000 (1,600 mcg/minute). Next, multiply the weight (75 kg) by the prescribed dose (5 mcg/kg/minute), and multiply the result (375 mcg/minute) by 60. This equals 22,500 mcg/hour. Calculate mL/hr by dividing 22,500 mcg/hour by 1,600 mcg/mL. The appropriate rate is 14 mL/hour.

(2) A rate of infusion of 16 mL/hour is not correct.

(3) A rate of infusion of 22.5 mL/hour is not correct.

(4) A rate of infusion of 37.5 mL/hour is not correct.

21. The answer is 105 mg

A client is prescribed doxorubicin 60 mg/m² as part of cancer therapy. The client is 5 ft 6 in tall, weighs 145 lb, and has a body surface area of 1.75 m². What is the correct dose that the nurse should administer the doxorubicin? Round your answer to the nearest whole number.

Category: Dosage calculation

Answer: 60 mg/m² $\times 1.75$ m² $= 105$ mg

22. The answer is 3

A client is admitted with sickle cell anemia and expresses concerns about becoming addicted to pain medicine. The nurse explains the difference between physical dependence, tolerance, and addiction. Which of these is associated with addiction?

Category: Pharmacological pain management

(1) Withdrawal symptoms when the drug is abruptly stopped are associated with physical dependence on a particular drug, not addiction.

(2) Withdrawal symptoms when the drug dose is reduced are associated with physical dependence on a particular drug, not addiction.

(3) CORRECT: Addiction is characterized by compulsive use of a drug for reasons other than therapeutic benefit.

(4) A state of adaptation is associated with tolerance to a particular drug, not addiction.

23. The answer is 2

A client has been prescribed amphetamine and dextro-amphetamine for attention-deficit/hyperactivity disorder (ADHD). The nurse explains that the client should be alert for which adverse reaction?

Category: Medication administration

(1) Adderall may be associated with weight loss, not weight gain.

(2) CORRECT: Adderall may be associated with depression.

(3) Adderall may be associated with agitation or restlessness, not somnolence.

(4) Adderall may be associated with tachycardia, not bradycardia.

24. The answer is 4, 2, 1, 3

The nurse administers a medication intramuscularly by Z-track method. Place the following steps in the appropriate order. **All options must be used.**

Category: Medication administration

(1) The third step in proper Z-track technique is to withdraw the needle.

(2) The second step in proper Z-track technique is to administer the drug IM.

(3) The last step in proper Z-track technique is to release the skin.

(4) The first step in proper Z-track technique is to displace the skin lateral to the injection site.

25. The answer is 2

A client admitted with chronic heart failure takes furosemide. Which statement, if made by the client, **best** demonstrates understanding of the side effects associated with furosemide?

Category: Medication administration

(1) Furosemide may be associated with hypotension.

(2) CORRECT: Furosemide may decrease potassium. Eating foods rich in potassium is advised. Bananas and apricots are good sources of dietary potassium.

(3) Furosemide may be associated with nocturia. It is best taken early in the morning.

(4) Furosemide may be taken without regard to timing of food intake.

26. The answer is 1

The nurse administers vancomycin 1 g every 12 hours. Which statement indicates that the client may be experiencing an ototoxic adverse reaction?

Category: Adverse effects/contraindications/side effects/interactions

(1) CORRECT: Tinnitus may indicate that ototoxicity is developing.

(2) A feeling that the IV is burning is not related to the development of ototoxicity.

(3) Itchiness of the skin is not related to the development of ototoxicity.

(4) The sensation of a bad taste in the mouth is not related to the development of ototoxicity.

27. The answer is 2

A client is prescribed lisinopril. Which instruction should the nurse give the client to minimize a potential adverse reaction of lisinopril?

Category: Expected actions/outcomes

(1) Eating fruits and vegetables high in iron will not minimize the side effects of lisinopril.

(2) CORRECT: The hypotensive effect of lisinopril may be reduced by rising slowly from a lying to a sitting position.

(3) Increasing fluid intake will not minimize the side effects of lisinopril.

(4) Avoiding aspirin-containing drugs will not minimize the side effects of lisinopril.

28. See explanation for answers

CORRECT OPTIONS: The client is at high risk for developing **hypovolemic shock**. The client has developed absolute hypovolemia due to **inadequate fluid intake** coupled with diuresis. **Excessive diuresis** occurs more commonly in older adult clients, clients with CKD, and clients taking nonsteroidal anti-inflammatory drugs (NSAIDs). The client's hypovolemia is evidenced by a falling blood pressure, weight loss, cool skin, pallor, faint pedal pulses, decreased urine output, and confusion. The client may not develop tachycardia in early shock due to taking a beta blocker and calcium channel blocker.

INCORRECT OPTIONS: The client is not at high risk for hyperkalemia, due to the potassium loss which has likely occurred with diuretic use. The client's temperature is normal and lung sounds are clear. Although the client has been ill, the client's symptoms and history are more consistent with volume loss than with worsening infection. Eating a low-sodium diet will not contribute to volume loss but will decrease the edema and fluid retention common in heart failure. Living in an independent living facility places the client at a higher risk of infection, not hypovolemia. Taking a beta blocker will not result in hypovolemia, hyperkalemia, or sepsis. The client's symptoms and vital sign findings do not suggest medication adverse effects; experiencing diuresis with furosemide is an expected medication effect. There are no symptoms of allergic reaction. While the client might have some nausea with a new medication, the client's medications are unchanged except for an increased dose of diuretic.

29. The answer is 2

The nurse administers doxorubicin IV push to a client with breast cancer. Which of these should the nurse explain is to be expected during therapy with doxorubicin?

Category: Expected actions/outcomes

(1) Burning at the IV site during administration is not a side effect of doxorubicin.

(2) CORRECT: A common side effect of doxorubicin is red-colored urine.

(3) Permanent alopecia is not a side effect of doxorubicin.

(4) Teeth discoloration is not a side effect of doxorubicin.

30. The answer is 1, 2, 4, and 5

The nurse prepares to infused total parenteral nutrition (TPN) to a client. Which actions are appropriate for the nurse to perform in TPN administration? (**Select all that apply.**)

Category: Parenteral/intravenous therapies

(1) CORRECT: Aseptic technique is observed during handling and administration of TPN to prevent infection.

(2) CORRECT: A designated filter is used in infusing TPN. The size and type of the filter depends on whether the TPN contains fat emulsion.

(3) A surgical mask may be worn by the client during central line dressing of the TPN catheter. It is not indicated when the nurse is administering the TPN.

(4) CORRECT: Labeling all IV tubings with the date and time is part of best practices in IV therapies.

(5) CORRECT: Checking the expiration date of TPN is an essential best practice. The nurse should also check the bag for leaks and obvious impurities.

[CHAPTER 10]

PHYSIOLOGICAL INTEGRITY: REDUCTION OF RISK POTENTIAL

Reduction of risk potential involves ways in which you can help to reduce the likelihood that clients will develop complications or health problems related to existing conditions, diagnostic tests, treatments, or other procedures.

On the NCLEX-RN® exam, you can expect 12 percent of the questions to relate to Reduction of Risk Potential. Exam content for this category includes, but is not limited to, the following areas:

- Changes/abnormalities in vital signs
- Diagnostic tests
- Laboratory values
- Potential for alterations in body systems
- Potential for complications of diagnostic tests/treatments/procedures
- Potential for complications from surgical procedures and health alterations
- System specific assessments
- Therapeutic procedures

Now let's review some of the most important concepts related to these subtopics.

Changes/Abnormalities in Vital Signs

You must be able to assess client vital signs and intervene when those vital signs are abnormal. Abnormal vital signs include fever, hypertension, bradycardia, and tachypnea.

In order to properly assess vital signs and recognize abnormalities, apply your knowledge of the client's pathophysiology. Evaluate invasive monitoring data, such as pulmonary artery pressure and intracranial pressure.

Diagnostic Tests

It is important to understand the general principles of specimen collection. Ideally, routine specimen collection should take place early morning before a client has any food or fluids. If fasting is required, it is usually for an 8- to 12-hour period prior to the test. Use standard precautions and aseptic techniques to protect yourself and your clients from infection.

Label specimens with the client's name, date, exact time of collection, and type of specimen. On the laboratory requisition slip, include the client's name, age, gender, room number, physician's name, possible diagnosis, tests requested, and any factors that might interfere with the test results. To avoid hemolysis, do not shake blood specimens unless instructed to do so.

All specimens should be sent to the lab promptly. Values, or test results, that fall within predetermined laboratory reference ranges are considered normal. Abnormal values are outside the reference range, and critical values are far enough outside of the reference range that they can cause immediate risk to the client. Critical values are called in to the nurse's station and should be acted on immediately. You may be responsible for informing the client's physician about these critical lab values.

You should understand the purpose of and preparation for a variety of diagnostic tests, such as the following:

- General
  - Biopsy
  - Computed tomography (CT) scan
  - Fluoroscopy
  - Magnetic resonance imaging (MRI)
  - Nuclear scan (radionuclide imaging or radioisotope scan)
  - Positron emission tomography (PET) scan
  - Ultrasonography
  - X-rays
- Respiratory
  - Bronchoscopy
  - Pulmonary function tests
  - Ventilation scan (pulmonary ventilation scan)
- Cardiovascular
  - Angiography (angiogram)
  - Cardiac catheterization
  - Echocardiography (echocardiogram)
  - Electrocardiography (electrocardiogram or ECG, EKG)
  - Holter monitoring
  - Stress/exercise tests
  - Venography (venogram), also called phlebography
- Renal/Urinary
  - Cystoscopy and cystography (cystogram)
  - Intravenous pyelography (IVP)
  - Retrograde pyelography (retrograde pyelogram)

- Neurological
    - Electroencephalography (electroencephalogram or EEG)
    - Myelography (myelogram)
- Musculoskeletal
    - Arthroscopy
    - Bone densitometry
- Gastrointestinal
    - Barium enema
    - Cholangiography
    - Cholecystography (oral)
    - Colonoscopy
    - Endoscopic retrograde cholangiopancreatography (ERCP)
    - Esophagogastroduodenoscopy
    - Gastric analysis
    - Gastrointestinal (GI) series
- Reproductive
    - Fetal nonstress test
    - Amniocentesis
    - Hysteroscopy
    - Mammography
    - Papanicolaou smear (Pap smear)
- Integumentary
    - Tuberculin skin test
    - Other skin tests (allergy)

Know how to compare client diagnostic findings with pretest results, and how to perform a variety of diagnostic tests, including:

- Oxygen saturation
- Glucose monitoring
- Testing for occult blood
- Gastric pH
- Urine specific gravity
- Arterial blood gases
- Serum electrolytes

You should also know how to perform an electrocardiogram. This test measures electrical activity of the heart and detects cardiac dysrhythmias and electrolyte imbalances. Electrodes are placed on the client's extremities and chest, and the electrical activity of the heart is recorded with each heartbeat.

Cardiac waveforms are recorded in 12 leads. There are no food and fluid restrictions on clients getting an electrocardiogram, and no preconsent is needed for the test. The client should be asked to lie down and to expose arms and legs for lead placement. It is your responsibility to make note of any medications the client is taking that might impact the test results. The client should be told to relax their muscles and to breathe normally during the procedure, which is painless.

In addition to performing an electrocardiogram on an adult, you should know how to perform fetal heart monitoring using computer-assisted auditory assessment. This involves inserting a fetal scalp electrode through the client's cervix and attaching it to the epidermis of the fetus. You should also be able to monitor the results of additional maternal and fetal diagnostic tests, including nonstress tests, an amniocentesis, and an ultrasound.

Laboratory Values

You must be familiar with a wide range of laboratory values, which include the following:

- Arterial blood gases, including pH, pO_2, pCO_2, SaO_2, and HCO_3
- Serum electrolytes
- Glucose studies, such as fasting blood glucose, random blood glucose, two-hour postprandial blood glucose, glucose tolerance test (GTT), and glycosylated hemoglobin (HgbA1C)
- Coagulation studies, such as prothrombin time (PT), international normalized ratio (INR), and activated partial thromboplastin time (APTT)
- Complete blood count (CBC), which includes hematocrit (Hct), hemoglobin (Hgb), RBC count and index, platelet count and mean volume, and white blood cell (WBC) count and differential
- Cardiovascular function studies, which include serum lipids, creatine kinase (CK) or creatine phosphokinase (CPK), lactic dehydrogenase (LDH), and troponins
- Thyroid function studies, such as thyroxine (T4), triiodothyronine (T3), and thyroid-stimulating hormone (TSH)
- Renal function studies, such as blood, urea, nitrogen (BUN) and serum creatinine
- Urinalysis, which includes the detection of nitrites and leukocyte esterase
- Liver function studies, such as alanine aminotransferase (ALT) or serum glutamic-pyruvic transaminase (SGPT), aspartate aminotransferase (AST) or serum glutamic-oxaloacetic transaminase (SGOT), bilirubin, and ammonia
- Pancreatic enzymes, such as amylase and lipase
- GI function studies, such as albumin, alkaline phosphatase, total protein, and uric acid
- Immune function studies, such as human immunodeficiency virus (HIV) test, CD4 T cell counts, CD4 to CD8 ratios, and viral load testing

You should know how to measure the amount of drug circulating in the client's bloodstream, usually before the scheduled daily dose of the drug. Trough levels are drawn when the dose is at its lowest, right before the next scheduled drug administration. Peak levels are drawn when the dose is at its highest (30 minutes after infusion). You must make sure drug levels remain within the proper therapeutic range. If you find an abnormal level, alert the prescribing physician immediately.

In addition to knowing laboratory values, and how to measure drug levels, you should be able to recognize deviations from normal values of the following:

- Albumin (blood)
- ALT (SGPT) (liver enzyme test)
- Ammonia
- AST (SGOT) (liver enzyme test)
- Bilirubin
- Bleeding time
- Calcium (total)
- Cholesterol (HDL and LDL)
- Creatinine
- Digoxin
- Erythrocyte sedimentation rate (ESR), to diagnose conditions associated with inflammation
- Lithium
- Magnesium
- Partial thromboplastin time (PTT) and APTT
- INR
- Phosphorous/phosphate
- Protein (total)
- PT (clotting)
- Urine (albumin, pH, WBC count, differential)

Know how to obtain blood specimens peripherally or through a central line. Also know how to obtain specimens other than blood for diagnostic testing. This includes procedures for getting specimens from wound cultures and stool and urine samples.

Monitor client laboratory values and provide clients with information about the purpose and procedures for prescribed laboratory tests.

Potential for Alterations in Body Systems

It is important to be able to compare current client data to baseline client data, particularly to evaluate symptoms of illness/disease. Identify client potential for aspiration (such as feeding tube, sedation, and swallowing difficulties), skin breakdown potential due to immobility, nutritional status or incontinence, and clients with an increased risk for insufficient vascular perfusion (such as clients with immobilized limbs, who are postsurgery, or who have diabetes). You should also be able to provide treatments and/or care in response.

Monitor client output for changes from baseline (nasogastric tube, emesis, stools, and urine) and educate clients about methods to prevent complications associated with activity level or diagnosed illness/disease (such as contractures, and foot care for clients with diabetes mellitus).

Potential for Complications of Diagnostic Tests/Treatments/Procedures

You must assess a client for complications or abnormal responses following a diagnostic test or procedure, such as monitoring the client for signs of bleeding. Know how to position clients to prevent complications following tests, treatments, and procedures, by, for example, elevating the head of the bed or immobilizing an extremity. When you see a complication, it is important to recommend a change in tests, procedures, and/or treatment prescriptions based on the client's response to the initial testing and treatment.

You should be able to insert an oral/nasogastric tube, and maintain tube patency. Be able to recognize potential circulatory complications (such as hemorrhage, embolus, and shock) and know how to intervene to manage them. Examples of measures you can take to manage, prevent, or lessen possible complications include restricting fluids or sodium, raising side rails of the client's bed, or implementing suicide precautions.

You also need to know how to provide care for clients undergoing electroconvulsive therapy. This includes monitoring the airway, assessing for side effects, and teaching the client about the procedure. You should be able to intervene to prevent aspiration, and to prevent potential neurological complications. Signs of neurological complications include foot drop, numbness, and tingling. Make sure to evaluate and document responses for all procedures and treatments.

Potential for Complications from Surgical Procedures and Health Alterations

Apply your knowledge of pathophysiology to monitor for complications from surgical procedures and health alterations. For example, you should recognize signs of thrombocytopenia. You should also evaluate the client's response to postoperative interventions aimed at preventing complications, such as reducing the risk of aspiration and promoting venous return and mobility.

System-Specific Assessments

Assess clients for abnormal peripheral pulses and neurological status after a procedure or treatment. Neurological status can be assessed by checking level of consciousness and evaluating muscle strength and mobility. You should also be able to assess clients for peripheral edema, hypoglycemia, and hyperglycemia.

It is also important to identify factors that could result in delayed wound healing and to implement appropriate treatment in response, and/or to notify the primary care provider.

Perform a risk assessment for sensory impairment, falls, level of mobility, and skin integrity. Once initial assessments are complete, perform focused assessments and reassessments based on initial findings.

Therapeutic Procedures

When caring for clients undergoing therapeutic procedures, assess client response to recovery from local, regional, or general anesthesia.

Educate clients about treatments and procedures, and home management and care. The education may include preoperative and/or postoperative instructions to clients and families.

Monitor a client before, during, and after a procedure or surgery, and provide preoperative and intra-operative care (positioning, maintaining sterile field, and operative assessment). To prevent further injury while moving a client with a musculoskeletal condition, for example, use the log-rolling technique or an abduction pillow.

Chapter Quiz

1. The nurse reviews the medical record of a client after surgery for removal of the parathyroid glands. The client reports difficulty swallowing and a feeling of "pins and needles." Which laboratory value is consistent with this finding?

   1. Decreased calcium.
   2. Increased lipase.
   3. Decreased potassium.
   4. Increased sodium.

2. A client is one day post-op for abdominal surgery. The nurse teaches the client techniques to reduce pain when moving, coughing, or deep breathing. Which client statement indicates to the nurse an accurate understanding of the information presented?

   1. "I can start exercising my limbs as soon as you medicate me."
   2. "I will just lie here for a few days until the pain goes away."
   3. "I will use the side rail for support when I move or turn."
   4. "I will ask for pain medication only when necessary."

3. The nurse answers a call light from a client who is 2 days post-op for abdominal surgery. The client states, "I coughed and heard this pop." The nurse assesses the surgical site and observes dehiscence of the wound. Which action should the nurse take **first**?

   1. Stay with the client and have a colleague notify the provider.
   2. Help the client to lie with the head slightly elevated and with knees bent.
   3. Apply warm, sterile normal saline soaks over the operative wound.
   4. Help the client to sit upright, and obtain a full set of vital signs.

4. The nurse admits a client who fell at home. The nurse assesses the client's cerebellar function. Which question should the nurse ask the client?

   1. "Who is the current president of the United States?"
   2. "Do you have trouble swallowing fluids or foods?"
   3. "Do you have any leg muscle pain?"
   4. "Do you have problems with balance?"

5. A client with a history of myasthenia gravis is admitted to the medical-surgical unit. Which test should the nurse expect to be prescribed for this client? **(Select all that apply.)**

   1. Tensilon test.
   2. Nerve conduction studies.
   3. Lumbar puncture.
   4. Electroencephalogram (EEG).
   5. Electromyography (EMG).

6. A client with a history of atherosclerosis reports abdominal tenderness during deep palpation. The nurse notices a pulsating mass in the periumbilical area. Which potential cause does the nurse suspect?

   1. Appendicitis.
   2. Abdominal aortic aneurysm.
   3. Acute cholecystitis.
   4. Paralytic ileus.

7. A client is in the emergency department with suspected deep vein thrombosis (DVT) of the left leg. The nurse starts IV heparin as prescribed. Which action is **least** likely to be included in the plan of care for this client?

   1. Ambulate the client as tolerated.
   2. Monitor activated partial thromboplastin time (aPTT).
   3. Administer analgesics as prescribed.
   4. Report any signs of bleeding to the provider.

8. The nurse cares for a client with a history of chronic liver disease and cirrhosis of the liver. Lab values reveal rising ammonia levels. Which treatment should the nurse question?

    1. High-carbohydrate diet.
    2. Protein 100 g/day.
    3. Neomycin sulfate.
    4. Potassium supplements.

9. The laboratory values of a client reveal the presence of hepatitis B surface antigens and hepatitis B antibodies. Which laboratory result should the nurse also expect to see? **(Select all that apply.)**

    1. Elevated serum albumin.
    2. Decreased serum globulin.
    3. Elevated serum transaminate (ALT and AST).
    4. Prolonged prothrombin time (PT).
    5. Decreased urine bilirubin.

10. The nurse assesses a client with Addison disease. The nurse expects to find which manifestation?

    1. Anorexia.
    2. Weight gain.
    3. Yellow skin coloration.
    4. A craving for sweets.

11. A client is having a tonic-clonic seizure. Which action should the nurse take **first**?

    1. Check the client's breathing.
    2. Remove objects from the client's surroundings.
    3. Place a tongue blade in the client's mouth.
    4. Restrain the client's arms.

Refer to the Case Study to answer the next six questions.

The nurse is providing care for an 89-year-old client in an ambulatory surgical center.

| Admission Notes | Nurse's Notes |

1215: The client is undergoing a colonoscopy for evaluation of changes in bowel pattern and habits that have been occurring over the past several months. The client has been NPO (nothing by mouth) since the previous evening and has completed a bowel prep using laxatives. The client has mild memory decline but has no cognitive impairments. The client lives with an adult child, is socially and physically active, and walks two miles every day. Additionally, the client has hearing and vision deficits and wears hearing aids and glasses.

Past history: Benign prostatic hyperplasia (BPH), hypertension, coronary artery disease (CAD), osteoarthritis. No allergies.

Admission Vital Signs	Results
BP	110/62 mmHg
Heart rate	88, regular
Respiratory rate	20, regular
Temperature (oral)	97.4° F (36.33° C)
Pulse oximetry	96% on room air

| Admission Notes | Nurse's Notes |

1300: Client received from colonoscopy. Peripheral IV intact at keep vein open (KVO) rate. Site without redness or edema.

Assessment	Client Finding
General	Calm, cooperative affect. Is not wearing glasses or hearing aids.
Neurological	Sleeping, rouses to voice stimuli, oriented to person and place. Needs reorienting to time and situation. Speech flow is slow, but understandable. Pupils equal round and reactive to light (PERRL).
Integument	Skin intact, pale, warm, and dry. Hands and feet are cool to touch. Dry oral mucous membranes. Decreased turgor.
Cardiovascular	S1 and S2 auscultated, regular rhythm, no murmurs. Capillary refill less than 2 seconds. 1+ radial pulses, equal.
Respiratory	Low pitched vesicular breath sounds bilaterally. Non labored breathing.
Abdomen	Soft, flat, nontender. Bowel sounds present × 4.
Musculoskeletal	Moves all extremities. Joint pain and stiffness in hips and knees bilaterally. Muscle strength 4/5 bilaterally.

Vital Signs	Results 1300
BP	90/60 mmHg
Heart rate	104, regular
Respiratory rate	20, regular
Temperature (oral)	97.6° F (36.4° C)
Pulse oximetry	95% on room air

12. The nurse is monitoring the client after the colonoscopy procedure. The nurse reviews the admission notes and documents nurse's notes and vital signs at 1300.

The nurse is concerned about which **4** assessment findings?

1. Joint pain and stiffness in hips and knees.
2. Blood pressure, 90/60 mmHg.
3. Heart rate 104.
4. Vision and hearing deficits.
5. Mild memory decline.
6. 1+ radial pulses.
7. Client age, 89.

Admission Notes   Nurse's Notes   Vital Signs

Vital Signs	1315	1330	1345
BP	88/60	86/58	82/56
Heart rate	110, regular	114, regular	120, regular
Respiratory rate	22, regular	24, regular	24, regular
Temperature (oral)		97.7° F (36.5° C)	
Pulse oximetry	94% on room air	94% on room air	94% on room air

13. The nurse continues to monitor the client's vital signs every 15 minutes.

    Complete the following sentence by choosing from the list of options.

    The client is most likely experiencing [Select from list 1] as evidenced by [Select from list 2] and [Select from list 3].

(1)	(2)	(3)
orthopnea	hypotension	S1 and S2, regular rhythm
hypovolemia	capillary refill less than 2 seconds	tachycardia
orthostatic hypotension	low pitched vesicular breath sounds	sleeping, rouses to voice stimuli

14. The nurse reports the client's vital signs to the physician.

    Drag the choices below to fill in each blank in the following sentence. Each choice will only be used once.

    The nurse determines that the client's vital signs indicate an increased risk for developing _____ [Select from the list], _____ [Select from the list], and _____ [Select from the list].

confusion
hyperactive reflexes
heart failure
pulmonary edema
hypovolemic shock
oliguria

15. The nurse plans care for the client. For each potential nursing goal, specify if the goal is indicated or not indicated in the client's plan of care.

Potential Nursing Goal	Indicated	Not Indicated
Restore vascular volume	○	○
Reduce injury from falls	○	○
Maintain oxygenation status	○	○
Reduce infection with antibiotics	○	○
Achieve normal vital signs	○	○

16. The nurse implements the care plan. Which action is included? **(Select all that apply.)**

    1. Administer and monitor 0.9% normal saline 500 mL fluid bolus intravenous (IV) as prescribed.
    2. Provide high flow oxygen per Venturi mask.
    3. Monitor for changes in capillary refill, peripheral pulses, and skin color and temperature.
    4. Report changes in mental status.
    5. Administer epinephrine as prescribed.
    6. Report changes in blood pressure, respirations, pulse rate, pulse rhythm, and pulse oximetry.
    7. Have client sit on side of bed and dangle feet prior to standing.
    8. Monitor EKG continuously.

17. The nurse prepares the client for discharge. For each assessment below, specify the client findings that indicate nursing care has been effective. Each assessment may support more than 1 client finding.

Assessment	Client Findings
Neurological	☐ Awake, oriented × 4. ☐ PERRL. ☐ Speech is fluid and is understandable.
Cardiovascular	☐ 2+ radial pulses, equal. ☐ Skin, warm, and dry. ☐ Sitting on the side of the bed with feet dangling, no dizziness.
Respiratory	☐ Lung sounds clear bilaterally. ☐ Slight dyspnea at rest. ☐ Chest expansion full and equal.
Vital Signs	☐ BP 108/70 mmHg. ☐ Heart rate, 90 regular. ☐ Respiratory rate, 24 regular.

18. A client is admitted to the hospital with a pressure injury involving full-thickness loss extending to the bone. The nurse documents the pressure injury as being at which stage?

   1. Stage 1.
   2. Stage 2.
   3. Stage 3.
   4. Stage 4.

19. A client diagnosed with Raynaud disease experiences an acute attack. The nurse should anticipate to find which assessment finding?

   1. Involuntary muscle contractions and twitching.
   2. Unilateral facial weakness and drooping mouth.
   3. Tingling of fingers and blanching at the fingertips.
   4. New onset of photophobia and double vision.

20. The provider prescribes a CT scan of the client's chest with IV contrast. Which finding in the client's history should the nurse report to the provider?

   1. Hypertension
   2. Allergy to shellfish.
   3. Urinary tract infection (UTI).
   4. Allergy to penicillin.

21. The nurse cares for a client with severe bone marrow depression due to chemotherapy. Which nursing diagnosis takes priority in the client's care plan?

   1. Imbalanced nutrition.
   2. Potential for infection.
   3. Pain.
   4. Potential for injury.

22. The nurse prepares to discharge a client after a sickle-cell anemia crisis. Which instruction should the nurse provide to the client to avoid future crises? **(Select all that apply.)**

   1. Limit fluid intake.
   2. Avoid strenuous exercise.
   3. Apply cold compresses to painful areas.
   4. Take pain medications as prescribed.
   5. Avoid tight clothing.

Refer to the Case Study to answer the next question.

The nurse is caring for an adult client on the medical surgical unit.

| History | Flow Sheets | Nurse's Notes |

The client was admitted 4 days ago with nausea, vomiting, fever, and abdominal pain. A computed tomography (CT) of the abdomen with contrast was performed and confirmed a ruptured appendix. The client underwent an exploratory laparotomy with appendectomy, then was admitted to the medical surgical unit. One day postoperatively, the client developed increasing abdominal pain, and another CT of the abdomen confirmed a large pelvic abscess. The client was taken to radiology and the abscess was drained under fluoroscopy. The client was placed on intravenous vancomycin 1 gram every 12 hours and piperacillin/tazobactam 3.375 g IV every 6 hours.

The client has no known medication or food allergies. Previous medical history includes a diagnosis of obesity, hypertension, and type 2 diabetes mellitus. The client's home medications include:

Home Medications	Dose	Route	Frequency
Lisinopril	20 mg	PO	Once daily
Amlodipine	5 mg	PO	Once daily
Metformin	500 mg	PO	Twice daily
Ibuprofen	400 mg	PO	Every 6–12 hours

| History | Flow Sheets | Nurse's Notes |

24 -Hour Intake and Output	Post Op Day 1	Post Op Day 2	Post Op Day 3
IV Fluids	3200 mL	2400 mL	2200 mL
IV Piggyback	300 mL	300 mL	300 mL
PO Intake	0	200 mL	110 mL
TOTAL Intake	**3500 mL**	**2900 mL**	**2610 mL**
Urine	2800 mL	2100 mL	1800 mL
NG Drainage	600 mL	100 mL/DC	0
Stool	0	0	× 6
TOTAL Output	**3400 mL**	**2200 mL**	**1800 + mL**

History	Flow Sheets	Nurse's Notes

The client is awake and alert. Orientation intact. Client is on a "no added carbohydrate soft diet," but appetite has been poor since nasogastric (NG) tube removed 2 days ago. The client reports nausea today and is taking nothing by mouth except for ice and sips of water with PO medications. All home medications except ibuprofen have been continued. IV 0.9% normal saline (NS) with 10 mEq KCl/L infusing at 100 mL/hour to left forearm. Skin warm, dry. Mucous membranes dry. Lung sounds clear, diminished in bases bilaterally. Clear S1 S2. Capillary refill 2 seconds. 1+ pulses in lower extremities bilaterally.

Abdomen firm, dressing intact to lower right quadrant with moderate amount serous drainage. Abdominal wound is open with packing. Dressing must be changed every 4–6 hours due to large amounts of drainage. No odor detected. Bowel sounds present throughout. Client voiding to urinal, dark amber urine. Client reports having loose, watery brown stools yesterday afternoon and evening. The client is receiving hydromorphone 2 mg IV every 4 hours PRN pain. Last medicated 1 hour ago.

23. The nurse reviews the client's history and flow sheets, and documents an assessment.

The nurse recognizes that the client is at high risk for developing acute kidney injury due to which factor? **(Select all that apply.)**

1. History of diabetes mellitus.
2. History of hypertension.
3. Taking metformin.
4. Receiving vancomycin IV.
5. History of taking ibuprofen.
6. Receiving contrast medium.
7. Taking lisinopril.
8. Obesity.
9. Having diarrhea.

24. The nurse performs an assessment on a client who has cirrhosis. Which signs and symptoms should the nurse expect to see? **(Select all that apply.)**

   1. Dull abdominal ache.

   2. Cyanosis.

   3. Poor tissue turgor.

   4. Bruises.

   5. Fruity breath.

25. The nurse prepares to administer a red blood cell transfusion to a client. Which statement is part of blood transfusion best practices?

   1. The client should be monitored for at least 1 hour after the start of the transfusion.

   2. The transfusion should be completed within 2 hours using an intravenous pump.

   3. The transfusion should be started within 30 minutes of the blood's arrival from the blood bank.

   4. The only solution that should be added to blood or blood components is 0.45% sodium chloride.

26. The nurse provides discharge teaching to a client after an acute attack of primary gout. Which foods should the nurse teach the client to avoid to prevent future attacks?

   1. Cauliflower, asparagus, and mushrooms.

   2. Anchovies, liver, and lentils.

   3. Cherries, strawberries, and blueberries.

   4. Cereal, pasta, and rice.

27. The nurse cares for a client who reports substernal pain radiating to the arm and jaw, shortness of breath, and a feeling of impending doom. The client had a stroke one month ago. The client's vital signs are blood pressure 146/72 mmHg, heart rate 128/minute, and respirations 36/minute. The 12-lead ECG reveals evolving acute myocardial infarction (MI). Which prescription should the nurse question?

   1. Beta-adrenergic blocker.

   2. Morphine for pain.

   3. IV nitroglycerin.

   4. Thrombolytic therapy.

28. The nurse performs a 12-lead ECG on a client who has come to the emergency department reporting chest pain. Where should the nurse place the electrode for lead V1?

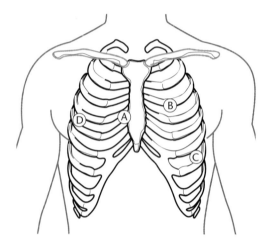

   1. A.

   2. B.

   3. C.

   4. D.

29. The nurse assesses a client admitted with a stroke. Which lobe of the cerebral hemisphere is involved in the control of voluntary muscle movement, including those necessary for speech and swallowing?

   1. Frontal.

   2. Parietal.

   3. Temporal.

   4. Occipital.

30. The nurse prepares to do the Heimlich maneuver on a client who is choking. Arrange the following steps in the order the nurse should perform them. **All options must be used.**

   1. Make a fist with one hand.

   2. Stand behind the client.

   3. Wrap the other arm around the client and grasp the fist with the hand.

   4. Place thumb toward the client, below the rib cage and above the waist, and wrap this arm around the client.

   5. Ask the client, "Are you choking?"

   6. Thrust upward 6–10 times.

Chapter Quiz Answers and Explanations

1. The answer is 1

The nurse reviews the medical record of a client after surgery for removal of the parathyroid glands. The client reports difficulty swallowing and a feeling of "pins and needles." Which laboratory value is consistent with this finding?

Category: Laboratory values

(1) CORRECT: Hypocalcemia is an indication of hypo-parathyroidism; symptoms include dysphagia and paresthesia.

(2) Lipase levels are not indicators of hypoparathyroidism. Lipase is increased in pancreatitis.

(3) Potassium levels are not indicators of hypoparathyroidism. Low potassium can be seen in diuretic use, vomiting, and diarrhea.

(4) Sodium levels are not indicators of hypoparathyroidism. Increased sodium is consistent with dehydration.

2. The answer is 3

A client is one day post-op for abdominal surgery. The nurse teaches the client techniques to reduce pain when moving, coughing, or deep breathing. Which client statement indicates to the nurse an accurate understanding of the information presented?

Category: Therapeutic procedures

(1) The client should wait until the medication has taken effect.

(2) The client should be encouraged and assisted to frequently move after surgery, unless clinically contraindicated.

(3) CORRECT: The client should use the side rail for support and move slowly and smoothly without sudden movement.

(4) The client should ask for pain medication as needed, such as prior to activity when pain is anticipated.

3. The answer is 1

The nurse answers a call light from a client who is 2 days post-op for abdominal surgery. The client states, "I coughed and heard this pop." The nurse assesses the surgical site and observes dehiscence of the wound. Which action should the nurse take **first**?

Category: Therapeutic procedures; Potential for complications of diagnostic tests/treatments/procedures; Potential for complications from surgical procedures and health alterations

(1) CORRECT: The nurse should stay with the client and have a colleague notify the health care provider first.

(2) The second thing the nurse should do is help the client lie with the head slightly elevated (low-Fowler position) with knees bent in to decrease abdominal tension and monitor the client's vital signs.

(3) The nurse should not place anything on the wound unless it has eviscerated, and then cover the extruding wound contents with warm, sterile normal saline soaks.

(4) The nurse would not help the client to sit up. Instead, the nurse would help the client to a low-Fowler position with knees bent in to decrease abdominal tension and monitor the client's vital signs. A set of vital signs should be obtained after the provider has been notified.

4. The answer is 4

The nurse admits a client who fell at home. The nurse assesses the client's cerebellar function. Which question should the nurse ask the client?

Category: System specific assessments

(1) This question will not help the nurse assess the client's cerebellar function, which is related to balance and coordination.

(2) Trouble swallowing fluids or foods is not related to cerebellar function.

(3) Muscle pain is not related to cerebellar function.

(4) CORRECT: The nurse evaluates cerebellar function by testing the client's balance and coordination.

5. The answer is 1, 2, and 5

A client with a history of myasthenia gravis is admitted to the medical-surgical unit. Which test should the nurse expect to be prescribed for this client? **(Select all that apply.)**

Category: Diagnostic tests; Potential for complications of diagnostic tests/treatments/procedures

(1) CORRECT: Myasthenia gravis produces sporadic but progressive weakness and abnormal fatigue in skeletal muscles. The Tensilon test confirms the diagnosis by temporarily improving muscle function after an IV injection of edrophonium or neostigmine (an anticholinesterase).

(2) CORRECT: Nerve conduction studies test for receptor antibodies.

(3) Lumbar puncture is a test used to diagnose multiple sclerosis, a result of progressive demyelination of the white matter of the brain and spinal cord. It is not indicated in myasthenia gravis.

(4) An EEG is a test used to diagnose multiple sclerosis, a result of progressive demyelination of the white matter of the brain and spinal cord. An EEG is also used to diagnose seizure or epilepsy. It is not indicated in myasthenia gravis.

(5) CORRECT: An EMG helps differentiate nerve disorders from muscle disorders.

6. The answer is 2

A client with a history of atherosclerosis reports abdominal tenderness during deep palpation. The nurse notices a pulsating mass in the periumbilical area. Which of these does the nurse suspect?

Category: System specific assessments; Potential for complications of diagnostic tests/treatments/procedures; Potential for complications from surgical procedures and health alterations

(1) Signs of appendicitis include loss of appetite, nausea, vomiting, fever, board-like abdominal rigidity, and increasingly severe abdominal spasm.

(2) CORRECT: Signs of abdominal aortic aneurysm include asymptomatic pulsating mass in the periumbilical area, possible systolic bruit over the aorta on auscultation, possible abdominal tenderness on deep palpation, and lumbar pain that radiates to the flank and groin (imminent rupture).

(3) Signs of acute cholecystitis include midepigastric or right upper quadrant pain radiating to the back or referred to the right scapula.

(4) Signs of paralytic ileus include severe abdominal distention, vomiting, and severe constipation.

7. The answer is 1

A client is in the emergency department with suspected deep vein thrombosis (DVT) of the left leg. The nurse starts IV heparin as prescribed. Which action is **least** likely to be included in the plan of care for this client?

Category: Potential for complications of diagnostic tests/treatments/procedures

(1) CORRECT: Treatment aims to prevent complications, relieve pain, and prevent recurrence. Due to risk for embolization, ambulation is not allowed until the provider approves walking.

(2) Monitoring the aPTT while receiving heparin infusion is an appropriate action to take. This will ensure that the aPTT therapeutic goal is achieved.

(3) Analgesics are an appropriate action to take.

(4) The nurse should report to the provider any signs of bleeding while the client is on heparin infusion.

8. The answer is 2

The nurse cares for a client with a history of chronic liver disease and cirrhosis of the liver. Lab values reveal rising ammonia levels. Which treatment should the nurse question?

Category: Laboratory values

(1) Adequate calorie intake (3,000 cal/day) in the form of glucose or carbohydrates helps prevent protein catabolism.

(2) CORRECT: Rising blood ammonia levels can result from cirrhosis, and hepatic encephalopathy follows. Protein is restricted to 40 g/day and increased up to 100 g/day as symptoms improve.

(3) Neomycin is administered to remove ammonia-producing substances from the GI tract and suppress bacterial ammonia production.

(4) Potassium supplements are administered to help correct alkalosis from increased ammonia levels.

9. The answer is 3 and 4

The laboratory values of a client reveal the presence of hepatitis B surface antigens and hepatitis B antibodies. Which laboratory result should the nurse also expect to see? **(Select all that apply.)**

Category: Laboratory values

(1) In viral hepatitis, serum albumin levels are low.

(2) In viral hepatitis, serum globulin levels are high.

(3) CORRECT: In viral hepatitis, serum transaminate levels are elevated.

(4) CORRECT: In viral hepatitis, prothrombin time is prolonged.

(5) In viral hepatitis, urine bilirubin levels are elevated.

10. The answer is 1

The nurse assesses a client with Addison disease. The nurse expects to find which manifestation?

Category: System specific assessments; Potential for alterations in body systems

(1) CORRECT: Anorexia is associated with Addison disease.

(2) Weight loss, not weight gain, is a sign of Addison disease.

(3) Bronze skin coloration (not yellow skin coloration) is a sign of Addison disease.

(4) A craving for salty foods (not sweets) is a sign of Addison disease.

11. The answer is 2

A client is having a tonic-clonic seizure. Which action should the nurse take **first**?

Category: Potential for complications of diagnostic tests/treatments/procedures; Therapeutic procedures

(1) This is not the first thing the nurse should do. When the seizure stops, the nurse should check for breathing and, if necessary, initiate rescue breathing.

(2) CORRECT: The nurse's first priority during a seizure is to protect the client from injury. To do this, the nurse must first remove objects from the surroundings and pad objects that cannot be removed.

(3) Placing an object in the client's mouth can cause injury.

(4) Restraining the client can cause injury.

12. The answer is 2, 3, 6, and 7

CORRECT OPTIONS: The nurse is concerned with abnormal clinical findings of **blood pressure 90/60 mmHg**, **heart rate 104**, and **1+ radial pulses**. The nurse recognizes normal aging has associated common physiological changes and as an older adult, an **89-year-old client** may have increased vulnerability to common clinical diseases and conditions, including fluid and electrolyte imbalances.

INCORRECT OPTIONS: The nurse is not concerned with the client's joint pain and stiffness in hips and knees, vision and hearing deficits, or mild decline in memory. Adults over 65 often have at least one chronic condition such as hypertension or diabetes; vision and hearing deficits are other common chronic conditions. A mild decline in memory is different from cognitive impairment such as delirium, dementia and depression. Joint pain and stiffness are findings consistent with the client's history of osteoarthritis.

13. See explanation for answers

CORRECT OPTIONS: The client is most likely experiencing **hypovolemia** as evidenced by **hypotension** and **tachycardia**. With aging, there is less percentage of body weight as water, increasing the risk of fluid volume deficit. Some conditions, including completing a bowel prep with the use of laxatives, especially in older adults, increases the risk for a serious fluid volume deficit. Hypotension can result from various causes, including loss of body fluids. Changes in blood pressure and pulse force and rate reflect hypovolemia.

INCORRECT OPTIONS: The client is not experiencing orthopnea or orthostatic hypotension. Orthopnea is dyspnea when supine and may be associated with heart failure, when excess fluid is present. Orthostatic hypotension is a decrease in blood pressure from lying to sitting or standing that can elicit dizziness and may occur with hypovolemia. There has been no change in the client's position.

Capillary refill less than 2 seconds and low pitched vesicular breath sounds are normal adult assessment findings for the cardiovascular and respiratory systems. Client findings of S1 and S2 and rousing to voice stimuli are also normal assessment findings.

14. The answer is 1, 5, and 6

CORRECT OPTIONS: The nurse recognizes that the client's low blood pressure increases the risk for developing **hypovolemic shock**, a serious condition of hypoperfusion in the body. Hypovolemic shock occurs when there is insufficient fluid volume in the vascular space needed for adequate tissue perfusion and cellular metabolism. Acute **confusion** and **oliguria** can occur as complications of inadequate perfusion to the brain and kidneys.

INCORRECT OPTIONS: Hyperactive reflexes are not associated with the client's vital signs of hypotension and tachycardia. Heart failure and pulmonary edema may occur as complications in conditions of excess intake or retention of fluids.

15. See explanation for answers

Indicated: The nurse plans goals to **restore vascular volume, reduce injury from falls, maintain oxygenation status**, and **achieve normal vital signs**. When hypotension is present due to fluid volume deficit and to maintain adequate tissue perfusion, restoring circulating volume with intravenous fluids is necessary. Reducing injury from falls is related to orthostatic hypotension, a decrease in blood pressure from positional changes, that may occur in older adults who have fluid volume deficit. Maintaining oxygenation status is essential to prevent hypoxemia. Hypotension can cause hypoperfusion to the vital organs, especially the heart, brain and kidneys. Achieving normal blood pressure, heart rate, and respiratory rate are goals relating to adequate tissue perfusion and homeostasis.

Not Indicated: Hypovolemia is caused by conditions of abnormal loss of body fluids, fluid shifts or inadequate intake. **Antibiotics** play an important role in treatment of *septic* shock, but they are not indicated for the client at this time.

16. The answer is 1, 3, 4, 6, 7, and 8

CORRECT OPTIONS: The nurse **administers intravenous (IV) therapy as prescribed for rapid fluid replacement** in hypovolemia. In clients with heart conditions, astute monitoring of the IV solution and flow rates is needed especially when giving large volumes. The nurse should **monitor for changes in capillary refill, peripheral pulses, and skin temperature** as these are indicators of tissue perfusion, vascular, and interstitial volume. **Changes in mental status** can reflect cerebral hypoperfusion related to hypotension. **Reporting changes in blood pressure, respirations, pulse rate, strength, rhythm, and pulse oximetry** are important aspects of cardiovascular assessment and can determine fluid responsiveness. Hypovolemia may cause **orthostatic hypotension**. The nurse should adjust the bed to a low position and have the client dangle feet prior to standing as fall prevention from dizziness. In the postanesthesia period, **continuous EKG monitoring** is recommended for clients who have a history of heart disease.

INCORRECT OPTIONS: The nurse does not provide high flow oxygen per the Venturi mask. It is more commonly used for clients who have chronic obstructive pulmonary disease (COPD) and need a low, constant oxygen concentration. Timely administration of IV fluids (or blood as needed) and oxygen administration by nasal cannula, or facemask are interventions to avoid hypoxemia caused by hypovolemic shock. Oxygen therapy is individualized to meet the client's needs. Epinephrine is the first treatment for anaphylactic shock, that is needed to oppose histamine release; it is not indicated for this client.

17. See explanation for answers

Neurological: The nurse recognizes effective nursing care as indicated by normal neurological client assessments of **awake**, **oriented** × 4 client, **PERRL**, and **speech that is fluid and understandable**.

Cardiovascular: **2+ radial pulses, equal** and **skin that is warm and dry** are normal assessment findings. The client is **not exhibiting dizziness when changing positions** from lying to sitting on the side of the bed, which would indicate orthostatic hypotension.

Respiratory: Respiratory findings of **clear lung sounds**, and **full, equal chest expansion** are normal adult assessment findings. INCORRECT OPTION: Slight dyspnea at rest is an abnormal clinical finding and should be documented and reported to the health care provider.

Vital Signs: Findings of **BP 108/70 mmHg** and **heart rate, 90 regular** are acceptable adult vital signs. INCORRECT OPTION: Respiratory rate of 24 is an abnormal clinical finding and should be documented and reported to the health care provider.

18. The answer is 4

A client is admitted to the hospital with a pressure injury involving full-thickness loss extending to the bone. The nurse documents the pressure injury as being at which stage?

Category: System specific assessments; Potential for complications of diagnostic tests/treatments/procedures

(1) Stage 1 pressure injury is intact skin with a localized area of nonblanchable erythema, which may appear different in darkly pigmented skin. This stage may be preceded by blanchable erythema or changes in sensation, temperature, or firmness. Color changes do not include purple or maroon discoloration; these may indicate a deep-tissue pressure injury.

(2) Stage 2 pressure injury involves partial-thickness loss of skin with exposed dermis. The wound bed is pink or red and moist. It is important to note that a stage 2 pressure injury may also present as an intact or ruptured serum-filled blister. Adipose (fat) is not visible and deeper tissues are not visible. Granulation tissue, slough, and eschar are not present.

(3) Stage 3 pressure injury involves full-thickness loss of skin, in which adipose is visible and granulation tissue and epibole (rolled wound edges) are often present. Slough and/or eschar may be visible.

(4) CORRECT: Stage 4 pressure injury involves full-thickness skin and tissue loss with exposed or directly palpable fascia, muscle, tendon, ligament, cartilage, or bone. Slough and/or eschar may be visible. Epibole, undermining, and/or tunneling often occur.

19. The answer is 3

A client diagnosed with Raynaud disease experiences an acute attack. The nurse should anticipate to find which assessment finding?

Category: System specific assessments

(1) Involuntary muscle contractions and twitching may be signs of amyotrophic lateral sclerosis (ALS).

(2) Unilateral facial weakness and drooping mouth are signs of Bell palsy.

(3) CORRECT: The cause of Raynaud disease is unknown; however, after exposure to cold or stress, the client typically experiences blanching of the skin at the fingertips and numbness and tingling of the fingers.

(4) Photophobia is not a symptom of Raynaud disease.

20. The answer is 2

The provider prescribes a CT scan of the client's chest with IV contrast. Which finding in the client's history should the nurse report to the provider?

Category: Potential for complications of diagnostic tests/treatments/procedures

(1) Hypertension is not a contraindication for a CT scan with IV contrast.

(2) CORRECT: A client with an allergy to iodine or shellfish may have an adverse reaction to the contrast medium.

(3) A UTI is not a contraindication for a CT scan with IV contrast.

(4) An allergy to penicillin is not a contraindication for a CT scan with IV contrast.

21. The answer is 2

The nurse cares for a client with severe bone marrow depression due to chemotherapy. Which nursing diagnosis takes priority in the client's care plan?

Category: Potential for complications of diagnostic tests/treatments/procedures

(1) Imbalanced nutrition is a health-threatening but not life-threatening problem.

(2) CORRECT: Because clients with bone marrow depression have a decrease in white blood cells (those cells that fight infection), risk for infection takes priority. Nursing diagnoses should be categorized in order of priority, with life-threatening problems addressed first, followed by health-threatening concerns.

(3) Pain may be a health-threatening problem, but typically is not life-threatening.

(4) The potential for injury is a health-threatening but not life-threatening problem.

22. The answer is 2, 4, and 5

The nurse prepares to discharge a client after a sickle-cell anemia crisis. Which instruction should the nurse provide to the client to avoid future crises? **(Select all that apply.)**

Category: Therapeutic procedures

(1) Clients should maintain a high fluid intake to prevent dehydration.

(2) CORRECT: Sickle-cell anemia clients should avoid strenuous exercise, which could provoke hypoxia.

(3) Clients should apply warm compresses to painful areas.

(4) CORRECT: Sickle-cell anemia clients should take pain medications as prescribed to provide effective pain management.

(5) CORRECT: Sickle-cell anemia clients should avoid tight clothing that restricts circulation.

23. The answer is 1, 2, 3, 4, 5, 6, 7, 8, and 9

CORRECT OPTIONS: The client is at high risk for the development of acute kidney injury (AKI). Prerenal causes of AKI include volume depletion without adequate fluid replacement. The client had an NG tube and now has **diarrhea** and a draining abdominal wound. The client's intake and output indicates the client is not receiving adequate intake to compensate for the gastrointestinal losses and draining wound. **Diabetes mellitus**, **hypertension**, and **obesity** are all risk factors for AKI. These conditions alter the structure and function of the kidneys and predispose them to injury. Taking several nephrotoxic agents can cause intrarenal failure. The client is receiving **vancomycin**, **metformin**, and **lisinopril** and has a history of taking **ibuprofen**. All four of these medications are considered nephrotoxic. **Contrast medium** is also nephrotoxic.

24. The answer is 1, 3, and 4

The nurse performs an assessment on a client who has cirrhosis. Which signs and symptoms should the nurse expect to see? **(Select all that apply.)**

Category: System specific assessments; Potential for alterations in body systems

(1) CORRECT: Signs and symptoms of cirrhosis include dull abdominal ache.

(2) Jaundice, not cyanosis, is a sign of cirrhosis.

(3) CORRECT: Signs and symptoms of cirrhosis include poor tissue turgor.

(4) CORRECT: Signs and symptoms of cirrhosis include bruises due to bleeding tendencies.

(5) Musty breath, not fruity breath, is a sign of cirrhosis.

25. The answer is 3

The nurse prepares to administer red blood cell transfusion to a client. Which statement is part of best practices in blood transfusion?

Category: Diagnostic tests; Potential for complications of diagnostic tests/treatments/procedures

(1) The client should be monitored for at least 15 minutes after the start of the transfusion.

(2) The transfusion needs to be completed within 4 hours, not 2 hours.

(3) CORRECT: The transfusion should be started within 30 minutes of removing the blood or blood components from the blood bank.

(4) The only solution that should be added to blood or blood components is 0.9% sodium chloride (normal saline solution).

26. The answer is 2

The nurse provides discharge teaching to a client after an acute attack of primary gout. Which foods should the nurse teach the client to avoid to prevent future attacks?

Category: Therapeutic procedures

(1) Cauliflower, asparagus, and mushrooms can be consumed unless contraindicated for a comorbid condition.

(2) CORRECT: A client with gout should avoid high-purine foods, such as anchovies, liver, sardines, and lentils.

(3) Cherries, strawberries, and blueberries can be consumed unless contraindicated for a comorbid condition.

(4) Cereal, pasta, and rice can be consumed unless contraindicated for a comorbid condition, such as diabetes.

27. The answer is 4

The nurse cares for a client who reports substernal pain radiating to the arm and jaw, shortness of breath, and a feeling of impending doom. The client had a stroke one month ago. The client's vital signs are blood pressure 146/72 mmHg, heart rate 128/minute, and respirations 36/minute. The 12-lead ECG reveals evolving acute myocardial infarction (MI). Which prescription should the nurse question?

Category: Changes/abnormalities in vital signs; Potential for complications of diagnostic tests/treatments/procedures

(1) Beta-adrenergic blockers are an appropriate treatment for evolving acute MI.

(2) Morphine for pain is an appropriate treatment for evolving acute MI.

(3) IV nitroglycerin (in clients without hypotension or bradycardia) is an appropriate treatment for evolving acute MI.

(4) CORRECT: Thrombolytic therapy is contraindicated in clients with a history of recent stroke (within the past 3 months).

28. The answer is 1

The nurse performs a 12-lead ECG on a client who has come to the emergency department reporting chest pain. Where should the nurse place the electrode for lead V1?

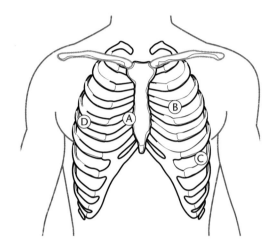

Category: Diagnostic tests

(1) CORRECT: Location A is correct. The V1 lead is placed at the fourth intercostal space to the right of the sternum. A 12-lead ECG measures electrical potential and helps make a definitive diagnosis of acute myocardial infarction. The six precordial leads—V1–V6—in combination with other leads, record potential in the horizontal plane.

(2) Location B is incorrect for the V1 lead.

(3) Location C is incorrect for the V1 lead.

(4) Location D is incorrect for the V1 lead.

29. The answer is 1

The nurse assesses a client admitted with a stroke. Which of these lobes of the cerebral hemisphere is involved in the control of voluntary muscle movement, including those necessary for speech and swallowing?

Category: System specific assessments

(1) CORRECT: The frontal lobe deals with higher levels of cognitive functions, such as reasoning and judgment. It also contains several cortical areas involved in the control of voluntary muscle movement, including those necessary for the production of speech and swallowing.

(2) The parietal lobe is associated with sensation, and is involved in writing and some aspects of reading.

(3) The temporal lobe is associated with auditory processing, olfaction, and word meaning.

(4) The occipital lobe is involved in vision.

30. The answer is 5, 2, 1, 4, 3, 6

The nurse prepares to do the Heimlich maneuver on a client who is choking. Arrange the following steps in the order the nurse should perform them. **All options must be used.**

Category: Therapeutic procedures

(1) The third step is to make a fist with one hand.

(2) The second step is to stand behind the client.

(3) The fifth step is to wrap the other arm around the client and grasp the fist with the hand.

(4) The fourth step is to place the thumb toward the client, below the rib cage and above the waist, and wrap this arm around the client.

(5) The first step is to ask the client, "Are you choking?"

(6) The last step is to thrust upward 6–10 times.

[CHAPTER 11]

PHYSIOLOGICAL INTEGRITY: PHYSIOLOGICAL ADAPTATION

Physiological adaptation involves managing and providing care for clients who may have a variety of acute, chronic, or life-threatening health conditions. To provide the proper care, you need to understand the client's stable/normal state (homeostasis), understand the internal and external factors that can influence or change it, and know how to help the client return to a stable state.

Understanding "normal" involves knowing the basics about all bodily systems, and knowing about the fluids and chemicals that keep the body functioning properly. In addition to knowing what a normal state looks like—in general and for each client—you also must know proper fluid and electrolyte balances and pH balance (water, sodium, potassium, calcium, magnesium, chloride, etc.). This is also a good time to remember the six elements of infection:

(1) Susceptible host

(2) Portal of entry

(3) Cause

(4) Reservoir

(5) Portal of exit

(6) Modes of transmission

It's important to know how to protect yourself and your client from infection and understand how to intervene to break the chain of infection. When a client is ill or injured, their body cannot respond quickly enough to internal or external events. Between your powers of observation and your understanding of pathophysiology, you should know how to determine whether there is a problem, identify the problem, and respond appropriately. This includes recognizing which body systems can be affected by the client's condition, being aware of each client's usual baselines and preexisting conditions, and incorporating that information to determine which care measures to try and whether they are effective.

On the NCLEX-RN® exam, you can expect approximately 13 percent of the questions to relate to Physiological Adaptation. Exam content for this subcategory includes, but is not limited to, the following areas:

- Alterations in body systems
- Fluid and electrolyte imbalances
- Hemodynamics
- Illness management
- Medical emergencies

- Pathophysiology
- Unexpected response to therapies

Now let's review some of the most important concepts related to these subtopics.

Alterations in Body Systems

Clients can experience a variety of alterations in body systems when they are ill. You should be able to monitor and assess these changes, and implement and explain appropriate interventions to clients.

You should understand the most common therapeutic activities, which include:

- Assessing tube drainage when a client has an alteration in a body system (such as whether the amount of fluid increased or decreased or whether the color of the fluid changed)
- Monitoring and maintaining a client on a ventilator
- Maintaining desired temperature using external devices
- Implementing and monitoring phototherapy
- Providing ostomy care
- Providing care to clients who have experienced a seizure
- Assisting with invasive procedures (central line placement, biopsy, debridement)
- Performing peritoneal dialysis
- Providing pulmonary hygiene (chest physiotherapy, spirometry)
- Performing oral nasopharyngeal suctioning
- Suctioning via an endotracheal or a tracheostomy tube
- Performing tracheostomy care
- Providing care for clients experiencing increased intracranial pressure

Providing wound care includes assisting in or performing dressing changes and removal of sutures or staples, monitoring wounds for signs and symptoms of infection, and promoting client wound healing through turning, hydration, nutrition, and skin care. In surgical cases, wound care may also include monitoring and maintaining devices and equipment used for drainage, such as chest tube suction.

It is important to identify signs of potential prenatal complications, and to provide care for clients experiencing complications from pregnancy, labor, and delivery (such as eclampsia, precipitous labor, or hemorrhage). You should also be able to assess a client's response to surgery and provide postoperative care.

In a more general sense, you should be able to educate clients about managing their health problem, whether it's a chronic illness such as diabetes or appropriate post-stroke care. Your efforts should promote progress toward recovery, and you should be able to evaluate whether the client has successfully achieved treatment goals.

Fluid and Electrolyte Imbalances

It is important to understand the concepts of fluid transport, capillary fluid movement, and the chemical regulation of fluid and electrolyte balances (hormones and peptides).

One of the most important elements is being able to identify the signs and symptoms of fluid or electrolyte imbalance in a client. In terms of fluids, this means identifying both dehydration and edema, knowing how to treat each one, and being able to teach the client how to prevent recurrence.

For example, a dehydrated client needs fluids, with no sugar, salt, or caffeine. If the client can take fluids orally, they should be delivered that way, but you should know when parenteral (IV) therapy is the right choice. Clients may also retain excess fluid; risk factors include age, surgery, cardiac or renal failure, and medications. A client with excess fluid should have fluid intake limited, protein intake increased, and excretion promoted, and should be carefully monitored for overcorrection.

Implement interventions to restore client fluid and/or electrolyte balance. Common electrolyte imbalances include the following:

- Hyponatremia and hypernatremia (sodium)
- Hypokalemia and hyperkalemia (potassium)
- Hypocalcemia and hypercalcemia (calcium)
- Hypomagnesemia and hypermagnesemia (magnesium)
- Hypochloremia and hyperchloremia (chlorine)
- Hypophosphatemia and hyperphosphatemia (phosphates)

Hemodynamics

Your responsibility in hemodynamic monitoring is to position the transducer at the level of the right atrium, level central venous pressure (CVP) of the pulmonary artery catheter transducer into this point during each shift and before each measurement, and maintain patency of the catheter with a constant small amount of fluid delivered under pressure.

Assess clients for decreased cardiac output, and identify cardiac rhythm strip abnormalities, such as sinus bradycardia, premature ventricular contractions, ventricular tachycardia, and fibrillation.

Monitor and maintain arterial lines, and connect and maintain pacing devices, including pacemakers, biventricular pacemakers, and implantable cardioverter defibrillators. You should also be able to initiate, maintain, and evaluate telemetry monitoring.

In addition to monitoring pacemakers and defibrillators, you should be able to intervene to improve client cardiovascular status through modifying an activity schedule and initiating a protocol to manage cardiac arrhythmias.

You should be able to provide care for clients with vascular access for hemodialysis, such as via an arteriovenous shunt, a fistula, or a graft.

Finally, apply your knowledge of pathophysiology to interventions in response to client abnormal hemodynamics, and provide clients with strategies to manage decreased cardiac output, such as frequent rest periods and limiting activities.

Illness Management

In addition to recognizing symptoms and helping to identify client health issues, it is important to implement interventions that help a client manage recovery from an illness. This includes applying your knowledge of each client's pathophysiology when determining which interventions are best.

When examining a client who is ill, examine and interpret data and know what information should be reported to the physician immediately. This means knowing a particular client's baseline values, identifying abnormal values or test results, and identifying critical values.

You play an important role in teaching clients how to manage their illnesses, so communicate appropriate and helpful information to clients with infectious illnesses such as AIDS, as well as chronic conditions such as asthma and diabetes. Evaluate and document client response to interventions, and promote continuity of care in illness management activities.

In terms of specific care, you should be able to perform gastric lavage and to administer oxygen therapy and evaluate client response.

Medical Emergencies

When a client appears to be experiencing a medical emergency, you should know how best to intervene. Although things are likely to happen very quickly, you should also be able to explain emergency interventions to the client, despite being in a pressure situation.

You should be able to perform a variety of emergency care procedures, including CPR, the Heimlich maneuver (abdominal thrusts), respiratory support, and use of an automated external defibrillator. You should also know how to provide emergency care for a wound disruption (evisceration or dehiscence). You should also be able to monitor and maintain a client on a ventilator. Once emergency procedures are implemented, evaluate and document client responses, such as restoration of breathing and return to normal pulse rate.

Nurses are typically expected to notify the clinician about unexpected responses and/or emergency situations.

Pathophysiology

It is important to understand the general principles of pathophysiology, including injury and repair, immunity, and cellular structure. You should also be able to identify and determine a client's health status based on pathophysiology.

Unexpected Response to Therapies

Most clients will respond to therapies in a predictable manner, but some will not. Assess clients for unexpected adverse responses to therapy (such as increased intracranial pressure or hemorrhage) and know how to intervene to counteract such complications.

Chapter Quiz

1. The nurse sets up an external warming device (Bair Hugger) for a client. The client's core temperature taken rectally is 91.4° F (33° C). Which action should the nurse perform?

   1. Active rewarming to increase the core temperature no more than 0.9° F (0.5° C) per hour.

   2. Active rewarming to increase the core temperature as quickly as possible.

   3. Active rewarming to increase the core temperature to 96.8° F (36° C).

   4. Active rewarming to increase the core temperature to 100.4° F (38° C).

2. The nurse prepares to cleanse a simple surgical wound on a client with a Jackson-Pratt drain adjacent to the incision site. Which cleansing steps should the nurse take?

   1. Cleanse the incision and drain sites while wearing standard clean gloves.

   2. Cleanse back and forth across the incision line and in a circular motion around the drain site.

   3. Cleanse the incision site and drain site together while wearing standard clean gloves.

   4. Cleanse the incision and drain sites using a sterile saline solution.

3. The nurse empties a Jackson-Pratt drain. The nurse has drained the fluid into a calibrated container and has placed the container on a level flat surface. The nurse measures 20 mL of bloody fluid. Arrange the following actions the nurse should take in sequential order. **All options must be used.**

   1. Dispose of the bloody drainage.

   2. Compress the evacuator completely.

   3. Replace the plug in the evacuator.

   4. Cleanse the plug with an alcohol wipe.

   5. Document the amount, odor, and consistency of the drainage.

4. The nurse receives a prescription from the provider to remove the client's sutures. Which action is **most** appropriate for the nurse to perform?

   1. Use gloves when removing sutures.

   2. Apply hydrogen peroxide gauze pads to cleanse the area first, then remove the sutures.

   3. Use sterile technique when removing sutures.

   4. Nothing, suture removal is outside of the nurse's scope of practice.

5. The nurse admits a client who receives continuous ambulatory peritoneal dialysis (CAPD). Which steps should be included in the client's plan of care?

   1. Maintain a permanent peritoneal catheter with flushes of 0.9% normal saline (0.9% NS) every 4–6 hours.

   2. Flush the CAPD catheter with heparin solution and obtain an IV pump in preparation for dialysate infusion.

   3. Ensure the dialysate is refrigerated until ready to infuse, and warm the dialysate to body temperature prior to exchange.

   4. Weigh the client at the same time every day, and use sterile technique while working with peritoneal dialysis catheter.

Refer to the Case Study to answer the next question.

The nurse is caring for a client admitted with acute myocardial infarction.

| Admission Notes | Nurse's Notes |

The client presented to the emergency department (ED) early this morning with acute onset of crushing chest pain that awakened the client during the night. Client was awake, alert, and fully oriented at admission. Vital signs in the ED: Temperature 99.3° F (37.4° C), pulse 98, respiratory rate of 18, and BP 148/96 mmHg. In the ED, the client was placed on a cardiac monitor, and blood samples obtained for evaluation of cardiac enzymes. The results indicated elevated creatine kinase (CK-MB), lactate dehydrogenase (LDH), and troponin levels. The client was diagnosed with an acute myocardial infarction. Because of recent oral surgery, the client was not eligible for thrombolytic therapy. The client was started on a nitroglycerin infusion and admitted to the Cardiac Care Unit (CCU).

| Admission Notes | Nurse's Notes |

CCU Day 2

Client lying supine in bed with head elevated. Client is lethargic and difficult to arouse; oriented to person and place only when roused. Current vital signs are temperature 99.9° F (37.7° C), pulse 88, respiratory rate of 30, and BP 88/60. Fine crackles present in both lung bases. Weak peripheral pulses with pale, cool skin noted. Client has had a 4 pound (1.81 kg) weight gain since admission. IV of 0.9% Normal Saline infusing at 50 mL/hour. Urine output for the past 24 hours is 600 mL. The client is prescribed a low sodium diet, but is eating less than 50% at each meal.

6. The nurse reviews the client's record and prepares to notify the physician of changes in the client's condition.

Complete the following sentence by choosing from the list of options.

The client is at **greatest** risk for developing [Select from list 1] due to [Select from list 2] and [Select from list 3].

(1)	(2)	(3)
kidney insufficiency	decreased preload	increased afterload
respiratory arrest	decreased peripheral resistance	increased kidney perfusion
heart failure	decreased cardiac contractility	increased cardiac conduction

7. A school-age client is discharged from the hospital with a tracheostomy. The parents received trachestomy care education. Which statement by one of the parents indicates understanding of correct procedure in tracheostomy care?

   1. "The cleansing and dressing of the stoma will be done at least every 24 hours."

   2. "It is not always necessary to suction before tracheostomy care."

   3. "The inner cannula should be changed by the provider or home health nurse."

   4. "Hydrogen peroxide is used to cleanse the stoma area."

8. The nurse prepares to suction a client with an endotracheal tube. After ventilating the client, which is the correct sequence of actions for the nurse to perform during suctioning?

   1. Apply suction, insert a sterile catheter, and withdraw while rotating the catheter.

   2. Insert a sterile catheter, begin to withdraw, apply suction, and continue to withdraw while rotating the catheter.

   3. Apply suction, insert a sterile catheter, and withdraw without rotating the catheter.

   4. Instill saline solution into the endotracheal tube, Insert a sterile catheter, begin to withdraw, and apply suction.

9. The nurse assesses a client with a parathyroid disease. The client is having abdominal cramping, positive Chovstek and Trousseau signs, and tingling in the extremities. These findings are consistent with an imbalance in which electrolyte?

   1. Hypermagnesemia.
   2. Hypomagnesemia.
   3. Hypercalcemia.
   4. Hypocalcemia.

10. The provider prescribes a 2-L daily fluid restriction for a client with heart failure. The nurse is totaling the client's fluid intake for the 8-hour shift. The client drank 5 oz of juice at breakfast, 2 oz of water with medications, 8 oz of soup at lunch, and 6 oz of milk with lunch. Intravenous fluids, flushes, and intravenous antibiotics for the shift were 400 mL. Urinary output was 300 mL, 100 mL, and 250 mL. What should the nurse document, in milliliters, as the total fluid intake for the shift?

    _____ mL

11. A client presents to the emergency department with shortness of breath, crackles in the bases and middle of the lung fields bilaterally, +2 pitting edema bilaterally of the lower extremities, and a weight increase of 6 lb (2.7 kg) in one week. The client's heart rate is 82 beats/minute and the blood pressure is 162/90 mmHg. The nurse administers 40 mg of furosemide intravenously as prescribed. Which finding indicates effectiveness of the furosemide?

    1. A heart rate of 58 beats/minute.
    2. A blood pressure of 100/52 mmHg.
    3. Urine output increase of 200 mL over the next hour.
    4. Diminished lung sounds bilaterally with crackles in the bases.

12. The nurse observes the following cardiac rhythm. Which is the correct interpretation of the client's cardiac rhythm?

    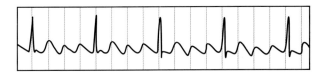

    1. Atrial fibrillation.
    2. Atrial flutter.
    3. Ventricular fibrillation.
    4. Third-degree atrioventricular block.

13. The nurse cares for a client with an arterial line (A-line). The nurse can utilize the A-line for which purposes?

    1. Monitoring blood pressure and heart rate, and infusing medications.
    2. Monitoring blood pressure and heart rate, and obtaining blood gases and other laboratory samples.
    3. Monitoring heart rate, obtaining arterial blood gases sample, and infusing medications.
    4. Obtaining blood gases and other laboratory samples, and infusing medications.

14. A client is admitted with a diagnosis of rapid atrial fibrillation. The nurse initiates telemetry monitoring. An alarm sounds at the central cardiac monitoring station indicating that the client is in what appears to be ventricular tachycardia. Which action should the nurse take **first**?

    1. Call a code blue.
    2. Silence the alarm and change the alarm parameters.
    3. Notify the health care provider of a change in rhythm.
    4. Assess the client and check lead placement.

15. The nurse cares for a client who is receiving dialysis through a subclavian central vein catheter. Which step should be included in the client's plan of care to prevent central line–associated bloodstream infection (CLABSI)?

    1. Perform hand hygiene prior to touching the dialysis catheter.
    2. Draw routine blood works from the dialysis catheter.
    3. Use the dialysis catheter for infusing intravenous antibiotics.
    4. Request a prescription for prophylactic intravenous (IV) antibiotics.

16. A client is brought into the emergency department by the client's spouse. The spouse tells the nurse that the client is confused, disoriented, and weak and has not been eating well. Which electrolyte imbalance correlates with the client's manifestations?

    1. Potassium (K^+) 3.8 mEq/L (3.8 mmol/L).
    2. Sodium (Na^+) 122 mEq/L (122 mmol/L).
    3. Magnesium (Mg^+) 1.9 mg/dL (0.95 mmol/L).
    4. Calcium (Ca^+) 9.5 mg/dL (2.4 mmol/L).

17. The nurse provides discharge instructions to a client going home on enoxaparin. Which response by the client indicates that the teaching was effective?

    1. "Prior to injection, I will rub the site with an alcohol wipe."
    2. "I will use the same site for each injection."
    3. "I will not pull back the plunger after inserting the needle."
    4. "After injection, I will massage the site to increase absorption of the meds."

18. The nursing home nurse finds a client down on the floor. The client is not responsive. Vital signs are: blood pressure 98/52 mmHg, heart rate 120/minute, respirations 28/minute, and oxygen saturation 94%. The client's medical record indicates a signed health care provider prescription that states "Do not resuscitate" and "Do not intubate" (DNR/DNI). Which action should the nurse take?

    1. Stay with the client and have another staff member call 911.
    2. Begin CPR and have another staff member call 911.
    3. Move the client into the bed and call the health care provider.
    4. Ask the family what they would like to have done for the client.

Refer to the Case Study to answer the next six questions.

The nurse in the clinic is interviewing an older adult client who reports fatigue, lethargy, anorexia, and swelling of feet and ankles.

┌─────────────────────┐
│ History and Physical │
└─────────────────────┘

The client is 70 years old with a history of type 1 diabetes mellitus (DM), hypertension, peripheral vascular disease (PVD), asthma, gastroesophageal reflux disease (GERD), and chronic kidney disease (CKD). The client's height is 66 inches (167.64 cm) and weight is 145 pounds (63.50 kg). The client's DM is managed with twice daily doses of regular and NPH insulin. The client is prescribed a calcium channel blocker and furosemide for management of hypertension. GERD is controlled with proton pump inhibitors and dietary changes including 6 small meals per day. On physical exam, the client is in no acute distress. There is 2+ pitting edema in the ankles. The client also describes decreased urine output.

19. The nurse reviews the client's history and physical, and sees the admitting diagnosis for the client is chronic kidney disease (CKD).

    Which finding does the nurse identify as a risk factor for the development of CKD in this client? **(Select all that apply.)**

    1. Diabetes mellitus.
    2. Asthma.
    3. Gastroesophageal reflux disease (GERD).
    4. Hypertension.
    5. Peripheral vascular disease.

┌─────────────────────┬──────────────────────┐
│ History and Physical │ Laboratory Results   │
└─────────────────────┴──────────────────────┘

Laboratory Test	Results	Interpretation
Sodium	150 mEq/L (150 mmol/L)	High
Potassium	7.4 mEq/L (7.4 mmol/L)	High
Chloride	112 mEq/L (112 mmol/L)	High
Blood Urea Nitrogen	30 mg/dL (10.71 mmol/L)	High
Creatinine	2.4 mg/dL (212 µmol/L)	High
Glucose	350 mg/dL (19.43 mmol/L)	High

20. The physician orders stat lab work. The nurse performs an assessment and reviews the lab results.

    For each client assessment finding, specify if the finding is consistent with hyperglycemia, hyperkalemia, or hypernatremia. **Each finding may support more than one abnormality. Each column must have at least 1 response option selected.**

Assessment Finding	Hyperglycemia	Hyperkalemia	Hypernatremia
Diarrhea	☐	☐	☐
Numbness and tingling (paresthesia)	☐	☐	☐
Elevated temperature	☐	☐	☐
Bradycardia	☐	☐	☐
Polydipsia	☐	☐	☐
Weakness	☐	☐	☐

21. Complete the following sentence by choosing from the list of options.

    The client is at risk for [Select from list 1] due to [Select from list 2].

(1)	(2)
hyperreflexia	elevated serum potassium
seizures	elevated serum sodium
cardiac dysrhythmias	elevated creatinine

22. Based upon the client's clinical presentation and laboratory results, the physician transfers the client to the hospital for treatment.

    Which medication does the nurse expect to be ordered for this client?

    1. Sodium polystyrene.
    2. Spironolactone.
    3. Methylprednisolone.
    4. Ibuprofen.

23. The nurse implements which nursing action at this time? **(Select all that apply.)**

    1. Place the client on a cardiac monitor.
    2. Maintain strict bedrest.
    3. Implement seizure precautions.
    4. Administer IV regular insulin and Dextrose 5%.
    5. Administer loop diuretics.
    6. Monitor urinary output.

24. Because of the client's history of chronic kidney disease, the nurse provides dietary teaching about foods high in potassium.

    Which **4** client statements indicate the need for further teaching?

    1. "Apples are a good choice of fruit for me."
    2. "It is okay to eat bananas."
    3. "I need to restrict adding table salt to my food."
    4. "I should limit tomatoes and potatoes in my diet."
    5. "I can eat eggs for breakfast."
    6. "Melons and oranges are high in potassium."
    7. "It is fine to use most salt substitutes."
    8. "I need to avoid red meat in my diet."

25. The nurse cares for a client who is six days postoperative and has a large midline abdominal incision that is not well approximated. The client reports a popping sensation in the abdominal area. Upon assessment, the nurse finds a small portion of the viscera to be protruding through the incision. Which action should the nurse take **first**?

    1. Do nothing; this is a normal finding for a large midline abdominal incision.
    2. Call the surgeon who operated on the client and notify of the findings.
    3. Place sterile dressings moistened with sterile normal saline (0.9% NS) over the viscera and hold in place with a sterile gloved hand.
    4. Place an abdominal binder, elevate the head of the bed no more than 20 degrees, and have the client recline with the knees bent.

26. The nurse cares for a client requiring mechanical ventilation. Which intervention should the nurse take to help prevent ventilator-associated pneumonia (VAP)? **(Select all that apply).**

    1. Reposition the client at least every 2 hours and maintain the head of the bed upright at 30–45 degrees.
    2. Promote nutrition with the use of a nasogastric tube and high-calorie feedings.
    3. Suction oral and pharyngeal secretions, and provide oral care at least every 2 hours.
    4. Assess the client for sedation reduction and weaning/extubation readiness.
    5. Perform hand hygiene before and after care of the client, and implement prophylactic intravenous antibiotic therapy.

27. The nurse receives report on four clients. Which client should the nurse examine **first**?

    1. A client with pancreatitis who is experiencing abdominal pain rated 4 on a 1–10 scale.
    2. A client who had a transurethral resection of the prostate (TURP) yesterday and is having a burning sensation upon urination.
    3. A client diagnosed with heart failure who has developed a new nonproductive cough and is restless.
    4. A client diagnosed with cellulitis of the left leg who reports redness and warmth of the left leg.

28. The nurse receives a prescription to give cefazolin to a client. The nurse notes that the client has an allergy to penicillin. The client reports a history of shortness of breath and itching after receiving penicillin. Which action is **most** appropriate for the nurse to take?

    1. Call the pharmacy to change the medication and notify the provider.
    2. Hold the medication and call the provider to double-check the prescription.
    3. Give the medication as prescribed since cefazolin is not a penicillin.
    4. After asking another nurse, give the medication as prescribed.

29. The nurse cares for a client admitted for gastrointestinal (GI) bleed. The provider has ordered the client to receive 2 units of packed red blood cells (PRBCs). Fifteen minutes after the start of the transfusion, the client reports chills, shortness of breath, and lumbar pain. Which should be the nurse's **first** action?

    1. Obtain vital signs and notify the provider of potential reaction.
    2. Slow the transfusion and reassess the client in 15 minutes.
    3. Stop the blood transfusion and infuse normal saline (NS) to keep the vein open (KVO).
    4. Administer PRN analgesic, apply oxygen at 2 L/minute, and provide an additional blanket.

30. The nurse receives report on a client with a right total knee arthroplasty who developed methicillin-resistant *Staphylococcus aureus* (MRSA) in the surgical incision. The client's blood urea nitrogen (BUN) is 14 mg/dL (5 mmol/L) and serum creatinine (Cr) is 0.9 mg/dL (79.56 μmol/L). A vancomycin peak and trough have been prescribed. The next dose of vancomycin is to be given on the nurse's shift. Which is the **most** appropriate action by the nurse?

    1. Draw a trough 30 minutes prior to dose and draw a peak 60 minutes after the vancomycin infusion.
    2. Draw a peak 30 minutes prior to dose and draw a trough 60 minutes after the vancomycin infusion.
    3. Hold the dose of vancomycin and notify the provider of the serum BUN and Cr levels.
    4. Give the dose of vancomycin as prescribed and draw the peak and trough with other evening labs.

Chapter Quiz Answers and Explanations

1. The answer is 1

The nurse sets up an external warming device (Bair Hugger) for a client. The client's core temperature taken rectally is 91.4° F (33° C). Which action should the nurse perform?

Category: Alterations in body systems

(1) CORRECT: The client is in moderate hypothermia with a core temperature of 91.4° F (33° C). This would indicate the need for an external warming device and other measures to increase core temperature.

(2) The core temperature should be brought up by no more than 0.9° F (0.5° C) per hour for treatment of moderate hypothermia.

(3) Active rewarming would be discontinued when the core temperature is greater than 95° F (35° C) to prevent hyperthermia.

(4) Active rewarming would be discontinued when the core temperature is greater than 95° F (35° C) to prevent hyperthermia.

2. The answer is 4

The nurse cleanses a simple surgical wound on a client with a Jackson-Pratt drain adjacent to the incision site. Which of these should the nurse do?

Category: Alterations in body systems

(1) The nurse should use a sterile/aseptic technique; standard clean gloves are not sufficient.

(2) The nurse will use a small circular motion along the wound edges, but cleanse from one end of the incision to the other. This is to prevent contamination and trauma to the wound.

(3) The drain site should be cleansed last, separately from the primary incision site, to prevent the risk of cross-contamination; standard clean gloves are not sufficient.

(4) CORRECT: The nurse will use a sterile/aseptic technique while cleansing and dressing the wound, including using sterile gloves, cotton-tipped applicators, sterile saline, and sterile dressings.

3. The answer is 4, 2, 3, 1, 5

The nurse empties a Jackson-Pratt drain. The nurse has drained the fluid into a calibrated container and has placed the container on a level flat surface. The nurse measures 20 mL of bloody fluid. Arrange the following actions the nurse should take in sequential order. **All options must be used.**

Category: Alterations in body systems

(1) The fourth thing the nurse would do is dispose of the bloody drainage, typically into a toilet. This would be done after closing the Jackson-Pratt drain to potentially infective agents and after resuming negative pressure (suction).

(2) The second thing the nurse would do is compress the evacuator completely.

(3) The third thing the nurse would do is replace the plug while the evacuator is compressed. This creates a negative pressure as the evacuator expands.

(4) The first thing the nurse would do is cleanse the plug with an alcohol wipe. This is to reduce the risk of infection.

(5) The last thing the nurse would do is document the process and drainage, including amount, consistency, color, odor, date, time, and client's tolerance of the procedure.

4. The answer is 3

The nurse receives an order from the provider to remove the client's sutures. Which action is **most** appropriate for the nurse to perform?

Category: Alterations in body systems

(1) To prevent incision contamination, this should be a sterile procedure. Wearing regular gloves is not sufficient.

(2) To prevent incision contamination, this should be a sterile procedure. This answer choice does not provide enough information to determine if proper sterile procedures are being followed.

(3) CORRECT: A sterile field is maintained, a sterile suture removal tray is used, and sterile gloves are applied.

(4) In many facilities, nurses do remove sutures and staples following a physician's order.

5. The answer is 4

The nurse admits a client who receives continuous ambulatory peritoneal dialysis (CAPD). Which of these should be included in the client's plan of care?

Category: Alterations in body systems

(1) The nurse would not flush a CAPD permanent peritoneal catheter with normal saline solution.

(2) The dialysate bag is raised to shoulder level and is infused by gravity into the peritoneal cavity after the dwell dialysate solution is drained. The CAPD catheter does not require a heparin flush.

(3) Dialysate for CAPD is not refrigerated but should be warmed to body temperature prior to infusion, if a warmer is available. Never use a microwave to warm the dialysate; this method creates an unpredictable temperature.

(4) CORRECT: The nurse would weigh the client at the same time daily. The nurse would use sterile technique and equipment when working with the peritoneal catheter to infuse and drain the dialysate, including having the client and nurse wear a surgical mask while the peritoneal catheter and hub are exposed.

6. See explanation for answers

CORRECT OPTIONS: Acute myocardial infarction, with significant cardiac tissue damage, is a risk factor for development of heart failure. Elevated cardiac enzymes correlate with this cardiac damage. **Heart failure** develops because of **decreased cardiac contractility** to meet the body's demands. **Afterload**, the peripheral resistance that the heart must pump against, increases with heart failure and can cause a precipitous drop in cardiac output. Compensatory mechanisms are activated in response to decreases in stroke volume and cardiac output. The sympathetic nervous system (SNS) releases epinephrine which leads to an increase in heart rate, increased myocardial contractility, and increased vasoconstriction. With decreasing cardiac output caused by a combination of decreased contractility and increased peripheral resistance, perfusion to all vital organs decreases as evidenced by confusion, pale cool skin, decreased urine output, and reduced amplitude of peripheral pulses.

INCORRECT OPTIONS: The client is at risk for kidney insufficiency if there is a decrease in cardiac output and kidney perfusion, but the development of heart failure is the greatest risk. There are no risk factors for development of respiratory arrest in this client at this time. Preload may decrease in the client with heart failure due to the heart muscle's inability to adequately pump the blood. Kidney perfusion is decreased in heart failure. Cardiac conduction is typically decreased, not increased, in the client with acute MI.

7. The answer is 4

A school-age client is discharged from the hospital with a tracheostomy. The parents received trachestomy care education. Which statement by one of the parents indicates understanding of correct procedure in tracheostomy care?

Category: Alterations in body systems

(1) The stoma should be cleaned and dressed at least every 8 hours and the ties every 24 hours; cleaning and dressing changes may be done more frequently to keep the dressing and ties dry to prevent infection.

(2) Suctioning the trachea and pharynx thoroughly before tracheostomy care keeps the area clean longer.

(3) The inner cannula can be cleaned and changed by the parents, and should be removed and cleaned at least every 8 hours.

(4) CORRECT: Hydrogen peroxide-soaked gauze pads or cotton-tipped applicators are used to clean the stoma area, followed by the use of sterile water-soaked gauze pads and cotton-tipped applicators to remove the hydrogen peroxide. The stoma area would then be dried using sterile gauze pads to reduce the risk of infection and irritation.

8. The answer is 2

The nurse prepares to suction a client with an endotracheal tube. After ventilating the client, which is the correct sequence of actions for the nurse to perform during suctioning?

Category: Alterations in body systems

(1) Suctioning on insertion unnecessarily decreases oxygen in the airway. Most clients will cough when the suction catheter touches the carina.

(2) CORRECT: The nurse would ventilate the client and insert the sterile catheter without applying suction. The nurse would then withdraw the catheter about 1 inch and apply suction while rotating the catheter.

(3) Suctioning on insertion unnecessarily decreases oxygen in the airway. Most clients will cough when the suction catheter touches the carina.

(4) Instilling saline solution into the endotracheal tube is harmful and no longer recommended. Failure to withdraw and rotate the catheter may result in damage to the tracheal mucosa.

9. The answer is 4

The nurse assesses a client with a parathyroid disease. The client is having abdominal cramping, positive Chovstek and Trousseau signs, and tingling in the extremities. These findings are consistent with an imbalance in which electrolyte?

Category: Fluid and electrolyte imbalances

(1) A person with hypermagnesemia would not exhibit all of these symptoms.

(2) A person with hypomagnesemia might exhibit a positive Chovstek sign but not the rest of the symptoms listed.

(3) A person with hypercalcemia would not exhibit all of these symptoms.

(4) CORRECT: Hypocalcemia can be demonstrated by abdominal cramping, tingling of the extremities, and tetany. Chovstek sign refers to an abnormal reaction to the stimulation of the facial nerve such that, when tapped at the masseter muscle, the facial muscles on the same side of the face contract, causing a brief twitching of the nose or lips. Chovstek sign can be seen in hypomagnesemia and hypocalcemia. Trousseau's sign of latent tetany is more sensitive than Chovstek sign in hypocalcemia, and may be positive before gross manifestations of hypocalcemia, specifically tetany and hyperreflexia. A blood pressure cuff is inflated to a pressure greater than the systolic pressure and held in place for 3 minutes. This causes the occlusion of the brachial artery, and the hypocalcemia and subsequent neuromuscular irritability will induce a muscle spasm of the client's hand and forearm.

10. The answer is 1,030 mL

The provider prescribes a 2-L daily fluid restriction for a client with heart failure. The nurse is totaling the client's fluid intake for the 8-hour shift. The client drank 5 oz of juice at breakfast, 2 oz of water with medications, 8 oz of soup at lunch, and 6 oz of milk with lunch. Intravenous fluids, flushes, and intravenous antibiotics for the shift were 400 mL. Urinary output was 300 mL, 100 mL, and 250 mL. What should the nurse document, in milliliters, as the total fluid intake for the shift?

Category: Fluid and electrolyte imbalances

The answer can be calculated as follows: 1 ounce is equal to 30 milliliters. Oral intake is 150 mL (because 5 oz × 30 mL = 150 mL) + 60 mL (because 2 oz × 30 mL = 60 mL) + 240 mL (because 8 oz × 30 mL = 240 mL) + 180 mL (because 6 oz × 30 mL = 180 mL) to equal 630 mL of oral intake. Add that to the intravenous fluids and antibiotics for a total intake of 1,030 mL (630 mL + 400 mL).

Intake consists of oral intake, intravenous intake, intake through any feeding tube, intravenous blood products, liquid medications, and flushes of any tubes or IV accesses. The nurse would not include urinary output in intake totals, because that is totaled separately under output. Output includes urine, diarrhea, emesis, wound drainage, and any gastric suction.

11. The answer is 3

A client presents to the emergency department with shortness of breath, crackles in the bases and middle of the lung fields bilaterally, +2 pitting edema bilaterally of the lower extremities, and a weight increase of 6 lb (2.7 kg) in one week. The client's heart rate is 82 beats/minute and the blood pressure is 162/90 mmHg. The nurse administers 40 mg of furosemide intravenously as prescribed. Which of these indicates effectiveness of the furosemide?

Category: Fluid and electrolyte imbalances

(1) A heart rate of 58 beats/minute could indicate a side effect of the medication rather than effectiveness. This significant drop in heart rate would be cause for alarm, especially after the administration of furosemide.

(2) A blood pressure of 100/52 mmHg could indicate a side effect of the medication rather than effectiveness. This significant drop in blood pressure would be cause for alarm, especially after the administration of furosemide.

(3) CORRECT: The nurse would expect an increase in urine output after the administration of furosemide. The client presented with signs and symptoms of hypervolemia or fluid overload, including shortness of breath, crackles in lung bases, and edema. Weight gain and hypertension can also be indicative of hypervolemia. The goal of treatment using furosemide is diuresis, with care not to send the client into hypovolemia.

(4) The nurse would expect to auscultate a reduction, if not elimination, of crackles in the lung bases. The nurse would also not expect diminished lung sounds, because this could indicate atelectasis and/or decreased air flow through the lungs. The goal would be baseline or clear lung sounds bilaterally, with minimal to no crackles in the lung bases upon auscultation.

12. The answer is 2

The nurse observes the following cardiac rhythm. Which of these is the correct interpretation of the client's cardiac rhythm?

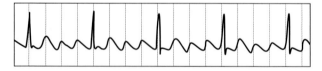

Category: Alterations in body systems

(1) The atrial rhythm would be irregular in atrial fibrillation. Coarse, chaotic, asynchronous waves would be present, and the atrial and ventricular rhythms would be grossly irregular and barely discernible with rates that vary.

(2) CORRECT: This is an atrial flutter rhythm—there are no identifiable P waves, and characteristic sawtooth flutter waves are present. The PR interval

is not measurable, and the atrial rate is regular and greater than the ventricular rate. This is expressed in a ratio; the example is 3:1, because there are 3 atrial beats for every 1 ventricular beat. The flutter waves should be able to be mapped across the rhythm strip. Flutter waves would mostly be visible with few occurring within the QRS and T waves. The subsequent flutter waves would occur on time.

(3) Ventricular fibrillation (VF) is characterized by atrial and ventricular rates and rhythms that cannot be determined, coarse and chaotic waves in coarse VF, and fine and chaotic waves in fine VF.

(4) Third-degree atrioventricular (AV) block, also known as complete heart block, is characterized by a regular rhythm, an independent atrial rate that is faster than the ventricular rate, an identifiable P wave that is normal and occurring without a QRS complex, and no PR interval.

13. The answer is 2

The nurse cares for a client with an arterial line (A-line). The nurse can utilize the A-line for which purpose?

Category: Hemodynamics

(1) Medications should never be infused through an arterial line.

(2) CORRECT: Arterial lines are used for monitoring blood pressure and heart rate, especially in clients requiring the use of vasopressor medications intravenously. They are also used for clients requiring frequent blood draws. The nurse may also draw arterial blood gases and other laboratory samples from the line, following the proper procedure. This saves the client from frequent arterial and venous draws.

(3) Medications should never be infused through an arterial line.

(4) Medications should never be infused through an arterial line.

14. The answer is 4

A client is admitted with a diagnosis of rapid atrial fibrillation. The nurse initiates telemetry monitoring. An alarm sounds at the central cardiac monitoring station indicating that the client is in what appears to be ventricular tachycardia. Which action should the nurse take **first**?

Category: Medical emergencies

(1) This would be premature on the part of the nurse. Assessment of the client may yield different information than what is reported by the monitor.

(2) Verify alarm limits with the physician, and only change parameters following an order from the physician.

(3) The nurse would first check the lead wires and assess the client to ensure that information given to the physician is accurate.

(4) CORRECT: Assess the client first, then the equipment for disconnections or malfunctions. Check lead placement to determine if the monitoring results are indeed accurate, and not due to interference or an artifact. If assessment of the client reveals true ventricular tachycardia, follow advance directives as established by the client, including, but not limited to, calling a code.

15. The answer is 1

The nurse cares for a client who is receiving dialysis through a subclavian central vein catheter. Which of these should be included in the client's plan of care to prevent central line–associated bloodstream infection (CLABSI)?

Category: Unexpected response to therapies

(1) CORRECT: All health care workers caring for this client should wash their hands with soap and water or an alcohol-based hand sanitizer before and after touching the dialysis catheter to prevent infection.

(2) Using the dialysis catheter for a purpose other than dialysis could jeopardize the access and increase the client's risk for CLABSI.

(3) Using the dialysis catheter for a purpose other than dialysis could jeopardize the access and increase the client's risk for CLABSI.

(4) Use of prophylactic antibiotics is not part of standard of care of dialysis catheters.

16. The answer is 2

A client is brought into the emergency department by the client's spouse. The spouse tells the nurse that the client is confused, disoriented, and weak and has not been eating well. Which electrolyte imbalance correlates with the client's manifestations?

Category: Fluid and electrolyte imbalances

(1) This lab value is within normal range. Normal range for potassium is 3.5–5 mEq/L (3.5–5 mmol/L).

(2) CORRECT: Symptoms of hyponatremia include confusion, disorientation, weakness, and poor appetite. The provider should be notified immediately of this critical level of sodium. Normal range for sodium is 135–145 mEq/L (135–145 mmol/L).

(3) This lab value is within normal range. Normal range for magnesium is 1.5–2.5 mEq/L (0.65–1.1 mmol/L).

(4) This lab value is within normal range. Normal range for calcium is 9–11 mg/dL (2.1–2.6 mmol/L) .

17. The answer is 3

The nurse provides discharge instructions to a client going home on enoxaparin. Which response by the client indicates that the teaching was effective?

Category: Illness management

(1) The area would be cleansed with an alcohol wipe, with care not to rub. Rubbing may cause damage to the skin and could contribute to formation of a hematoma.

(2) Sites for injection should be rotated, focusing on areas that have an easily accessible, fatty, subcutaneous layer. This is also minimizes tissue damage from repeated injections, which may affect absorption.

(3) CORRECT: Aspiration, or pulling back the plunger after needle insertion, can cause damage to small capillaries and blood vessels and can lead to hematoma formation and bleeding.

(4) Massaging the area postinjection may cause damage to the skin and could contribute to hematoma formation.

18. The answer is 1

The nursing home nurse finds a client down on the floor. The client is not responsive. Vital signs are: blood pressure 98/52 mmHg, heart rate 120/minute, respirations 28/minute, and oxygen saturation 94%. The client's medical record indicates a signed health care provider prescription that states "Do not resuscitate" and "Do not intubate" (DNR/DNI). Which of these should the nurse do?

Category: Medical emergencies

(1) CORRECT: The nurse should have another staff member call 911, gather paperwork, and contact the primary provider to notify of the transfer while the nurse stays with the client to continue to assess for any change in condition.

(2) The client has a pulse and is breathing spontaneously at this point, so initiation of CPR would be contraindicated. If the client would no longer have a pulse and/or stop breathing, CPR would not be initiated due to the DNR/DNI status of the client. Unless the client has advance directives that indicate no emergency treatment or no hospitalization, the nurse should continue reasonable and necessary treatment and nursing care up to the point of resuscitation and intubation. This includes calling 911 for emergency assistance.

(3) The nurse would not move the client from the floor because the client may have experienced a fracture or head trauma during the unwitnessed fall.

(4) Family notification would take place after emergency services are requested (or prescribed).

19. The answer is 1 and 4

CORRECT OPTIONS: Chronic kidney disease (CKD) is the progressive loss of kidney function. The most common causes of CKD are **diabetes mellitus** and **hypertension** due to damage to the glomerulus caused by vascular injury and uncontrolled hyperglycemia.

INCORRECT OPTIONS: Asthma and GERD are not risk factors for the development of CKD. Clients with CKD may develop peripheral vascular disease, but it does not cause CKD.

20. See explanation for answers

Hyperglycemia: Clinical manifestations of hyperglycemia, similar to hypernatremia, include **elevated temperature**, increased thirst (**polydipsia**), tachycardia, and **weakness**. Clinical manifestations develop secondary to fluid losses associated with the effects of elevated glucose on renal function.

Hyperkalemia: **Bradycardia**, sinus arrest, heart block, and ventricular dysrhythmias are associated with hyperkalemia. Clinical manifestations of hyperkalemia include **diarrhea** that is caused by increased intestinal mobility, as well as **paresthesias** and **weakness** caused by changes in nerve conduction.

Hypernatremia: Clinical manifestations of hypernatremia include **elevated temperature**, tachycardia, **polydipsia**, and **weakness**. The clinical manifestations are associated with water losses that lead to elevated sodium levels.

21. See explanation for answers

CORRECT OPTIONS: An elevated potassium level affects the cardiac conduction system. **Cardiac dysrhythmias secondary to hyperkalemia** are potentially life threatening. These dysrhythmias are typically observed when the **potassium levels** exceed 6 mEq/L (6 mmol/L). Electrocardiogram (ECG) changes include narrow, peaked T waves, ST depression, and shortening of the QT. If hyperkalemia is not treated, it may progress to cardiac arrest.

INCORRECT OPTIONS: The client's elevated sodium level is not consistent with hyperreflexia or seizures, and cardiac dysrhythmias are not directly related to an elevated creatinine level.

22. The answer is 1

CORRECT OPTION: **Sodium polystyrene** lowers serum potassium levels by causing an exchange of sodium for potassium in the gastrointestinal tract that leads to excretion of potassium.

INCORRECT OPTIONS: Spironolactone is a potassium-sparing diuretic and is not indicated as it may further increase the potassium levels. Corticosteroids (e.g., methylprednisolone) are not indicated for treatment of hyperkalemia as they lead to potassium retention. Nonsteroidal anti-inflammatory medications, like ibuprofen, may increase serum potassium by decreasing the renal excretion of potassium.

23. The answer is 1, 4, 5, and 6

CORRECT OPTIONS: **Placing the client on a cardiac monitor** is indicated due to the risk of cardiac dysrhythmias. The **IV administration of regular insulin with dextrose** leads to the shifting of potassium into the cells, particularly in hyperkalemia secondary to metabolic acidosis. **Loop diuretics** are potassium-wasting diuretics and lead to increased urinary excretion of potassium. The **urinary output must be monitored** for potential kidney insufficiency, which can further exacerbate hyperkalemia.

INCORRECT OPTIONS: There is no indication for limiting activity, and hyperkalemia does not increase the risk of seizures.

24. The answer is 2, 3, 7, and 8

CORRECT OPTIONS: Foods high in potassium, such as **bananas**, should be avoided. **Table salt** is composed of sodium chloride and is not contraindicated with hyperkalemia. **Most salt substitutes are composed of potassium**, so are contraindicated for this client. **Red meat** is not high in potassium.

INCORRECT OPTIONS: Apples and eggs can be included in a low potassium diet. Tomatoes, potatoes, oranges, beans, dried fruit, and starchy vegetables like winter squash are high in potassium and should be limited or avoided.

25. The answer is 3

The nurse cares for a client who is six days postoperative and has a large midline abdominal incision that is not well approximated. The client reports a popping sensation in the abdominal area. Upon assessment, the nurse finds a small portion of the viscera to be protruding through the incision. Which action should the nurse take **first**?

Category: Medical emergencies

(1) This is not a normal finding for a large midline abdominal incision.

(2) It is very important for someone to stay with the client due to the anxiety that the client will be feeling. The surgeon must be notified, and possible surgery could ensue, but this is not the first thing the nurse would do.

(3) CORRECT: This medical emergency is known as wound dehiscence with evisceration. The nurse would saturate sterile dressings with normal saline and hold the dressings over the viscera, which is most likely part of the bowel loop.

(4) The nurse should attempt to minimize any additional stress on the incision by having the client lie in a low Fowler position with knees bent. An abdominal binder is used in the prevention of dehiscence, not in the treatment of evisceration.

26. The answer is 1, 3, and 4

The nurse cares for a client requiring mechanical ventilation. Which interventions should the nurse take to help prevent ventilator-associated pneumonia (VAP)? **(Select all that apply).**

Category: Unexpected responses to therapies

(1) CORRECT: The standard of care is to reposition the client at least every 2 hours using lateral and horizontal positioning techniques. The head of the bed should be raised 30–45 degrees unless contraindicated. This helps reduce aspiration of both secretions and gastric contents.

(2) A nasogastric tube can lead to sinusitis, which increases the likelihood of the client developing VAP. The use of an orogastric tube to aid in feeding and/or gastric decompression is recommended over the use of a nasogastric tube.

(3) CORRECT: Oral care should be done at least every 2 hours. The removal of excess secretions is also an important element in the reduction of VAP. These secretions can cause aspiration, and can also be a perfect moist breeding ground for infection.

(4) CORRECT: A reduction in the duration of mechanical ventilation and/or a reduction in sedation to assess readiness of weaning have been shown to decrease the development and incidence of VAP. No alteration in medication or weaning/extubation should be attempted without an order from the physician. The nurse can be proactive and encourage the progression of weaning through assessment and subsequent discussions with the physician.

(5) Although proper hand hygiene and the use of gloves have been shown to reduce the risk of VAP, prophylactic intravenous antibiotic therapy is not recommended. A broad-spectrum antibacterial oral rinse (chlorhexidine) has been used in conjunction with thorough oral care with good results.

27. The answer is 3

The nurse receives report on four clients. Which client should the nurse examine **first**?

Category: Illness management

(1) The client with mild to moderate pain related to pancreatitis is not as critical as the client with potential acute pulmonary edema.

(2) The client with the burning sensation post-TURP is not as critical. This is a common finding with this procedure/diagnosis.

(3) CORRECT: The new nonproductive cough and restlessness could indicate acute pulmonary edema. The nurse would assess this client first, focusing on lung and heart sounds. Acute pulmonary edema is seen in heart disease, circulatory overload (from transfusions and infusions), and lung injuries; postanesthesia; and in other ediologies that can generate fluid in the alveoli that impedes gas

exchange. This situation can quickly escalate into a medical emergency, so the nurse should assure oxygenation and implement measures to decrease pulmonary congestion.

(4) The client with the redness related to cellulitis is not as critical. This is a common finding with this procedure/diagnosis.

28. The answer is 2

The nurse receives a prescription to give cefazolin to a client. The nurse notes that the client has an allergy to penicillin. The client states he becomes short of breath and itches after receiving penicillin. Which action is **most** appropriate for the nurse to take?

Category: Unexpected response to therapies

(1) The provider should be made aware of this allergy before the client receives the medication. In some instances, the provider will confirm the prescription, depending on the severity of the past reaction to penicillin or cephalosporins. More often, the provider will change to a different class of antibiotic. It is a decision for the provider to make, not the pharmacist or the nurse.

(2) CORRECT: The nurse would call the provider and double-check this prescription.

(3) Cefazolin is not a penicillin; it's a first-generation cephalosporin, which can cause a reaction in clients with penicillin allergies.

(4) It is for the provider to decide whether to change the medication, not the nurse.

29. The answer is 3

The nurse cares for a client admitted for gastrointestinal (GI) bleed. The provider has ordered the client to receive 2 units of packed red blood cells (PRBCs). Fifteen minutes after the start of the transfusion, the client reports chills, shortness of breath, and lumbar pain. Which should be the nurse's **first** action?

Category: Unexpected response to therapies

(1) Vital signs should be obtained and the provider notified after treatment is discontinued. The unit in question should not be restarted, and any other units that were issued should not be implemented.

(2) Just slowing the infusion will not resolve the issue of an allergic reaction to the treatment.

(3) CORRECT: The symptoms of chills, shortness of breath, and back pain could indicate an acute hemolytic reaction. This medical emergency requires swift action on the part of the nurse, including immediately discontinuing the blood infusion. The nurse removes all the existing tubing, replaces it with new tubing hydrating the client with normal saline, and notifies the health care provider. It is essential for the nurse to save the unit of blood in question along with the original tubing used for the transfusion for testing.

(4) Treating the symptoms will not resolve the issue of an allergic reaction to the treatment.

30. The answer is 1

The nurse receives report on a client with a right total knee arthroplasty who developed methicillin-resistant *Staphylococcus aureus* (MRSA) in the surgical incision. The client's blood urea nitrogen (BUN) is 14 mg/dL (5 mmol/L) and serum creatinine (Cr) is 0.9 mg/dL (79.56 μmol/L). A vancomycin peak and trough have been prescribed. The next dose of vancomycin is to be given on the nurse's shift. Which is the **most** appropriate action by the nurse?

Category: Illness management

(1) CORRECT: The nurse would expect to draw a trough 30 minutes prior to the third dose of vancomycin and draw a peak 60 minutes after infusion is complete. The provider prescribes this set of labs to be drawn, or the prescription is part of a hospital protocol for clients receiving vancomycin intravenously.

(2) Drawing a peak 30 minutes prior to dose and drawing a trough 60 minutes after infusion would yield an inaccurate result.

(3) The BUN and Cr levels that are given in this scenario are within normal limits.

(4) Giving the dose of vancomycin as prescribed and drawing the peak and trough with other evening labs would yield an inaccurate result.

THE PRACTICE TEST

PRACTICE TEST

> **Directions**: This practice test consists of 150 exam-style questions. Allot 5 hours of uninterrupted time to take the practice test. For each fill-in-the-blank question, write in the correct answer. For each drag-and-drop ordered response question, write the number of each step in the sequence in which the steps should be performed. For each item of the remaining question types, HIGHLIGHT the option or options that best answer the question.

1. The nurse is interviewing a client who is receiving treatment for obsessive-compulsive disorder (OCD). Which is the **most** important question for the nurse to ask this client?

   1. "Do you find yourself forgetting simple things?"
   2. "Do you find it difficult to focus on a given task?"
   3. "Do you have trouble controlling upsetting thoughts?"
   4. "Do you experience feelings of panic in a closed area?"

2. The nurse on a postpartum unit is preparing 4 clients for discharge. It would be **most** important for the nurse to refer which client for home care?

   1. A primipara client who delivered a 7-lb (3.2 kg) infant 2 days ago.
   2. A multipara client who delivered a 9-lb (4 kg) infant by cesarean section 2 days ago.
   3. A multipara client who delivered 1 day ago and is reporting cramping.
   4. A client who delivered by cesarean section and is reporting burning on urination.

3. A client is telling the nurse about personal thought patterns. Which statement by the client would validate the diagnosis of schizophrenia?

   1. "I can't get the same thoughts out of my head."
   2. "I sometimes feel on top of the world, then suddenly down."
   3. "Sometimes I look up and wonder where I am."
   4. "It's clear that this is an alien laboratory and I am in charge."

4. A nursing team consists of an RN, an LPN/LVN, and an unlicensed assistive personnel (UAP). The nurse should assign which client to the LPN/LVN?

   1. A client with a diabetic ulcer that requires a dressing change.
   2. A client diagnosed with cancer who is reporting bone pain.
   3. A client with terminal cancer being transferred to hospice home care.
   4. A client with a fracture of the right leg who asks to use the urinal.

5. The nurse is leading an inservice program about management issues. The nurse would intervene if another nurse made which statement?

   1. "It is my responsibility to ensure the signed consent form is in the client's medical record before the surgical procedure."

   2. "It is my responsibility to witness the signature of the client on the consent form before the surgical procedure."

   3. "It is my responsibility to provide a detailed description of the surgical procedure."

   4. "It is my responsibility to answer client questions prior to the surgical procedure."

6. The nurse in the newborn nursery has just received hand-off report. Which client should the nurse see **first**?

   1. A 2-day-old client who is lying quietly alert with a heart rate of 185 beats/minute.

   2. A 1-day-old client who is crying and has a bulging anterior fontanel.

   3. A 12-hour-old client whose respirations are 45 breaths/minute and irregular while being held.

   4. A 5-hour-old client whose hands and feet appear blue bilaterally during sleep.

Refer to the Case Study to answer the next six questions.

The nurse provides care in the emergency department (ED) for a young adult client with a diagnosis of type 1 diabetes.

Admission Notes	Nurse's Notes

The client is a student athlete on a university soccer team. The client was brought to the emergency department (ED) by a teammate after the afternoon soccer practice. The teammate described the client as walking with an unsteady gait, shaky, sweating and "seemed confused." The teammate observed that the client is wearing a diabetic alert medical identification arm band.

Client records from the university health clinic indicate the client was diagnosed with type 1 diabetes 6 months ago at age 19. The client's basal-bolus insulin plan consists of multiple daily injections with frequent self-monitoring of glucose. The client's injections include a rapid-acting (bolus) insulin before meals and a long-acting (basal) insulin at nighttime for background metabolic needs. The client is in transition to an insulin pump delivery system.

Vital Signs	Results
Blood pressure	110/64
Pulse	120 bpm, regular
Respiratory rate	20, regular
Temperature (oral)	97.6° F (36.44° C)
Pulse oximetry	97% on room air
Body Mass Index (BMI)	21 kg/m² (normal)

Admission Notes	Nurse's Notes

The client is rousable to verbal stimuli and opens eyes. The client is able to answer questions appropriately, but responses are slow. The client states, "I have a dull headache." The client has confusion as to place, events, and time of the last food and insulin dose. Head is normocephalic, nontender. Pupils equal, round, reactive to light. Skin pale, cool, diaphoretic, with elastic turgor. Moist oral mucous membranes. Apical heart rate 120, regular, no murmurs; 2+ radial pulses equal, bilaterally; capillary refill less than 2 seconds; no dependent edema. Chest expansion equal. Soft, vesicular lung sounds throughout with absence of adventitious lung sounds. Abdomen soft, flat and non tender, with bowel sounds present throughout. Client moves all extremities spontaneously. No tremors noted.

7. The nurse reviews the admission notes and documents nurse's notes.

For each client finding below, specify whether the nurse recognizes the finding as concerning or not concerning.

Client Finding	Concerning	Not Concerning
Skin pale, cool, diaphoretic.	○	○
Headache.	○	○
Shaky and unsteady gait.	○	○
Absence of adventitious lungs sounds.	○	○
Pulse 120, regular.	○	○
Blood pressure 110/64.	○	○
Confused.	○	○

8. The nurse performs a capillary blood glucose test and obtains results of 57 mg/dL (3.16 mmol/L).

Complete the following sentence by choosing from the list of options.

The nurse identifies the client is most likely experiencing symptoms of ⌊ Select from list 1 ⌋ that may occur when there is ⌊ Select from list 2 ⌋ and ⌊ Select from list 3 ⌋.

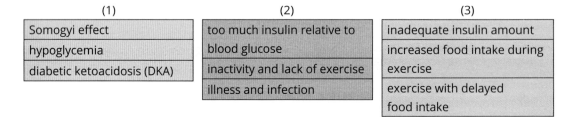

(1)	(2)	(3)
Somogyi effect	too much insulin relative to blood glucose	inadequate insulin amount
hypoglycemia		increased food intake during exercise
diabetic ketoacidosis (DKA)	inactivity and lack of exercise	
	illness and infection	exercise with delayed food intake

9. Due to the client's low blood glucose, the nurse's **priority** consideration is the client's risk to develop which complication?

1. Hypokalemia.
2. Osmotic diuresis.
3. Seizures.
4. Hypovolemia.

10. The nurse plans care to manage the client's low blood glucose. Select **3** goals the nurse includes.

1. Replace electrolytes.
2. Achieve normal blood glucose.
3. Reduce risk for injury from low blood glucose.
4. Restore fluid balance.
5. Promote self-care efforts to balance food, activity, and insulin.
6. Educate about weight loss.

11. The nurse provides treatment for the client's low blood glucose. Which action is appropriate? **(Select all that apply.)**

1. Give carbohydrates containing fat, such as candy bars or cookies.
2. Obtain blood glucose 15 minutes after administering 15 grams of fast-acting carbohydrate.
3. Administer 15 grams of fast-acting carbohydrate, such as 6 ounces regular soda, 4–6 ounces orange juice, or 1 tablespoon honey.
4. Prepare a continuous insulin drip and administer as prescribed.
5. Prepare to administer 25–50 mL of 50% dextrose intravenous if client becomes unconscious.
6. Administer potassium chloride to correct electrolyte imbalance.
7. Prepare 1 mg of glucagon intramuscular if client cannot swallow or has no intravenous access.
8. If blood glucose is < 70 mg/dL (3.9 mmol/L) after 15 grams of fast-acting carbohydrate, repeat 15 grams of fast-acting carbohydrate.

12. The nurse prepares the client for discharge. Highlight the client findings in the table that indicate the nursing actions have been effective.

Assessment	Client Findings
Statements	"I understand my glucose can stay low for several hours after I finish soccer practice or a game."
	"I should always check my blood glucose more frequently when I exercise."
Vital Signs	Pulse 88 bpm, regular
	Respirations 28 and deep
Lab work	Blood glucose, 102 mg/dL (5.66 mmol/L)
Neurologic	Headache
	Dizziness when standing
	Coherent thoughts with smooth flow to speech
Respiratory	Fruity odor to breath

13. The nurse is caring for clients in the outpatient clinic. Which phone call should the nurse return **first**?

    1. A client diagnosed with hepatitis A who states, "My arms and legs are itching."
    2. A client with a cast on the right leg who states, "I have a funny feeling in my right leg."
    3. A client diagnosed with osteomyelitis of the spine who states, "I am so nauseous that I can't eat."
    4. A client diagnosed with rheumatoid arthritis who states, "I am having trouble sleeping."

14. The nursing team consists of 1 RN, 2 LPN/LVNs, and 3 unlicensed assistive personnel (UAPs). The RN should care for which client?

    1. A client with a chest tube who is ambulating in the hallway.
    2. A client with a colostomy who requires colostomy irrigation assistance.
    3. A client with a right-sided stroke who requires assistance with bathing.
    4. A client who is refusing medication to treat cancer of the colon.

15. A 1-day-old client diagnosed with intrauterine growth restriction has a high-pitched, shrill cry and appears restless and irritable. The nurse also observes fist-sucking behavior. Based on this data, which action should the nurse take **first**?

    1. Gently massage the client's back every 2 hours.
    2. Tightly swaddle the client in a flexed position.
    3. Schedule feeding times every 3 to 4 hours.
    4. Encourage eye contact with the client during feedings.

16. A client with suicidal ideation who was admitted to the psychiatric unit for treatment and observation a week ago suddenly appears cheerful and motivated. The nurse should be aware of which possible cause of the change in behavior?

    1. The client is likely sleeping well because of the medication.
    2. The client has made new friends and has a support group.
    3. The client may have finalized a suicide plan.
    4. The client is no longer depressed due to treatment.

17. The nurse is caring for a client who reports an off-white vaginal discharge with a curdlike appearance. The nurse observes the discharge and vulvular erythema. It would be **most** important for the nurse to ask which question?

    1. "Do you have diabetes insipidus?"
    2. "Are you sexually active?"
    3. "What kind of birth control do you use?"
    4. "Do you take cough medicine?"

18. The nurse is caring for a client at 37 weeks' gestation who has a history of type 1 diabetes mellitus. The client states, "I am so thrilled that I will be breastfeeding my baby." Which response by the nurse is **best**?

    1. "You will probably require less insulin while you breastfeed."
    2. "You will initially require more insulin after the baby is born."
    3. "You will be able to take an oral antidiabetic agent instead of insulin."
    4. "You will likely require the same dose of insulin that you require now."

19. The nurse is caring for a client who had a thyroidectomy 6 hours ago for treatment of Graves disease. The nurse would be **most** concerned if which response was observed?

1. The client's vital signs include: blood pressure 138/82 mmHg, pulse 84 beats/minute, and respirations 16 breaths/minute.

2. The client supports the head and neck to turn head to right.

3. The client spontaneously flexes the wrist when the blood pressure cuff is inflated during blood pressure measurement.

4. The client becomes drowsy and reports a sore throat.

Refer to the Case Study to answer the next six questions.

The nurse is caring for a pregnant client who was admitted 2 hours ago to the labor/delivery (L/D) unit.

| History | Laboratory Studies |

Client is a 41-year-old primigravida at 34 weeks gestation. Client presented for a routine obstetric appointment today and reported increasing peripheral edema and daily headaches unresolved with the use of acetaminophen. The client's obstetrician evaluated the client. Findings included 2+ pretibial edema, a BP of 158/90, and weight gain of 11 lbs (4.98 kg) since previous office visit 2 weeks ago. Reflexes 3+ and brisk without clonus. Urine sample evaluated in provider's office revealed 2+ protein via dipstick. Client history significant for smoking 6–8 cigarettes daily, obesity with a pre-gravid body mass index (BMI) of 32. The client has consumed 2 servings of decaffeinated soda daily throughout pregnancy. Remainder of past medical history and obstetric history are unremarkable.

Plan: Draw Complete Blood Count (CBC) and Comprehensive Metabolic Panel (CMP). Admit to labor and delivery.

| History | Laboratory Studies |

Laboratory Test	Result 1000	Range
RBC	4.1 million/mm^3 (4.1 × 10^{12}/L)	normal
WBC	6,700 /mm^3 (6.7 × 10^9/L)	normal
Hemoglobin	11.5 g/dL (115 g/L)	low
Hematocrit	33% (0.33)	low
Platelets	100,000/mm^3 (100 × 10^9/L)	low
Blood urea nitrogen (BUN)	22 mg/dL (8.2 mmol/L)	high
Creatinine	1.5 mg/dL (132.6 µmol/L)	high
AST	22 units/L (22 U/L)	high
ALT	24 units/L (24 U/L)	high
LDH	99 units/L (99 U/L)	high
Serum uric acid	6.7 mg/dL (398.5 mmol/L)	high

20. The nurse reviews the client's history and laboratory results.

Highlight tokenized information in the client's history that **most** concerns the nurse. Tokenized options are enclosed in boxes.

Client is a 41-year-old primigravida at 34 weeks gestation. Client presented for a routine obstetric appointment today and reported increasing peripheral edema and daily headaches unresolved with the use of acetaminophen. The client's obstetrician evaluated the client. Findings included 2+ pretibial edema, a BP of 158/90, and weight gain of 11 lbs (4.98 kg) since previous office visit 2 weeks ago. Reflexes 3+ and brisk without clonus. Urine sample evaluated in provider's office revealed 2+ protein via dipstick. Client history significant for smoking 6 – 8 cigarettes daily, obesity with a pre-gravid body mass index (BMI) of 32. The client has consumed 2 servings of decaffeinated soda daily throughout pregnancy. Remainder of past medical history and obstetric history are unremarkable.

21. The nurse recognizes which client finding is consistent with pre-eclampsia?
(Select all that apply.)

1. Hypertension.
2. Proteinuria.
3. Peripheral edema.
4. Headaches with visual changes.
5. Low platelets.
6. Hyperreflexia.
7. Impaired liver functions.
8. Maternal age less than 20 or more than 40 years.

22. Complete the following sentence by choosing from the list of options.

The nurse knows that pre-eclampsia increases the client's risk for developing [Select from list 1] due to [Select from list 2] and associated [Select from list 3].

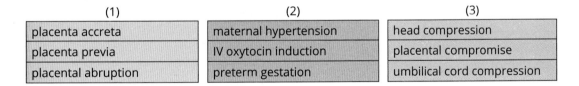

(1)	(2)	(3)
placenta accreta	maternal hypertension	head compression
placenta previa	IV oxytocin induction	placental compromise
placental abruption	preterm gestation	umbilical cord compression

| History | Laboratory Studies | Nurse's Notes |

1030: Client admitted to room. Client reports frontal headache 6/10 on pain scale, with some photophobia and scotomas. Intermittently nauseated with vague, generalized abdominal discomfort. 20 gauge IV catheter inserted in right forearm × 1 attempt; lactated ringer (LR) solution infusing at 100 mL/hr. Magnesium sulfate 4 gm/100 mL 0.9% normal saline (NS) piggybacked into IV line infusing at 1 g/hour (25 mL/hr). Client placed on external fetal monitor. Mild uterine irritability observed. Fetal heart rate (FHR) ranging 120–150 bpm with moderate variability and no decelerations noted.

1230: Client re-evaluated by physician and lab results discussed with client and significant other. BP remains elevated and labs indicate fetus will need to be delivered. Decision made to induce labor with IV oxytocin and manage blood pressure with IV magnesium sulfate. Cervix 1 centimeter dilated, 30% effaced, firm consistency with vertex presenting at –3 station and membranes intact. FHR baseline 120–140 with moderate variability and no decelerations noted.

1300: IV oxytocin initiated per protocol at 3 milliunits/minute. FHR baseline remains 120–140 bpm with moderate variability and no decelerations.

1330: Client having mild uterine contractions every 4 minutes with spontaneous rupture of membranes and blood-tinged fluid observed. IV oxytocin rate at 6 milliunits/minute. Client reporting left upper quadrant abdominal pain. Abdomen rigid. FHR baseline at 100–110 bpm, minimal variability with intermittent late decelerations.

| History | Laboratory Studies | Nurse's Notes | Vital Signs |

Assessment	1030	1230	1330
Blood pressure	160/90 mmHg	166/90 mmHg	172/100 mmHg
Pulse	82 bpm	84 bpm	90 bpm
Respirations	18/minute	20/minute	24/minute
Temperature	97.9° F (36.6° C)	97.9° F (36.6° C)	98.2° F (36.7° C)
Reflexes	3+, no clonus	3+, no clonus	3+, no clonus

23. The nurse monitors the client's vital signs and documents the client's care over the next several hours. The nurse recognizes the client is exhibiting signs and symptoms associated with placental abruption.

For each client finding below, specify the potential nursing intervention that would be appropriate for the care of the client. Each finding supports 1 potential nursing intervention.

Finding	Potential Nursing Interventions
FHR decreased with late decelerations.	Select... ▾
	Apply anti-embolism stockings.
	Place client in Trendelenburg position.
	Administer oxygen by mask.
Pink-tinged amniotic fluid.	Select... ▾
	Monitor maternal vital signs every 5–10 minutes.
	Anticipate massive vaginal bleeding.
	Massage the uterus.
Focal uterine pain and rigidity.	Select... ▾
	Discontinue magnesium infusion.
	Stop oxytocin infusion.
	Administer PO pain medication.

24. The nurse notifies the physician, and the client is prepared to undergo an emergency Cesarean birth under general anesthesia.

Complete the following sentences by choosing from the list of options.

The nurse understands the indication for this client to undergo an emergency Cesarean birth is [Select from list 1]. It would be a **priority** for the nurse to notify the [Select from list 2]. The nurse will [Select from list 3].

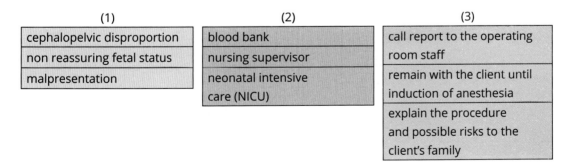

(1)	(2)	(3)
cephalopelvic disproportion	blood bank	call report to the operating room staff
non reassuring fetal status	nursing supervisor	remain with the client until induction of anesthesia
malpresentation	neonatal intensive care (NICU)	explain the procedure and possible risks to the client's family

25. The client delivers a viable newborn, who is transported to the neonatal intensive care unit (NICU). The nurse is caring for the client 2 hours after the delivery. IV oxytocin and IV magnesium sulfate are infusing.

For each assessment finding below, specify whether the finding indicates the client's condition has improved, not changed, or declined.

Assessment Finding	Improved	No Change	Declined
Blood pressure 158/92	○	○	○
Pulse 76	○	○	○
Respirations 16	○	○	○
Hematocrit 29% (0.29)	○	○	○
Platelets 95,000/mm^3 (95 × 10^9/L)	○	○	○
Serum uric acid 6.4 mg/dL (380.7 mmol/L)	○	○	○
Headache mild, 3/10 on pain scale	○	○	○
Reflexes 3+ without clonus	○	○	○

26. A client is admitted who reports severe pain in the right lower quadrant of the abdomen. Which action should the nurse take to assist the client with pain relief?

    1. Encourage rhythmic, shallow breathing.
    2. Massage the right lower quadrant of the abdomen.
    3. Apply a warm heating pad to the client's abdomen.
    4. Position client for comfort using pillows.

27. The nurse is preparing a client for peritoneal dialysis. Which action should the nurse take **first**?

    1. Assess access for a bruit and a thrill.
    2. Warm the dialysate solution.
    3. Position client on the left side.
    4. Insert an indwelling urinary catheter.

28. The nurse is teaching an older adult client with right leg weakness how to use a cane. Which behavior by the client indicates that the teaching was effective?

    1. The client holds the cane with the right hand, moves the cane forward followed by the right leg, and then moves the left leg.
    2. The client holds the cane with the right hand, moves the cane forward followed by the left leg, and then moves the right leg.
    3. The client holds the cane with the left hand, moves the cane forward followed by the right leg, and then moves the left leg.
    4. The client holds the cane with the left hand, moves the cane forward followed by the left leg, and then moves the right leg.

29. The nurse is helping an unlicensed assistive personnel (UAP) provide a bed bath to a comatose client who is incontinent. The nurse should intervene if which action is noted?

    1. The UAP answers the phone while wearing gloves.
    2. The UAP log-rolls the client to provide back care.
    3. The UAP places an incontinence pad under the client.
    4. The UAP positions client on the left side, head elevated.

30. A client is brought to the emergency department for treatment after being found on the floor by a family member. X-rays reveal a displaced subcapital fracture of the left hip. When comparing the legs, the nurse would most likely make which observation?

    1. The client's left leg is shorter than the right leg and externally rotated.
    2. The client's left leg is longer than the right leg and internally rotated.
    3. The client's left leg is shorter than the right leg and adducted.
    4. The client's left leg is longer than the right leg and is abducted.

31. The nurse is discharging a client from an inpatient alcohol treatment unit. Which statement by the client's family member indicates to the nurse that the family member is coping adaptively?

    1. "He will do well if I keep him engaged in his favorite activities."
    2. "My focus is learning how to live my life."
    3. "I am glad that our problems are behind us."
    4. "I'll make sure that the children don't give him any problems."

32. A client with a history of alcohol use disorder is brought to the emergency department in an agitated state. The client is vomiting and diaphoretic, and states that it has been 5 hours since the last drink. The nurse would expect to administer which medication?

1. Chlordiazepoxide.
2. Disulfiram.
3. Methadone.
4. Naloxone.

33. The nurse is caring for a client diagnosed with end-stage colon cancer. The spouse of the client says, "We have been married for so long. I am not sure how I can go on now." What is the **most** appropriate response by the nurse?

1. "It sounds like your children will be there to help during your time of grieving."
2. "I know this is difficult. Tell me more about what you are feeling now."
3. "Think about the pain and suffering your spouse has endured lately."
4. "I will call the hospice nurse to discuss your spouse's condition with you."

34. The nurse is teaching an older adult client how to use a standard walker. Which client behavior indicates that the nurse's teaching was effective?

1. The client slowly pushes the walker forward 12 inches (30 cm), then takes small steps forward while leaning on the walker.
2. The client lifts the walker, moves it forward 10 inches (25 cm), and then takes several small steps forward.
3. The client supports weight on the walker while advancing it forward, then takes small steps while balancing on the walker.
4. The client slides the walker 18 inches (46 cm) forward, then takes small steps while holding onto the walker for balance.

35. After receiving hand-off report, the nurse should see which client **first**?

1. A client in sickle cell crisis experiencing an IV infiltration.
2. A client with leukemia receiving a red blood cell transfusion.
3. A client scheduled for an elective bronchoscopy.
4. A client reporting a leaking colostomy appliance.

36. The nurse is calculating the IV flow rate for a postoperative client. The client is to receive 3,000 mL of lactated Ringer solution IV infused over 24 hours. The IV administration set has a drop factor of 10 drops per milliliter. The nurse should regulate the client's IV administration set to deliver how many drops per minute?

1. 18.
2. 21.
3. 35.
4. 40.

37. A client diagnosed with emphysema becomes restless and confused. Which step should the nurse take next?

1. Encourage pursed-lip breathing.
2. Measure the client's temperature.
3. Assess the client's potassium level.
4. Increase oxygen flow rate to 5 L/minute.

38. The nurse is caring for a client one day after an abdominal-perineal resection for rectal cancer. The nurse should question which prescription?

1. Remove nasogastric tube if audible bowel sounds.
2. Irrigate the colostomy every 8 hours for 2 days.
3. Cover the stoma site with petrolatum gauze.
4. Administer meperidine 50 mg IM for postoperative pain.

39. The nurse is caring for a client 4 hours after intracranial surgery. Which action should the nurse take immediately?

    1. Instruct the client to deep breathe, cough, and expectorate into a tissue.
    2. Position the client in a left lateral position with the neck flexed.
    3. Perform passive range-of-motion exercises every 2 hours.
    4. Use a turning sheet under the client's head to midthigh to reposition in bed.

40. A pediatric client with a congenital heart defect is admitted with a diagnosis of heart failure. Digoxin 0.12 mg by mouth daily is prescribed for the client. The bottle contains 0.05 mg of digoxin in 1 mL of solution. Which amount of digoxin should the nurse administer to the child?

    1. 1.2 mL.
    2. 2.4 mL.
    3. 3.5 mL.
    4. 4.2 mL.

41. The nurse is caring for a client with cervical cancer. The nurse notes that the radium implant has become dislodged. Which action should the nurse take **first**?

    1. Grasp the implant with a sterile hemostat and carefully reinsert it into the client.
    2. Wrap the implant in a blanket and place it behind a lead shield until reimplantation.
    3. Ensure the implant is picked up with long-handled forceps and placed in a lead container.
    4. Obtain a dosimeter reading on the client and report it to the health care provider.

Refer to the Case Study to answer the next six questions.

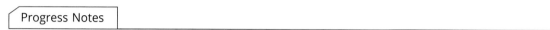

The nurse is caring for an adult client in the primary care clinic.

Progress Notes

Initial Clinic Visit

1500: Client reports cough, sore throat, nasal drainage, and headache for 5 days. Has been using over-the-counter antihistamines to manage symptoms and sleep without interruption. Viral respiratory cultures are negative. Prescribed azithromycin 500 mg PO once daily for 3 days, starting today.

Clinic Visit 3 Days Later

1030: Client reports worsening cough, headache, and new onset shortness of breath since last clinic visit. Started antibiotic therapy at home but reports "not feeling well" the last 2 days and is unable to take anything by mouth, including antibiotics. Client is alert and oriented × 3. Lungs sounds are clear at left lung fields but coarse crackles noted at the right lung base. S1 and S2 heart sounds heard, no murmur or gallop noted. Skin is warm to the touch and appears flushed, capillary refill >3 seconds.

Vital Signs	Result
HR	112 beats/minute
BP	98/56 mmHg
RR	24 breaths/minute
Pulse oximetry	89% on room air
Temperature	101.6° F (38.7° C) (temporal)

1100: Client transferred to hospital for further evaluation and treatment.

42. At 1145, the client is admitted to the medical surgical unit for evaluation of upper respiratory infection with worsening of symptoms. The nurse reviews the client's progress notes from the clinic.

Highlight tokenized client findings that are clinically significant and concerning. Tokenized options are enclosed in boxes.

1030: Client reports worsening cough, headache, and new onset shortness of breath since last clinic visit. Started antibiotic therapy at home but reports "not feeling well" the last 2 days and inability to take anything by mouth, including antibiotics. Client is alert and oriented × 3. Lungs sounds are clear to left lung fields but coarse crackles noted to the right lung base. S1 and S2 heart sounds heard, no murmur or gallop noted. Skin is warm to the touch and appears flushed, capillary refill >3 seconds.

43. For which complication is the client at greatest risk? **(Select all that apply.)**

1. Septic shock.
2. Urinary tract infection.
3. Pneumonia.
4. Airway obstruction.
5. Anaphylaxis.

44. Drag the choices below to fill in each blank in the following sentence. Each choice will only be used once.

It is important for the nurse to monitor the client for signs of poor tissue perfusion, such as decreased _____ [Select from the list], _____ [Select from the list], and _____ [Select from the list].

urine output
level of consciousness
hematocrit
temperature
creatinine
pulse oximetry

Progress Notes | Nursing Assessment

Body System	Findings 1145
Neurological	Alert and oriented × 3.
Eye, Ear, Nose, and Throat (EENT)	Admitted for worsening upper respiratory infection. Reports sore throat, nasal drainage, and headache.
Pulmonary	Reports cough and shortness of breath. Coarse crackles to bilateral lung bases.
Cardiovascular	S1 and S2 heart sounds heard, no murmur or gallop noted. Skin is warm to the touch and appears flushed, capillary refill >3 seconds. Peripheral pulses bounding and equal bilaterally.
Gastrointestinal	Reports inability to take anything by mouth the last 2 days due to nausea.
Genitourinary	Reports not having voided all day. When prompted client voids 20 mL clear, dark urine.
Musculoskeletal	Full range of motion against resistance.

45. The nurse completes an assessment of the client and documents findings.

For each body system below, specify the potential nursing intervention that is appropriate for the care of the client. Each body system supports 1 potential nursing intervention.

Body System	Potential Nursing Interventions
Respiratory	Select... ▾
	Place supplemental oxygen via nasal cannula.
	Perform nasotracheal suctioning.
	Obtain ventilation/perfusion (V/Q) scan.
Cardiovascular-Respiratory	Select... ▾
	Obtain echocardiogram.
	Elevate head of bed 45°.
	Administer 500 mL IV fluid bolus.
Genitourinary	Select... ▾
	Obtain urine specific gravity.
	Encourage toileting every 2 hours.
	Insert indwelling urinary catheter.

Progress Notes | Nursing Assessment | Orders

Physician's Orders

- Vital signs every 1 hour.
- Insert indwelling urinary catheter.
- Monitor intake and output; notify physician if urine output is < 30 mL per hour.
- Lactated Ringer (LR) bolus 500 mL IV over 1 hour.
- Following bolus, infuse LR at 75 mL IV per hour
- Initiate oxygen therapy and titrate to maintain pulse oximetry >92%.
- Obtain laboratory tests: serum lactate, complete blood count (CBC), blood culture and sensitivity (C&S), and sputum C&S.
- Administer piperacillin/tazobactam 3.375 g IV every 6 hours.
- Acetaminophen 325 mg PO every 4 hours PRN temperature >100.5° F (38.1° C).

46. The nurse reviews the physician's orders.

Which physician's order does the nurse perform **first**?

1. Obtain blood and sputum culture and sensitivity (C&S).
2. Administer piperacillin/tazobactam 3.375 g IV.
3. Administer acetaminophen 325 mg PO.
4. Insert indwelling urinary catheter.

47. The nurse performs the ordered interventions and assesses the client 2 hours later.

For each assessment finding below, specify whether the finding indicates the client's condition has improved, not changed, or declined.

Assessment Finding	Improved	No Change	Declined
BP 108/66 mmHg	○	○	○
RR 20 bpm	○	○	○
Urine output 35 mL/hour	○	○	○
Coarse crackles to bilateral lung bases	○	○	○
Pulse oximetry 96% on 2 L via nasal cannula	○	○	○

48. The nurse is caring for clients in the emergency department of an acute care facility. Four clients have been admitted in the last 20 minutes. Which admission should the nurse see **first**?

 1. A client with chest pain unrelieved by nitroglycerin.
 2. A client with third-degree burns to the face.
 3. A client with a fractured left hip.
 4. A client reporting epigastric pain.

49. The nurse is caring for clients on the pediatric unit. A client with second- and third-degree burns on the right thigh is being admitted. The nurse should assign the new client to which roommate?

 1. A client with chickenpox.
 2. A client with asthma.
 3. A client who developed acute diarrhea after antibiotics.
 4. A client with methicillin-resistant *Staphylococcus aureus*.

50. The nurse is teaching a client about elastic stocking use. Which statement by the client indicates to the nurse that teaching was successful?

 1. "I will wear the stockings until I'm told to remove them."
 2. "I should wear the stockings even when I am asleep."
 3. "Every 4 hours I should remove the stockings for a half-hour."
 4. "I'll put on stockings before I get out of bed in the morning."

51. A client is ordered 1,000 mL of 5% dextrose in half normal saline solution IV to infuse over 8 hours. The IV administration set tubing delivers 15 drops per milliliter. The nurse should regulate the flow rate so it delivers how many drops of fluid per minute?

 1. 15.
 2. 31.
 3. 45.
 4. 60.

52. A client is to receive 3,000 mL of normal saline solution IV infused over 24 hours. The IV administration set tubing delivers 15 drops per milliliter. The nurse should regulate the flow rate so that the client receives how many drops of fluid per minute?

 1. 21.
 2. 28.
 3. 31.
 4. 42.

53. The nurse is supervising the care of a client receiving parenteral nutrition through a single-lumen central venous access device (CVAD). The nurse would be **most** concerned if which step in client care was observed?

 1. The client receives insulin through the single-lumen CVAD.
 2. A mask is placed on the client during the site dressing change.
 3. The client's dressing is changed daily using sterile technique.
 4. The client is weighed 2 or 3 times per week in the morning.

54. The nurse is caring for clients in the outpatient clinic. A client reports weakness and numbness in the legs. The client's vital signs include: blood pressure 120/60 mmHg, pulse 86 beats/minute, and respiratory rate 20 breaths/minute. The client denies any pain but appears anxious to the nurse. It would be **most** important for the nurse to ask which question?

1. "Have you recently fallen or suffered a physical injury?"
2. "Have you recently had a viral infection, such as a cold?"
3. "Have you recently taken any over-the-counter medication?"
4. "Have you experienced any headaches over the past week?"

55. A client diagnosed with anorexia nervosa is admitted to the hospital. Which statement by the client requires immediate follow-up by the nurse?

1. "My gums bled this morning."
2. "I'm getting fatter every day."
3. "Nobody likes me, I'm so ugly."
4. "I feel dizzy and weak today."

56. A client is admitted to the hospital for treatment of *Pneumocystis jiroveci* pneumonia and Kaposi's sarcoma secondary to human immunodeficiency virus (HIV). The client informs the nurse about a personal decision to become an organ donor. Which response by the nurse is **best**?

1. "What does your family think about your decision?"
2. "You will help many people by donating your organs."
3. "Would you like to speak to an organ donor coordinator?"
4. "Your illness prevents you from becoming an organ donor."

57. The nurse is caring for a client 5 hours after a pancreatectomy for cancer of the pancreas. The nurse observes minimal drainage from the nasogastric (NG) tube. It is **most** important for the nurse to take which action?

1. Notify the health care provider.
2. Monitor vital signs every 15 minutes.
3. Assess the NG tube for kinking.
4. Replace the NG tube immediately.

58. The nurse is caring for a client who was involved in a motor vehicle accident one day ago. The client has a double-lumen tracheostomy tube with a cuff. Which action should the nurse perform?

1. Change tracheostomy dressing every 8 hours and as needed.
2. Change the tracheostomy ties every 48 hours.
3. Maintain the inner cannula in place at all times.
4. Push the outer cannula back in if it accidentally dislodges.

59. The nurse is assisting the health care provider with removal of a chest tube. Which instruction should the nurse give to the client before chest tube removal?

1. "Exhale and bear down."
2. "Hold your breath for 5 seconds."
3. "Inhale and exhale rapidly."
4. "Cough as hard as you can."

60. The nurse is preparing discharge teaching for a client with a new colostomy. The nurse knows teaching was successful when the client chooses which menu option?

1. Sausage, sauerkraut, baked potato, and fresh fruit.
2. Cheese omelet with bran muffin and fresh pineapple.
3. Pork chop, mashed potatoes, turnips, and salad.
4. Baked chicken, boiled potato, cooked carrots, and yogurt.

61. The nurse is teaching a client how to breastfeed her newborn. The nurse knows that teaching has been successful if the client makes which statement?

1. "My baby's weight should equal the birth weight in 5 to 7 days."
2. "My baby should have at least 6 to 8 wet diapers per day."
3. "My baby will sleep at least 6 hours between feedings."
4. "My baby will feed for about 10 minutes per feeding."

62. A client is admitted to the telemetry unit for evaluation of reported chest pain. Eight hours after admission, the client's cardiac monitor shows ventricular fibrillation. The health care provider defibrillates the client. The nurse understands that the purpose of defibrillation is to accomplish which goal?

1. Increase cardiac contractility, preload, and cardiac output.
2. Depolarize cells allowing SA node to recapture pacing role.
3. Reduce the degree of cardiac ischemia and acidosis.
4. Provide electrical energy for depleted myocardial cells.

63. A client is brought to the emergency department reporting chest pain. The nurse assesses the client. Which symptom would be **most** characteristic of an acute myocardial infarction (MI)?

1. Intermittent, localized epigastric pain.
2. Sharp, localized, unilateral chest pain.
3. Severe substernal pain radiating down the left arm.
4. Sharp, burning chest pain moving from place to place.

64. A client is admitted with diagnoses of deep vein thrombosis (DVT) and pulmonary embolism. A continuous heparin infusion is prescribed. Five days after receiving the infusion continuously, which finding **most** concerns the nurse?

1. Potassium level increases from 4 to 5 mEq/L (4 to 5 mmol/L).
2. The client states, "I just found out that I'm pregnant."
3. Platelet count drops to 135,000/mm^3 (135 × 10^9/L).
4. Aspartate aminotransferase (AST) level 20 U/L (0.33μkat/L).

65. A client returns to the clinic 2 weeks after hospital discharge. The client is taking warfarin sodium 2 mg PO daily. Which statement by the client to the nurse indicates that further teaching is necessary?

1. "I take an antihistamine before bedtime."
2. "I take aspirin whenever I have a headache."
3. "I put on sunscreen whenever I go outside."
4. "I take an antacid if my stomach gets upset."

66. To enhance the percutaneous absorption of nitroglycerin ointment, it would be **most** important for the nurse to select a site with which characteristic?

1. Muscular.
2. Near the heart.
3. Nonhairy.
4. Bony prominence.

67. A client newly diagnosed with major neurocognitive disorder (NCD) due to Alzheimer disease is admitted to the unit. Which action by the nurse is **best**?

1. Place the client in a semi-private room away from the nurses' station.
2. Ask family members to wait in the waiting room during admission process.
3. Assign a different nurse daily to care for client.
4. Ask the client to state the current date.

68. The nurse in the postpartum unit is caring for a client who delivered her first child the previous day. While assessing the client, the nurse notes multiple varicosities on the client's lower extremities. Which action should the nurse perform?

1. Teach the client to rest in bed when the baby sleeps.
2. Encourage early and frequent ambulation.
3. Apply warm soaks for 20 minutes every 4 hours.
4. Perform passive range-of-motion exercises 3 times daily.

Refer to the Case Study to answer the next six questions.

The nurse is caring for an older adult client in the intermediate care unit.

| Nurse's Notes | Vital Signs | Laboratory Results |

1100: Client admitted with a diagnosis of chronic obstructive pulmonary disease (COPD) exacerbation. Client has used home oxygen at 3 L/minute by nasal cannula for 3 years but reports increased dyspnea over the last several days. Client increased portable oxygen to 6 L/minute (O_2 6 L/min). At this time, the client is lethargic but alert and oriented × 3. Client reports shortness of breath at rest and copious amounts of thick, tan sputum. Visual assessment reveals labored breathing and tripod positioning. Lung sounds with wheezes bilaterally. S1 and S2 heart sounds heard, no murmur or gallop noted. Vital signs obtained and admission laboratory tests completed. Respiratory therapy obtaining arterial blood gases (ABGs). Physician notified.

| Nurse's Notes | Vital Signs | Laboratory Results |

Vital Sign	Result 1100
HR	106 bpm
BP	126/72 mmHg
RR	20 bpm
Pulse oximetry	84% on O_2 6 L/minute by nasal cannula
Temperature	98.6° F (38° C) (temporal)

| Nurse's Notes | Vital Signs | Laboratory Results |

Laboratory Test	Result (SI Units)	Interpretation
Arterial Blood Gas (ABG): pH	7.32	Low
ABG: pCO_2	65 mmHg (8.64 kPa)	High
ABG: HCO_3	22 mEq/L (22 mmol/L)	Normal
ABG: pO_2	60 mmHg (7.98 kPa)	Low
Red Blood Cell (RBC) Count	4.2 million/mm³ (4.2×10^{12}/L)	Normal
Hemoglobin	14.8 g/dL (148 g/L)	Normal
Hematocrit	44% (0.44)	Normal
White Blood Cell (WBC) Count	16,200/mm³ (16.2×10^9/L)	High

69. The nurse assesses the client, obtains the client's vital signs, and reviews the admission laboratory results.

    Which laboratory finding requires follow-up? **(Select all that apply.)**

    1. ABG: pH 7.32.
    2. ABG: pCO_2 65 mmHg (8.64 kPa).
    3. ABG: HCO_3 22 mEq/L (22 mmol/L).
    4. ABG: pO_2 60 mmHg (7.98 kPa).
    5. Hematocrit 44% (0.44).
    6. WBC 16,200/mm^3 (16.2 × 10^9/L).

70. For each finding, specify if the finding is consistent with hypercapnia or hypoxemia. Each finding may support more than one disease process. **Each column must have at least 1 response option selected.**

Assessment Finding	Hypercapnia	Hypoxemia
ABG: pH 7.32	☐	☐
ABG: pCO_2 65 mmHg (8.64 kPa)	☐	☐
ABG: pO_2 60 mmHg (7.98 kPa)	☐	☐
Client is lethargic	☐	☐

71. Complete the following sentence by choosing from the list of options.

    The client is at highest risk for developing [Select from list 1] due to the client's [Select from list 2] level.

(1)
metabolic acidosis
respiratory acidosis
metabolic alkalosis
respiratory alkalosis

(2)
pO_2
HCO_3
pCO_2
WBC

72. For each finding below, specify the potential nursing intervention that is appropriate for the nurse to include in the client's plan of care. Each finding may support more than 1 potential nursing intervention.

Finding	Potential Nursing Interventions
Wheezes to bilateral lung fields	☐ Administer a long-acting beta$_2$ agonist (LABA) ☐ Prepare client for computed tomography (CT) scan of the chest
pO$_2$ 60 mmHg (7.98 kPa)	☐ Elevate head of bed (HOB) 45° ☐ Place client on continuous pulse oximetry
pCO$_2$ 65 mmHg (8.64 kPa)	☐ Teach pursed-lip breathing ☐ Administer intravenous sodium bicarbonate
Copious amounts of thick, tan sputum	☐ Administer an expectorant ☐ Check gag reflex twice per shift

Nurse's Notes	Vital Signs	Laboratory Results	Orders

Physician's Orders

- Continuous pulse oximetry monitoring.

- Oxygen via venturi face mask, titrate to maintain pulse oximetry >88%.

- Sputum culture and sensitivity (C&S).

- Repeat ABGs this evening.

- Computed tomography (CT) of chest today.

- Medication therapy:

  - Salmeterol 50 mcg via inhaler twice daily.

  - Fluticasone 88 mcg via inhaler twice daily.

  - Guaifenesin 400 mg PO every 4 hours.

73. The nurse receives and reviews the latest physician's orders.

Which education does the nurse provide to the client regarding inhaled medications? **(Select all that apply.)**

1. Gargle and rinse with lukewarm water following salmeterol use.
2. Administer salmeterol prior to fluticasone.
3. You may notice increased heart rate after salmeterol administration.
4. Salmeterol will help remove excessive, thick mucus from the respiratory tract.
5. As soon as you inhale the medication, breath out slowly.
6. Your inhaled medications should never be abruptly discontinued.

74. The nurse assesses the client after implementation of the physician's orders.

Highlight the client assessment findings that indicate improvement.

Assessment	Assessment Findings
Neurologic	Client awake and alert. Oriented × 3.
Cardiovascular	S1 and S2 heart sounds heard, no murmur or gallop noted. HR 98 bpm and BP 120/76 mmHg.
Respiratory	Client denies shortness of breath at rest. Auscultation of lung sounds reveals wheezes bilaterally, RR 20 bpm. Pulse oximetry 92% on oxygen per 50% venturi mask.

75. The nurse is caring for a client who sustained a left femur fracture in a bicycle accident. A cast is applied. The nurse knows that which exercise would be **most** beneficial for this client?

1. Passive exercise of the affected limb.
2. Quadriceps setting of the affected limb.
3. Active range-of-motion exercises of unaffected limb.
4. Passive exercise of the upper extremities.

76. A client is to receive 35 mg/hr of intravenous aminophylline. The nurse mixes 350 mg of aminophylline in 500 mL in dextrose 5% in water. At which rate should the nurse infuse this solution?

1. 20 mL/hr.
2. 35 mL/hr.
3. 50 mL/hr.
4. 70 mL/hr.

77. The nurse is inserting an IV catheter into a client's left arm. Suddenly the client exclaims, "It feels like an electric shock is going all the way down my arm and into my hand!" Which action will the nurse take **first**?

1. Instruct the client to take slow, deep breaths.
2. Remove the catheter from the client's left arm.
3. Tell the client this is a common response to IV insertion.
4. Withdraw the catheter slightly and then push it forward.

78. The nurse is caring for a group of clients. The nurse knows that it is **most** important for which client to receive their scheduled medication on time?

1. A client diagnosed with myasthenia gravis receiving pyridostigmine bromide.
2. A client diagnosed with bipolar disorder receiving lithium carbonate.
3. A client diagnosed with tuberculosis receiving isoniazid.
4. A client diagnosed with Parkinson disease receiving levodopa.

79. A school-age client is admitted to the hospital for evaluation for a kidney transplant. During the initial assessment, the nurse learns that the client received hemodialysis for 3 years due to stage 5 kidney disease. The nurse knows that the illness can interfere with this client's achievement of which stage of personality development?

1. Intimacy.
2. Trust.
3. Industry.
4. Identity.

80. The nurse is assessing a client with a history of Addison disease who has received steroid therapy for several years. The nurse should expect the client to exhibit which changes in appearance?

1. Buffalo hump, girdle-obesity, gaunt facial appearance.
2. Skin tanning, mucous membrane discoloration, weight loss.
3. Emaciation, nervousness, breast engorgement, hirsutism.
4. Truncal obesity, purple striations on the skin, moon face.

81. The nurse is caring for a client who reports being beaten and sexually assaulted by a friend. Which action will the nurse take **first**?

1. Encourage the client to notify the family's legal counsel.
2. Request a consult with a psychiatric health care provider.
3. Remain with the client during the physical examination.
4. Clean and dress wounds before the physical examination.

82. The nurse is preparing discharge instructions for a client who underwent cataract surgery with lens implantation. Which point should the nurse include in the discharge teaching?

1. Importance of reporting a scratchy feeling in the eye.
2. Lie on the side of the affected eye the night after surgery.
3. Wipe eye with a single gesture from outer canthus inward.
4. Avoid lifting objects that weigh more than 15 lb (6.8 kg).

83. A client is preparing to take a 1-day-old infant home from the hospital. The nurse discusses the test for phenylketonuria (PKU) with the client. The nurse's teaching should be based on an understanding that the test is **most** reliable in which circumstance?

1. After a source of protein has been ingested.
2. After the meconium has been excreted.
3. After the danger of hyperbilirubinemia has passed.
4. After the effects of delivery have subsided.

84. The nurse is caring for a client who receives a balanced complete formula through an enteral feeding tube. The nurse knows that the **most** common complication of an enteral tube feeding is which of these?

1. Edema.
2. Diarrhea.
3. Hypokalemia.
4. Vomiting.

85. A client is brought to the emergency department bleeding profusely from a stab wound in the left chest area. Vital signs are: blood pressure 80/50 mmHg, pulse 110 beats/minute, and respiratory rate 28 breaths/minute. The nurse should expect which potential problem?

1. Hypovolemic shock.
2. Cardiogenic shock.
3. Neurogenic shock.
4. Septic shock.

86. A client is admitted to the hospital for surgical repair of a detached retina in the right eye. In planning care for this client postoperatively, the nurse should encourage the client to do undertake which action?

1. Perform self-care activities.
2. Maintain patches over both eyes.
3. Limit movement of both eyes.
4. Refrain from excessive talking.

Refer to the Case Study to answer the next question.

The home health nurse is providing care for an older adult client diagnosed with hypertension, diabetes mellitus type 2, chronic kidney disease (CKD), and coronary artery disease.

| Physician's Notes | Orders | Visit Notes |

Tuesday: Client in clinic today. Accompanied by spouse. Reports increasing fatigue and periods of confusion. At time of examination, client is alert and oriented × 4. Pupils equal and reactive. Grips strong and equal bilaterally. Moving all extremities well. Denies chest pain. S1 S2 clear. Apical pulse irregular. Lungs clear, abdomen soft with active bowel sounds × 4 quadrants. Pulses 2+ in upper extremities, 1+ in lower extremities. Results of complete blood count (CBC), coagulation profile, electrolytes within normal limits. Client monitors blood glucose at home twice daily, and results have been within prescribed limits. Vital signs: BP 184/94; HR 88, irregular; RR 16; SpO_2 95% on room air. Afebrile. Client reports daily blood pressure measurements have been higher the last few weeks. Denies headache. Denies changes in diet or activity. Reviewed client's home medications:

Medication	Dose	Route	Frequency
Atorvastatin	20 mg	PO	Once daily
Losartan	25 mg	PO	Twice daily
Carvedilol	12.5 mg	PO	Twice daily
Hydrochlorothiazide	25 mg	PO	Once daily
Glipizide	5 mg	PO	Once daily

| Physician's Notes | Orders | Visit Notes |

Physician's Orders

- Increase carvedilol to 25 mg PO twice daily.
- Home health for skilled nursing for disease management and medication teaching.
- Home health telehealth monitor for blood pressure daily.
- Notify office for systolic BP > 200 mmHg or < 100 mmHg or HR < 60 bpm.
- Return to office in 4 weeks.

Physician's Notes	Orders	Visit Notes

Visit 1 (Wednesday):

Assessment complete. Medication teaching complete for all home medications. Telehealth set up for client to transmit daily blood pressures to office. Client verbalizes understanding of new dosage of carvedilol and importance of blood pressure monitoring. Client's spouse fills pill box each week and takes client's blood pressure daily. Nurse to see client weekly. Next visit planned for next Wednesday.

Client Call (Friday):

Spouse calls office to report client has fallen twice since the nurse visited on Wednesday. Client is not hurt or in pain, and spouse was able to get client up. However, spouse reports concern because the client seems very "off balance" when getting up from the bed or toilet. Client denies headache, blurred vision, or difficulty moving or speaking. Telehealth blood pressure readings have been between 138/70–150/80 mmHg and HR has been 72–80 bpm each morning since client's admission. PRN visit planned for tomorrow morning.

87. The home health nurse reviews the client's history and physical and visit notes, and prepares to make a PRN visit to the client over the weekend.

    Complete the following sentences by choosing from the list of options.

    The nurse is very concerned the client [Select from list 1]. It is a priority for the nurse to [Select from list 2]. The nurse will teach the client to [Select from list 3]. It is also important for the nurse to instruct the client to [Select from list 4].

(1)	(2)	(3)	(4)
has a urinary tract infection (UTI)	notify the physician immediately	change positions slowly	limit fluid intake
could be seriously injured in a fall	teach the client's spouse how to take a blood pressure	take all medications on an empty stomach	eat plenty of sodium-rich foods
should be admitted to an assisted living facility	assess the client's sitting and standing blood pressures	skip a dose of hydrochlorothiazide if feeling dizzy	closely monitor the blood glucose

88. An infant is brought to the pediatrician's office for a well-baby visit. During the examination, congenital subluxation of the left hip is suspected. The nurse would expect to see which symptom?

    1. Lengthening of the limb on affected side.
    2. Deformities of the foot and ankle.
    3. Asymmetry of the gluteal and thigh folds.
    4. Plantar flexion of the foot.

89. After 2 weeks of receiving lithium therapy, a client in the psychiatric unit becomes depressed. Which evaluation of the client's behavior by the nurse would be **most** accurate?

    1. The treatment plan is not effective; the client requires a larger dose of lithium.
    2. This is an abnormal response to lithium therapy; the client should stop the lithium immediately.
    3. This is a normal response to lithium therapy; the client should be monitored for suicidal behavior.
    4. The treatment plan is not effective; the client requires an antidepressant.

90. The nurse is supervising care at an adult day-care center. Four meal choices are available to the residents. The nurse should ensure that a resident on a low-cholesterol diet receives which meal?

    1. Egg custard and boiled liver.
    2. Fried chicken and potatoes.
    3. Hamburger and French fries.
    4. Grilled salmon and green beans.

Refer to the Case Study to answer the next question.

The nurse is caring for a 65-year-old client in the cardiac care unit.

History and Physical | Nurse's Notes

History: Client admitted 3 days ago for a scheduled coronary artery bypass graft (CABG) ×3 vessels. No complications intraoperatively, recovered in the ICU overnight. Client transferred out of the intensive care unit (ICU) the following day to the cardiac care unit. Chest tubes were removed this morning. History of coronary artery disease, hypertension, hyperlipidemia, and osteoarthritis.

Body System	Findings
Neurological	Alert and oriented ×3.
Eye, Ear, Nose, and Throat (EENT)	Normocephalic, denies sore throat, nasal congestion, or vision changes. No swelling or drainage visualized.
Pulmonary	Denies shortness of breath and cough. Lung sounds clear throughout.
Cardiovascular	Irregular heart rhythm auscultated. Denies chest pain. Skin is warm to the touch, capillary refill < 3 seconds. No edema and peripheral pulses 2+, equal bilaterally.
Gastrointestinal	Denies nausea, bowel sounds active ×4 quadrants. Reports bowel movement (BM) prior to admission.
Genitourinary	Indwelling catheter discontinued this morning, has been voiding without complications.
Musculoskeletal	Full range of motion against resistance. Sitting in the bedside recliner, at this time.

History and Physical | **Nurse's Notes**

1300: Client is sitting at bedside. Reports "racing" heartbeat and feeling faint. Irregular heart rhythm auscultated.

Vital Sign	Result
HR	146 beats/min
BP	118/76 mmHg
RR	16 breaths/min
Pulse oximetry	96% on room air
Temperature (temporal)	98.8° F (37.1° C)

91. The nurse is reviewing the client's assessment data to prepare the client's plan of care.

Complete the diagram by choosing from the choices below to specify what condition the client is most likely experiencing, 2 actions the nurse takes to address that condition, and 2 parameters the nurse monitors to assess the client's progress.

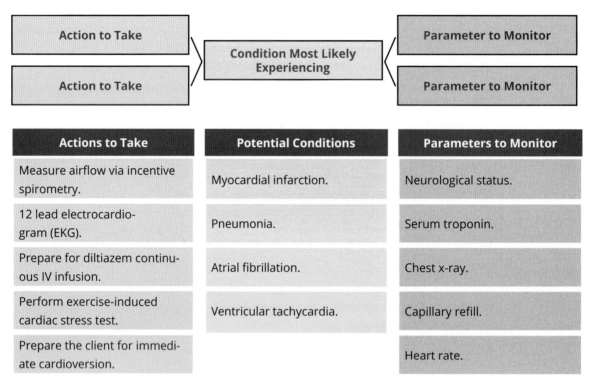

Actions to Take	Potential Conditions	Parameters to Monitor
Measure airflow via incentive spirometry.	Myocardial infarction.	Neurological status.
12 lead electrocardiogram (EKG).	Pneumonia.	Serum troponin.
Prepare for diltiazem continuous IV infusion.	Atrial fibrillation.	Chest x-ray.
Perform exercise-induced cardiac stress test.	Ventricular tachycardia.	Capillary refill.
Prepare the client for immediate cardioversion.		Heart rate.

92. The nurse is teaching a primigravid client how to measure the frequency of uterine contractions. The nurse should explain to the client that the frequency of uterine contractions is determined by which approach?

   1. By timing from the beginning of one contraction to the end of the next contraction.
   2. By timing from the beginning of one contraction to the end of the same contraction.
   3. By the number of contractions that occur within a given period of time.
   4. By the strength of the contraction at the peak of the contraction.

93. The nurse is teaching a woman who is receiving estrogen replacement therapy. Which statement by the nurse indicates that the nurse is aware of the possible complications of estrogen therapy?

   1. "Take an analgesic before you take estrogen, because estrogen may cause discomfort."
   2. "Make sure you keep your clinic appointments, especially your gynecologic checkup."
   3. "Increase your fluid intake, because estrogen promotes diuresis and weight loss."
   4. "You need to increase roughage in your diet to avoid constipation."

94. Several days after being admitted for depression, a client is observed sitting alone in the clients' dining room. The nurse notes that the client has not finished the meal. Which action is **most** appropriate?

   1. Allow the client to eat alone until more comfortable eating with other clients.
   2. Ask the client's family to bring in some of the client's favorite foods.
   3. Order small, frequent meals and sit with the client during meals in the dining room.
   4. Do not focus on eating behaviors; appetite will improve over time.

95. A client receives 10 units of isophane insulin subcutaneously every morning at 0800. At 1600, the nurse observes that the client is diaphoretic and slightly confused. The nurse takes which action **first**?

   1. Obtain the client's vital signs.
   2. Check urine for glucose and ketones.
   3. Give 6 oz (180 mL) of skim milk.
   4. Contact the health care provider.

96. Prior to the client undergoing a scheduled intravenous pyelogram (IVP), the nurse reviews the client's health history. It would be **most** important for the nurse to obtain the answer to which question?

   1. Does the client have any difficulty voiding?
   2. Does the client have any allergies to shellfish or iodine?
   3. Does the client have a history of constipation?
   4. Does the client have a history of frequent headaches?

97. Parents bring their child to the primary health care provider for suspected chickenpox. The nurse knows the rash characteristic of chickenpox can be described as which of the following?

   1. Maculopapular.
   2. Small, irregular red spots with minute bluish-white centers.
   3. Round or oval erythematous scaling patches.
   4. Petechiae.

98. The nurse is caring for a client admitted for a possible herniated intervertebral disk. The health care provider prescribed ibuprofen and cyclobenzaprine hydrochloride to be given as needed for pain. Several hours after admission, the client reports pain. Which action will the nurse take **first**?

    1. Give the client ibuprofen to promptly manage the pain.
    2. Ask the health care provider which medication to give first.
    3. Gather more information from the client about the pain.
    4. Allow the client some time to rest to see if the pain subsides.

99. During visiting hours the nurse finds a visitor unconscious on the floor of a client's room. Which nursing assessment findings indicate the need for cardiopulmonary resuscitation (CPR)?

    1. Shallow respirations and thready pulse.
    2. Rapid respirations and slow, weak pulse.
    3. Gasping respiration and pulselessness.
    4. Pupillary changes and rapid pulse.

100. A client is transferred to a long-term care facility after a stroke. The client has right-sided paralysis and dysphagia. The nurse observes an unlicensed assistive personnel (UAP) preparing the client to eat lunch. Which situation would require an intervention by the nurse?

    1. The client remains in bed in the high Fowler position.
    2. The client's head and neck are positioned slightly forward.
    3. UAP places food in the back of the mouth on unaffected side.
    4. UAP adds tap water to the pudding to help client swallow.

101. A parent with 4 children calls the clinic for advice on how to care for the oldest child, who has developed chickenpox. Which statement by the parent indicates a need for further teaching?

    1. "I should keep my child home until vesicles have crusted."
    2. "I can use calamine lotion if needed."
    3. "I should remove the crusts so the skin can heal."
    4. "I can use mittens if scratching becomes a problem."

102. The nurse is teaching a woman who comes to the clinic at 32 weeks' gestation with a diagnosis of pregnancy-induced hypertension (PIH). Which statement by the client indicates to the nurse that further teaching is required?

    1. "Lying in bed on my left side is likely to increase my urinary output."
    2. "If the bed rest works, I may lose a pound or two in the next few days."
    3. "I should be sure to maintain a diet that has a good amount of protein."
    4. "I will have to keep my room darkened and not watch much television."

103. The nurse is evaluating the care provided to a client hospitalized for treatment of adrenal crisis. Which change would indicate to the nurse that the client is responding favorably to medical and nursing treatment?

    1. The client's urinary output has increased.
    2. The client's blood pressure has increased.
    3. The client has experienced weight loss.
    4. The client's peripheral edema has decreased.

104. After completing an assessment, the nurse determines that a client is exhibiting early symptoms of a dystonic reaction related to the use of an antipsychotic medication. Which action by the nurse would be **most** appropriate?

1. Reality-test with the client and assure the client that physical symptoms are not real.
2. Teach the client about common side effects of antipsychotic medications.
3. Explain to the client that there is no treatment that will relieve these symptoms.
4. Notify the health care provider to obtain a prescription for IM diphenhydramine.

105. A client has undergone vagotomy with antrectomy for treatment of a duodenal ulcer. Postoperatively, the client develops dumping syndrome. Which statement by the client indicates to the nurse that further dietary teaching is necessary?

1. "I should eat bread with each meal."
2. "I should eat smaller meals more frequently."
3. "I should lie down after eating."
4. "I should avoid drinking fluids with my meals."

Refer to the Case Study to answer the next question.

The nurse is caring for a 48-year-old client in the emergency department.

Nurse's Notes	Laboratory Results

1100: Client admitted with chest pain. Electrocardiogram (EKG) on arrival shows no deviations from normal. Sublingual nitroglycerin administered. Troponin I drawn via venipuncture.

Vital Sign	Result
HR	98 beats/min
BP	148/86 mmHg
RR	16 breaths/min
Pulse oximetry	92% on room air
Temperature	98.8° F (37.1° C) (temporal)
Pain	8/10 heavy, aching pressure to sternum

1105: Client has ongoing chest pain. Repeat dose of sublingual nitroglycerin administered.

Vital Sign	Result
HR	98 beats/min
BP	126/74 mmHg
RR	16 breaths/min
Pulse oximetry	96% on room air
Temperature	98.8° F (37.1° C) (temporal)
Pain	4/10 pressure to sternum

1110: Chest pain relieved with the second dose of nitroglycerin. Prepare for transfer to the inpatient cardiac unit for management of non-ST elevated myocardial infarction (NSTEMI).

Vital Sign	Result
HR	94 beats/min
BP	116/72 mmHg
RR	15 breaths/min
Pulse oximetry	96% on room air
Temperature	98.8° F (37.1° C) (temporal)
Pain	0/10

Nurse's Notes	Laboratory Results

Laboratory Test	Result (SI Units)	Interpretation
Troponin I	0.8 ng/mL (0.8 µg/L)	High

106. The nurse reviews the client's vital signs and laboratory results.

Complete the following sentence by choosing from the list of options.

The nurse expects the troponin I to [Select from list 1] due to [Select from list 2].

(1)	(2)
increase	ongoing ischemia
decrease	permanent cellular damage
fluctuate	restoration of perfusion

107. The nurse is caring for a client diagnosed with bipolar disorder. The client paces endlessly in the halls and makes hostile comments to other clients. The client resists the nurse's attempts to move the client to a room in the unit. Which action by the nurse is **most** important?

    1. Offer the client fluids every hour.
    2. Inform the client about unit rules.
    3. Administer haloperidol IM.
    4. Encourage the client to rest.

108. The nurse is caring for an Rh-negative client who has delivered an Rh-positive child. The mother states, "The doctor told me about RhoGAM, but I'm still a little confused." Which response by the nurse is **most** appropriate?

    1. "RhoGAM is given to your child to prevent the development of antibodies."
    2. "RhoGAM is given to your child to supply the necessary antibodies."
    3. "RhoGAM is given to you to prevent the formation of antibodies."
    4. "RhoGAM is given to you to encourage the production of antibodies."

109. The nurse is teaching a client diagnosed with osteoarthritis. The client asks how to effectively decrease pain and stiffness in the joints before beginning the daily routine. Which instruction should the nurse give the client?

    1. "Perform isometric exercises for at least 10 minutes."
    2. "Do range-of-motion exercises, then apply ointment to joints."
    3. "Take a warm bath, and then rest for a few minutes."
    4. "Perform stretching exercises for all muscle groups."

110. The nurse is caring for a client receiving paroxetine. It is **most** important for the nurse to report which information to the health care provider?

    1. The client reports no appetite change.
    2. The client reports recently being started on digoxin.
    3. The client reports applying sunscreen to go outdoors.
    4. The client reports driving the car to work.

111. A pediatric client is seen in a clinic for treatment of attention-deficit/hyperactivity disorder (ADHD). Medication has been prescribed for the client along with family counseling. The nurse is teaching the parents about the medication and discussing parenting strategies. Which statement by the parents indicates that further teaching is necessary?

    1. "We will give the medication at night so it doesn't decrease appetite."
    2. "We will provide a regular routine for sleeping, eating, working, and playing."
    3. "We will establish firm but reasonable limits on behavior."
    4. "We will reduce distractions and external stimuli to help concentration."

Refer to the Case Study to answer the next question.

The nurse in the clinic is caring for a client with a history of anemia.

| History | Visit Note | Laboratory Results |

The client is a young adult female with a history of unusually heavy menstrual periods. The clinical presentation included fatigue and decreased energy. A diagnostic workup included a complete blood count (CBC) and serum ferritin level. The client was diagnosed with iron-deficiency anemia and prescribed ferrous sulfate 325 mg orally three times a day. Follow up appointment in 8 weeks.

| History | Visit Note | Laboratory Results |

Client being seen today for evaluation of anemia. Client reports fatigue and weakness have increased over the last two weeks. Client states, "I stopped taking the ferrous sulfate three weeks ago because it upset my stomach." Lab work repeated.

| History | Visit Note | Laboratory Results |

Test	Result Visit 1	Interpretation	Result Visit 2	Interpretation
White Blood Cells (WBC)	5,000/mm^3 (5×10^{12}/L)	Normal	4,400/mm^3 (4.4×10^{12}/L)	Normal
Hemoglobin (Hgb)	9.2 g/dL (92 g/L)	Low	8.8 g/dL (88 g/L)	Low
Hematocrit (Hct)	28% (0.28)	Low	27% (0.27)	Low
Red Blood Cells (RBC)	3.9 million/mm^3 (3.9×10^{12}/L)	Low	3.78 million/mm^3 (3.78×10^{12}/L)	Low
Platelets	282,000/mm^3 (282×10^9/L)	Normal	290,000/mm^3 (290×10^9/L)	Normal
Ferritin	60 ng/mL (100 µg/L)	Low	54 ng/mL (84 µg/L)	Low

112. The nurse reviews the client's lab work and assesses the client.

Which assessment finding is consistent with the client's lab results? **(Select all that apply.)**

1. Weight gain.
2. Dizziness.
3. Exercise intolerance.
4. Yellow sclera.
5. Shortness of breath.

6. Craving ice.
7. Polyuria.
8. Brittle fingernails.
9. Stomatitis.

113. The nurse is teaching a client undergoing a paracentesis for treatment of cirrhosis. The client asks about positioning for the procedure. Which description by the nurse would be **most** appropriate?

1. Sitting with the lower extremities well supported.
2. Side-lying with a pillow between the knees.
3. Prone with the head turned to the left side.
4. Dorsal-recumbent with a pillow at the back of the head.

114. A client is calling the suicide prevention hotline to report a personal suicide plan. Which question should the nurse ask **first**?

1. "What has happened to cause you to want to end your life?"
2. "Tell me the details of the plan you developed to kill yourself?"
3. "When did you start to feel as though you wanted to die?"
4. "Do you want me to prevent you from killing yourself?"

115. A client is admitted for treatment of hypovolemic shock. The health care provider prescribes normal saline solution IV to infuse at 125 mL/hr and central venous pressure (CVP) readings every 4 hours. Sixteen hours after admission, the client's CVP reading is less than 2 mmHg. Which evaluation of the client's fluid status by the nurse would be **most** accurate?

1. The client has received enough fluid.
2. The client's fluid status remains unaltered.
3. The client has received too much fluid.
4. The client requires additional IV fluid.

116. A client hospitalized for treatment of delusions tells the nurse, "I'm head of the hospital system working undercover to gather information on client abuse." Which statement by the nurse to the client is **best** initially?

1. "Tell me what you mean about being head of the hospital system and gathering client abuse information."
2. "I think you should share this story with the other clients at dinnertime and see what they say."
3. "You are not the head of the hospital system; you are an accountant under treatment for a mental disorder."
4. "It worries me when you say these things; it means you are not responding to the medication."

117. The nurse is caring for a client in labor. The nurse palpates a firm, round form in the uterine fundus, small parts on the client's right side, and a long, smooth, curved section on the left side. Based on these findings, the nurse should anticipate auscultating the fetal heart in which of the following locations?

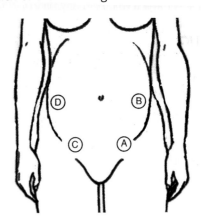

1. A.
2. B.
3. C.
4. D.

118. A client admitted with a diagnosis of pneumonia is receiving gentamicin. For this client, which laboratory values would be **most** important for the nurse to monitor?

    1. Blood urea nitrogen and creatinine.
    2. Hemoglobin and hematocrit.
    3. Sodium and potassium.
    4. Prothrombin time and bleeding time.

119. The nurse is preparing a client newly diagnosed with Addison disease for discharge. Which statement by the client indicates a need for further instruction from the nurse?

    1. "I understand that I will need lifelong cortisone therapy."
    2. "When stressed, I will need to decrease my medication."
    3. "I must take precautions to prevent injuring myself."
    4. "I should always carry a medical identification card."

120. The nurse is assessing a client newly diagnosed with initial-stage chronic glomerulonephritis. Which finding should the nurse expect to see? **(Select all that apply.)**

    1. Hypotension.
    2. Proteinuria.
    3. Severe anemia.
    4. Hematuria.
    5. Azotemia.
    6. Nausea.

121. The nurse is caring for a client who underwent a lumbar spinal fusion for a herniated intervertebral disk. To promote comfort and minimize complications, the nurse tells the client to **avoid** which activity?

    1. Bending the knees when lying on one side.
    2. Sitting for longer than 20 minutes at a time.
    3. Using an extra firm mattress.
    4. Sitting in a hardback chair.

122. The nurse is preparing a client for surgery. When obtaining informed consent, the nurse should **initially** take what action?

    1. Explain the risks, benefits, and alternatives to the procedure.
    2. Tell the client that a signature is needed for all surgeries.
    3. Witness the client's signature on the informed consent form.
    4. Assess whether client understands procedure enough to give consent.

Refer to the Case Study to answer the next question.

The nurse is caring for a postoperative adult client following an exploratory laparotomy due to a bowel obstruction.

> Nurse's Notes

Day of Surgery

Client presented to the Emergency Department with nausea and vomiting for 24 hours. Abdominal x-rays confirmed a bowel obstruction, and the client underwent emergency surgery. On arrival to the unit, the client is alert and oriented. Temperature is 98.2° F (36.8° C), pulse rate 90 beats/minute, respirations 18, and BP 130/78. Bilateral breath sounds diminished in the bases. 18-gauge right forearm IV infusing Lactated Ringer (LR) at 75 mL/hour. Nasogastric (NG) tube to low intermittent suction. Indwelling urinary catheter draining pale yellow urine to bedside bag. Client is utilizing patient-controlled analgesia (PCA) pump with morphine. Reports incisional pain 3 on 0–10 scale. Dressing to the lower abdomen is dry and intact.

Postoperative Day 3

Client is awake and alert, stating that abdominal pain is 7 on a 0–10 scale. The PCA morphine pump is piggybacked into client's infusing IV line, and the client demonstrates understanding of how to use the pump. Respiratory rate 24 to 30 breaths/minute. Breaths are shallow and client states, "It hurts if I take a big breath." Breath sounds reveal scattered rhonchi in the upper lobes with diminished breath sounds in lower lobes bilaterally. Client is expectorating moderate amounts of thick, yellowish-green sputum. Temperature 102.7° F (39.3° C), pulse rate 120–140 beats minute, BP 140/88. IV LR at 50 mL/hr intact to right arm, site without redness or edema. NG tube discontinued 16 hours ago. Client has diminished bowels sounds × 4 quadrants and is tolerating small amounts of clear liquids. Indwelling urinary catheter discontinued earlier this shift. No void at this time. Client is encouraged to use the incentive spirometer but has refused over the past 24 hours due to abdominal pain. Client is allowed up and out of bed but remains in bed due to pain. Physician notified of client's current respiratory status and vital signs.

123. Complete the following sentence by choosing from the list of options.

The client is at risk for developing [Select from list 1] due to [Select from list 2] and [Select from list 3].

(1)	(2)	(3)
pneumothorax	shallow respirations	having a urinary catheter
pneumonia	elevated pulse	use of a PCA pump
ileus	elevated blood pressure	decreased ambulation

124. The nurse is preparing to administer heparin sodium to a client diagnosed with thrombophlebitis. The nurse should ensure that which agent is available if the client develops a significant bleeding problem?

    1. Phytonadione.
    2. Fresh frozen plasma.
    3. Protamine sulfate.
    4. Reteplase.

125. The nurse finds a client sitting on the bathroom floor. The nurse assesses the client, obtains assistance, and assists the client back to bed. The nurse notifies the health care provider and completes an incident report. Which is the **most** appropriate nursing action?

    1. Document in medical record that incident report was filed.
    2. Make a copy of the incident report for the nurse manager.
    3. Document the incident in the client's medical record.
    4. Place the incident report in the client's medical record.

126. The nurse is performing an initial post-operative assessment on a client who has a chest tube attached to a water seal drainage system. The nurse should immediately intervene for which observation?

    1. There are no dependent loops in the chest tube.
    2. The chest tube remains unclamped.
    3. Water seal drainage system is above client's chest.
    4. Fluid level in water seal chamber is at 2 cm.

127. The nurse is caring for a client diagnosed with terminal cancer in the client's home. The nurse knows that which ethical principle **best** supports keeping client and family care consistent with the nurse's professional code of ethics?

    1. Virtues.
    2. Fidelity.
    3. Beneficence.
    4. Justice.

128. Prior to administering a tuberculin (Mantoux) skin test, the nurse in an outpatient clinic is educating a client suspected of having tuberculosis (TB). The nurse determines that the client understands the teaching when the client gives which response?

    1. "I know the test will tell me how long I've been infected with TB."
    2. "This test will tell me if I can spread TB to other people."
    3. "I will need to come back and have a nurse look at the site in a week."
    4. "The test will tell us if I've ever been infected with TB bacteria."

129. A client diagnosed with metastatic breast cancer is admitted with neutropenic fever. The client informs the nurse of the personal decision to not receive cardiopulmonary resuscitation. The nurse explains that this information can be outlined in an advance directive. The nurse understands that which regulation addresses the client's right to identify treatment desires in advance?

    1. Patient's Bill of Rights.
    2. Patient Self-Determination Act.
    3. Health Insurance Portability and Accountability Act.
    4. Americans with Disabilities Act.

130. A non-English-speaking client is being discharged after having a central venous access device (CVAD) inserted. Which description **best** summarizes the nurse's role in advocating for the client?

    1. The nurse uses a translator to help provide discharge instructions.
    2. The nurse provides the client with written discharge instructions.
    3. The nurse ensures the client has transportation home upon discharge.
    4. The nurse provides discharge instructions in a private room.

131. A nurse is caring for a client with a new colostomy. Which activity **best** describes the nurse's role as an advocate for the client?

    1. Ensuring the skin is dry before re-adhering the pouch.
    2. Teaching the client how to care for the ostomy pouch.
    3. Providing a family member with a list of foods to avoid.
    4. Explaining that adjustment to an ostomy takes time.

132. A client was admitted to a rehabilitation center after hip replacement surgery. During an episode of confusion, the client became a danger to self and required vest restraint application. The nurse knows that which implementation is also considered a form of restraint? **(Select all that apply.)**

    1. Administering haloperidol to a combative client.
    2. Raising all of the side rails on the client's hospital bed.
    3. Assigning unlicensed assistive personnel (UAP) to sit with client.
    4. Fastening a bed sheet tightly across the client's chest.
    5. Clipping a tray across the front of the client's wheelchair.

133. A client has an unsteady gait and requires assistance with ambulation. The nurse decides to use a gait belt. Which step should the nurse take when using a gait belt? **(Select all that apply.)**

    1. Secure the gait belt loosely around the client's waist.
    2. Twist the upper body when positioning the client.
    3. Remove gait belt from the client immediately after use.
    4. Place the gait belt over the client's clothes with the clip positioned in front.
    5. Walk in front of the client who is wearing the gait belt.

134. A pediatric client with acute otitis media has been prescribed ofloxacin ear drops. The nurse knows that which statement by the parent demonstrates an understanding of how to properly administer the ear drops?

    1. "I can stop giving the ear drops as soon as my child's fever is gone."
    2. "I should give the drops directly on the eardrum to help get rid of the infection quickly."
    3. "I should warm the ear drops before giving them by wrapping the bottle in my hand."
    4. "I should have my child lie flat while I administer the ear drops."

135. A client recently diagnosed with hypertension has been taking furosemide 40 mg PO twice daily. During a clinic appointment, the client reports new onset muscle weakness and abdominal cramping. Blood samples are drawn for laboratory analysis. The nurse knows which result is the best explanation for the symptoms experienced by the client?

    1. Potassium 3 mEq/L (3 mmol/L).
    2. Creatinine 1.2 mg/dL (106.1 µmol/L).
    3. Fasting glucose 105 mg/dL (5.8 mmol/L).
    4. Total calcium 10 mg/dL (2.5 mmol/L).

Refer to the Case Study to answer the next question.

The nurse in the emergency department (ED) is providing care to a middle aged adult client.

| Admission Notes | Nurse's Notes |

The client presents to the ED with difficulty breathing. Denies chest pain, temperature, or leg swelling. Over the past few days, dyspnea has increased with a dry cough, which occurs periodically during the day with a notable increase at night. The client has a history of asthma since adolescence, and has had occasional episodes during adulthood. Using a rescue inhaler every day for the last three days and symptoms are not improving. Client states, "Several weeks ago I ran out of my controller inhaler and I didn't get the prescription refilled." The client reports two weeks ago had a sore throat, runny nose, and nasal congestion and used over the counter medicines to treat symptoms.

Past History: Asthma, hypertension, hyperlipidemia, obesity, gastroesophageal reflux disease (GERD), obstructive sleep apnea. Non smoker. No known allergies.

Family history: Father died at age 60 from myocardial infarction.

Current home medications:

Medication	Dose	Route	Frequency
Albuterol multi dose inhaler (MDI)	2 puffs	inhaled	4-6 hours PRN dyspnea
Fluticasone propionate (MDI)	2 puffs	inhaled	twice daily
Atorvastatin	40 mg	oral	daily
Omeprazole	20 mg	oral	daily
Lisinopril	20 mg	oral	daily

| Admission Notes | Nurse's Notes |

Assessment: Client is alert, oriented × 4, slightly anxious. Pale, warm skin, slight sweating on face. Frequent coughing and dyspnea. Some difficulty speaking, completes sentences using short words. Diminished breath sounds bilaterally with expiratory wheezes in upper and lower lungs, no crackles. No tension in neck muscles. Client placed on oxygen 2L/min per nasal cannula. S1 and S2 auscultated, regular, no murmurs. Abdomen, soft with normoactive bowel sounds × 4. Moves all extremities.

Vital Signs	Results
BP	158/94 mmHg
Pulse	104, regular
Respiratory rate	28, labored
Temperature (oral)	98.4° F (36.88° C)
Pulse oximetry (continuous)	90% to 91% on 2L/min oxygen per nasal cannula

136. The nurse reviews the admission notes and assesses the client.

Complete the diagram by choosing from the choices below to specify what condition the client is most likely experiencing, 2 actions the nurse takes to address that condition, and 2 parameters the nurse monitors to assess the client's progress.

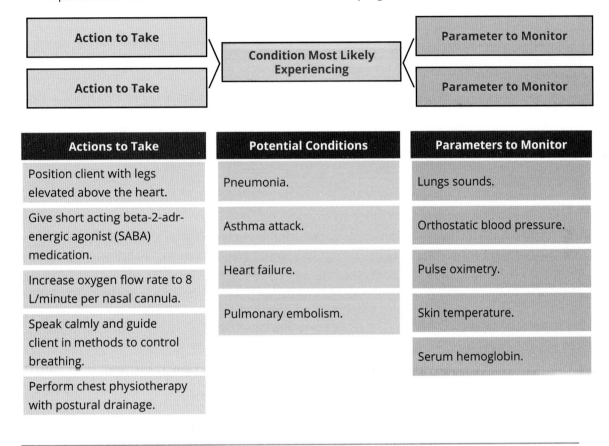

Actions to Take	Potential Conditions	Parameters to Monitor
Position client with legs elevated above the heart.	Pneumonia.	Lungs sounds.
Give short acting beta-2-adrenergic agonist (SABA) medication.	Asthma attack.	Orthostatic blood pressure.
Increase oxygen flow rate to 8 L/minute per nasal cannula.	Heart failure.	Pulse oximetry.
Speak calmly and guide client in methods to control breathing.	Pulmonary embolism.	Skin temperature.
Perform chest physiotherapy with postural drainage.		Serum hemoglobin.

137. Which pediatric client should the nurse provide assessment and intervention for **first**?

    1. A client who has suddenly developed hives on the trunk.
    2. A stable client who is receiving mechanical ventilation.
    3. A client who reports mild difficulty breathing after femur fracture repair.
    4. A client whose apnea alarm sounds with an oxygen saturation level of 82%.

138. The nurse is assigning rooms for a group of clients. The nurse knows that which client requires an airborne infection isolation room?

    1. A client with *Pneumocystis jiroveci* pneumonia.
    2. A client with suspected rubeola.
    3. A client with meningococcal pneumonia.
    4. A client with suspected seasonal influenza.

139. In the event of a fire, the nurse should should take which action **first**?

    1. Leave the building.
    2. Attempt to get clients out of immediate danger.
    3. Work to contain the fire.
    4. Extinguish the fire with a fire extinguisher.

140. The nurse is conversing with a client about a prescribed blood transfusion. It is clear to the nurse that the client does not understand the risks involved with the transfusion. Which intervention **best** supports the nurse's responsibility in the informed consent process?

    1. Tell client that blood transfusion carries few risks.
    2. Inform prescribing health care provider that client needs further explanation of associated risks.
    3. Have another health care professional witness the client's signature on the informed consent form.
    4. Describe alternative treatments to blood transfusion.

141. The nurse is caring for a celebrity who may have sustained a career-changing injury. When asked by coworkers about the status of the client, the nurse refuses to discuss the client's condition. Which ethical principle **best** supports the nurse's action?

    1. Justice.
    2. Beneficence.
    3. Confidentiality.
    4. Accountability.

Refer to the Case Study to answer the next question.

The nurse in the cardiology clinic is providing care for a client with a diagnosis of carotid atherosclerosis.

| History | Diagnostic Results |

The client is an older adult who presented to the emergency department (ED) over the weekend with right-sided facial drooping, right arm and hand weakness, and slurred speech. The symptoms resolved within 30 minutes of admission to the ED, and the client was diagnosed with a transient ischemic attack (TIA). Computed tomography (CT) scan of the head was negative. The client reported two other episodes of right hand tingling and numbness and loss of balance over the past 3 months. The client did not seek treatment for these episodes. Client refused to be admitted to the hospital and was discharged with a cardiology clinic appointment. The client is being seen in clinic today for discussion of lab work and carotid ultrasound results.

The client is retired and lives with a spouse and adult child. The client smokes 1 pack of cigarettes per day. Weight 220 lb (99.8 kg) and height 70 inches (180.3 cm) with a BMI of 30.7 (obese). The client and spouse walk around their neighborhood in the evenings. The client also has diagnoses of hypertension, type 2 diabetes, and migraine headaches. Home medications include:

- Lisinopril 20 mg PO daily.
- Amlodipine 10 mg PO daily.
- Metformin 500 mg PO twice daily with meals.
- Acetaminophen 500 mg PO every 6 hours PRN headache.

| History | Diagnostic Results |

Laboratory Test	Result	Interpretation
Sodium	140 mEq/L (140 mmol/L)	Normal
Potassium	3.4 mEq/L (3.4 mmol/L)	Low
Calcium	8.8 mg/dL (2.2 mmol/L)	Normal
Chloride	98 mEq/L (98 mmol/L)	Normal
Glucose (fasting)	88 mg/dL (4.88 mmol/L)	Normal
Creatinine	1.1 mg/dL (83.88 µmol/L)	Normal
Carbon dioxide (CO2)	24 mEq/L (24 mmol/L)	Normal
Blood urea nitrogen (BUN)	10 mg/dL (3.57 mmol/L)	Normal
Hemoglobin A_{1c}	6.8% (0.068)	High
Cholesterol (total)	234 mg/dL (6.06 mmol/L)	High
Cholesterol, high-density (HDL)	40 mg/dL (1 mmol/L)	Low
Cholesterol, low-density (LDL)	122 mg/dL (3.16 mmol/L)	High
Triglycerides	312 mg/dL (3.53 mmol/L)	High

Carotid Doppler Ultrasound	
Result	**Interpretation**
Right: Images of the right distal common carotid artery show plaque with some calcification.	35% stenosis
Left: Images of the left distal common carotid artery show plaque with moderate calcification.	54% stenosis

142. The nurse is reviewing the client's history and diagnostic tests to prepare the client's plan of care.

Complete the diagram by choosing from the choices below to specify the condition for which the client is at **high** risk, 2 treatments the nurse anticipates for the client, and 2 parameters which the nurse should monitor.

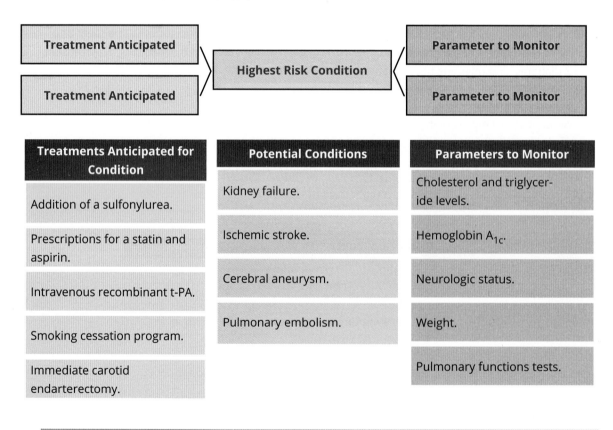

Treatment Anticipated
Treatment Anticipated

Highest Risk Condition

Parameter to Monitor
Parameter to Monitor

Treatments Anticipated for Condition	Potential Conditions	Parameters to Monitor
Addition of a sulfonylurea.	Kidney failure.	Cholesterol and triglyceride levels.
Prescriptions for a statin and aspirin.	Ischemic stroke.	Hemoglobin A_{1c}.
Intravenous recombinant t-PA.	Cerebral aneurysm.	Neurologic status.
Smoking cessation program.	Pulmonary embolism.	Weight.
Immediate carotid endarterectomy.		Pulmonary functions tests.

143. The charge nurse is preparing assignments on a medical unit. For this shift, there are several LPN/LVNs, several RNs, and one unlicensed assistive personnel (UAP). Which assignment by the charge nurse is appropriate? **(Select all that apply.)**

    1. The UAP is assigned to bathe all clients that cannot self-bathe.
    2. An LPN/LVN is assigned initial assessment on a newly-admitted client.
    3. An LPN/LVN is assigned clients needing prescribed oral medications and vital sign measurements.
    4. The RNs are assigned clients that require IVP medication administration.
    5. An LPN/LVN is assigned a client requiring the insertion of an indwelling urinary catheter.

144. The nurse is educating new nursing staff members about client safety on the pediatric unit. Which comment by a new staff member **best** demonstrates that teaching has been successful?

    1. "A toddler may be transported to the car by wheelchair when discharged, and then the parents are responsible for how the child is transported home in the family car."
    2. "School-aged children do not require booster seats if they weigh less than 80 lb (36.3 kg), and they do not require bicycle helmets if they weigh more than 80 lb (36.3 kg)."
    3. "Medications can be left at the bedside for pediatric clients, so the parents can dispense them when needed."
    4. "Medications and cleaning supplies must be stored in a locked, child-proof cabinet at all times."

145. The nurse is calling a client after discharge to follow-up regarding care of the newborn. The client reports that the newborn's eyes look yellow. Which is the **most** appropriate response by the nurse?

    1. "How often are you nursing your baby?"
    2. "Are you breastfeeding or bottle feeding?"
    3. "What was your baby's last bilirubin level?"
    4. "Has your baby been seen by the pediatrician?"

146. The nurse is assessing a client who begins to have a grand mal seizure for the first time. Which action does the nurse take **first**?

    1. Protect client's airway.
    2. Restrain the client.
    3. Record the duration of the seizure.
    4. Notify the health care provider.

147. A new staff nurse working on the intensive care unit is concerned about the client's status. The client's blood pressure, heart rate, and oxygen saturation level have progressively decreased. The nurse discusses the client's condition with the charge nurse. The charge nurse says, "Don't worry, the client always does that." Which action should the nurse take?

    1. Call the nursing supervisor for assistance.
    2. Wait and see how the client progresses.
    3. Take the advice of the experienced nurse.
    4. Discuss this with other nurses on the unit.

148. The nurse on a surgical unit has just received hand-off report for assigned clients. Which client should the nurse see **first**?

    1. A client awaiting discharge after surgical repair of an arm fracture.
    2. A client using a continuous passive motion machine after knee replacement surgery.
    3. A client who developed new oxygen requirements and wheezing after abdominal surgery.
    4. A client whose blood pressure is elevated one day after hip replacement surgery.

149. The nurse is working on a unit that is equipped with bar-code technology. Which method by the nurse is **best** when using this technology?

1. Rely solely on bar-code technology for safer medication administration practices.
2. Rely on nursing judgment, decision-making, and bar-code technology
3. Never give a medication that bar-code technology identifies as "incorrect medication."
4. Override bar-code technology when it identifies "incorrect medication" and administer it.

150. The nurse is working at a skilled nursing facility. The nurse witnesses a client getting up from a sitting position on the floor. When the nurse asks the client what happened, the client responds, "I fell." Which documentation should the nurse record in the incident report?

1. Client fell on the floor and there was no injury noted.
2. Client fell on floor landing in a sitting position on the floor.
3. Client found on flood but was able to get up without assistance. Client most likely slipped or tripped.
4. Client found on floor and reported, "I fell." Assessment findings reveal no injury; health care provider notified.

YOUR PRACTICE TEST SCORES

The test included in this book is designed to provide practice answering exam-style questions along with a review of nursing content. Your results on this test indicate where you are *now*. It is *not* designed to predict your ability to pass the NCLEX-RN® exam.

- If you scored 70 percent or better, you have a good understanding of essential nursing content, and you are able to utilize the critical thinking skills required to answer exam-style questions.

- If you scored 60 to 69 percent, you have areas of essential nursing content that need further review, or you may need continued work to master the critical thinking skills needed to correctly answer exam-style questions.

- If you scored 59 percent or less, you need concentrated study of nursing content and continued practice utilizing the critical thinking skills required to be successful on the NCLEX-RN® exam.

If you are looking for additional preparation materials for the NCLEX-RN® exam, Kaplan has live online and self-placed courses to prepare you for the NCLEX-RN® exam. These courses are designed to develop both your knowledge of the nursing content as well as your critical thinking skills. And Kaplan has courses specifically designed to fit *your* lifestyle and budget. Learn more at: **kaptest.com/nclex**

ANSWER KEY

1.	**3**	38.	**2**	76.	**3**	114.	**2**
2.	**4**	39.	**4**	77.	**2**	115.	**4**
3.	**4**	40.	**2**	78.	**1**	116.	**1**
4.	**1**	41.	**3**	79.	**3**	117.	**1**
5.	**3**	42.	**See explanation**	80.	**4**	118.	**1**
6.	**1**	43.	**1 and 3**	81.	**3**	119.	**2**
7.	**See explanation**	44.	**See explanation**	82.	**4**	120.	**2 and 4**
8.	**See explanation**	45.	**See explanation**	83.	**1**	121.	**2**
9.	**3**	46.	**1**	84.	**2**	122.	**4**
10.	**2, 3, and 5**	47.	**See explanation**	85.	**1**	123.	**See explanation**
11.	**2, 3, 5, 7, and 8**	48.	**2**	86.	**3**	124.	**3**
12.	**See explanation**	49.	**2**	87.	**See explanation**	125.	**3**
13.	**2**	50.	**4**	88.	**3**	126.	**3**
14.	**4**	51.	**2**	89.	**3**	127.	**2**
15.	**2**	52.	**3**	90.	**4**	128.	**4**
16.	**3**	53.	**3**	91.	**See explanation**	129.	**2**
17.	**3**	54.	**2**	92.	**3**	130.	**1**
18.	**1**	55.	**4**	93.	**2**	131.	**2**
19.	**3**	56.	**4**	94.	**3**	132.	**1, 2, 4, and 5**
20.	**See explanation**	57.	**3**	95.	**3**	133.	**3 and 4**
21.	**1, 2, 3, 4, 5, 6, 7, and 8**	58.	**1**	96.	**2**	134.	**3**
		59.	**1**	97.	**1**	135.	**1**
22.	**See explanation**	60.	**4**	98.	**3**	136.	**See explanation**
23.	**See explanation**	61.	**2**	99.	**3**	137.	**4**
24.	**See explanation**	62.	**2**	100.	**4**	138.	**2**
25.	**See explanation**	63.	**3**	101.	**3**	139.	**2**
26.	**4**	64.	**3**	102.	**4**	140.	**2**
27.	**2**	65.	**2**	103.	**2**	141.	**3**
28.	**3**	66.	**3**	104.	**4**	142.	**See explanation**
29.	**1**	67.	**4**	105.	**1**	143.	**1, 3, 4, and 5**
30.	**1**	68.	**2**	106.	**See explanation**	144.	**4**
31.	**2**	69.	**1, 2, 4, and 6**	107.	**3**	145.	**2**
32.	**1**	70.	**See explanation**	108.	**3**	146.	**1**
33.	**2**	71.	**See explanation**	109.	**3**	147.	**1**
34.	**2**	72.	**See explanation**	110.	**2**	148.	**3**
35.	**1**	73.	**2, 3, and 6**	111.	**1**	149.	**2**
36.	**2**	74.	**See explanation**	112.	**2, 3, 5, 6, 8, and 9**	150.	**4**
37.	**1**	75.	**2**	113.	**1**		

PRACTICE TEST ANSWERS AND EXPLANATIONS

1. The answer is 3

The nurse is interviewing a client who is receiving treatment for OCD. Which is the **most** important question for the nurse to ask this client?

Reworded Question: What are the signs and symptoms of obsessive-compulsive disorder?

Strategy: "Most important" indicates there may be more than one correct response.

Needed Info: OCD is characterized by a history of obsessions and compulsions. Obsessions are recurrent and persistent thoughts, ideas, impulses, or images that are experienced as intrusive and senseless. The client may know that the thoughts are ridiculous or morbid but cannot stop, forget, or control them. Compulsions are repetitive behaviors performed in a certain way to prevent discomfort and neutralize anxiety.

Category: Assessment/Psychosocial Integrity

(1) "Do you find yourself forgetting simple things?"—should be used to assess client with suspected cognitive disorder

(2) "Do you find it difficult to focus on a given task?"—assesses for disorders that disrupt the ability to concentrate, such as depression

(3) "Do you have trouble controlling upsetting thoughts?"—CORRECT: one feature of OCD is the client's inability to control intrusive thoughts that repeat over and over

(4) "Do you experience feelings of panic in a closed area?"—appropriate for client with suspected panic disorder related to closed spaces or claustrophobia

2. The answer is 4

The nurse on a postpartum unit is preparing 4 clients for discharge. It would be **most** important for the nurse to refer which client for home care?

Reworded Question: Who is the most unstable client?

Strategy: Think ABCs.

Needed Info: Need to meet the client's needs. Physical stability is the nurse's first concern. Most unstable client should be seen first.

Category: Implementation/Safe and Effective Care Environment/Management of Care

(1) A primipara client who delivered a 7-lb (3.2 kg) infant 2 days ago—stable situation, no indication of problems with the client or infant

(2) A multipara client who delivered a 9-lb (4 kg) infant by cesarean section 2 days ago—stable situation, no indication of problems with the client or infant

(3) A multipara client who delivered 1 day ago and is reporting cramping—stable client, cramping due to uterine contraction

(4) A client who delivered by cesarean section and is reporting burning on urination—CORRECT: unstable client, indicates urinary tract infection, requires follow-up

3. The answer is 4

A client is telling the nurse about personal thought patterns. Which statement by the client would validate the diagnosis of schizophrenia?

Reworded Question: What behaviors or thought patterns characterize schizophrenia?

Strategy: Consider each answer in turn. Which is relevant to schizophrenia?

Needed Info: Schizophrenia is generally characterized by delusions (grandiose, religious, paranoid, nihilistic, or delusions of reference or influence), confusion, hallucinations, and illusions (misinterpretations of real external stimuli).

Category: Assessment/Psychosocial Integrity

(1) "I can't get the same thoughts out of my head."—recurrent, intrusive thoughts are characteristic of obsessive-compulsive disorder

(2) "I sometimes feel on top of the world, then suddenly down."—rapid, changing moods are characteristic of the manic phase of bipolar disorder

(3) "Sometimes I look up and wonder where I am."—confused, disoriented thoughts are characteristic of cognitive disorders

(4) "It's clear that this is an alien laboratory and I am in charge."—CORRECT: illogical, disorganized thoughts are typical of schizophrenia

4. The answer is 1

A nursing team consists of an RN, an LPN/LVN, and a UAP. The nurse should assign which client to the LPN/LVN?

Reworded Question: Which client is an appropriate assignment for the LPN/LVN?

Strategy: Think about the skill level involved in each client's care.

Needed Info: LPN/LVN: assists with implementation of care; performs procedures; differentiates normal from abnormal; cares for stable clients with predictable conditions; has knowledge of asepsis and dressing changes; administers medications (varies with educational background and state nurse practice act).

Category: Planning/Safe and Effective Care Environment/Management of Care

(1) A client with a diabetic ulcer that requires a dressing change—CORRECT: stable client with an expected outcome

(2) A client with cancer who is reporting bone pain—requires assessment; RN is the appropriate caregiver

(3) A client with terminal cancer being transferred to hospice home care—requires nursing judgment; RN is the appropriate caregiver

(4) A client with a fracture of the right leg who asks to use the urinal—standard, unchanging procedure; assign to the UAP

5. The answer is 3

The nurse is leading an inservice about management issues. The nurse would intervene if another nurse made which statement?

Reworded Question: What are the nurse's responsibilities regarding obtaining informed consent?

Strategy: Think about each answer. Does it describe the nurse's responsibility for consent?

Needed Info: Requirements: capacity-age (adult), competent, voluntary; information must be given in understandable form. Legal responsibility: primary health care provider's responsibility to get the consent form signed; when a nurse witnesses a signature it means there's reason to believe the client is informed about upcoming treatment.

Category: Evaluation/Safe and Effective Care Environment/Management of Care

(1) "It is my responsibility to ensure the signed consent form is in the client's medical record before the surgical procedure"—describes the nurse's responsibility

(2) "It is my responsibility to witness the signature of the client on the consent form before the surgical procedure."—witnessing the signature indicates that the nurse saw the client sign the form; describes the nurse's responsibility

(3) "It is my responsibility to provide a detailed description of the surgical procedure."—CORRECT: the health care provider performing the procedure should explain the procedure in detail

(4) "It is my responsibility to answer client questions prior to the surgical procedure."—describes the nurse's responsibility

6. The answer is 1

The nurse in the newborn nursery has just received hand-off report. Which infant should the nurse see **first**?

Reworded Question: Which infant is most unstable?

Strategy: Remember ABCs (airway, breathing, circulation).

Needed Info: Need to meet client's needs. Physical stability of client is nurse's first concern. Most unstable client should be seen first.

Category: Evaluation/Safe and Effective Care Environment/Management of Care

(1) A 2-day-old client lying quietly alert with a heart rate of 185 beats/minute—CORRECT: infant has tachycardia; normal resting rate is 120–160 beats/minute; requires further investigation

(2) A 1-day-old client crying, with a bulging anterior fontanel—crying causes increased intracranial pressure, which causes the fontanel to bulge

(3) A 12-hour-old client being held; the respirations are 45 breaths/minute and irregular—normal respiratory rate is 30–60 breaths/minute with apneic episodes

(4) A 5-hour-old whose hands and feet appear blue bilaterally during sleep—acrocyanosis normally occurs for 2–6 hours after delivery due to poor peripheral circulation

7. See explanation for answers

Concerning: The nurse recognizes findings of **pale, cool, and diaphoretic skin**; a **headache**; a **shaky, unsteady gait**; a **pulse of 120**; and **confusion** as abnormal clinical findings for a young adult client.

Not Concerning: The **absence of adventitious lung sounds** (e.g., crackles, wheezes) is considered a normal clinical finding. A **blood pressure of 110/64** is within an acceptable adult range.

8. See explanation for answers

CORRECT OPTIONS: The nurse identifies the client is most likely experiencing symptoms of **hypoglycemia** (i.e., low blood glucose). Hypoglycemia, defined as a blood glucose less than 70 mg/dL (39 mmol/L), may occur when there is **too much insulin relative to blood glucose** and **exercise without food or delayed food.** Low blood glucose produces symptoms (e.g., sweating, tachycardia, shakiness) from the release of epinephrine and norepinephrine. A deficit of glucose impairs the central nervous system and deprives the brain of glucose that produces symptoms such as confusion and unsteady gait.

INCORRECT OPTIONS: The Somogyi effect occurs when nocturnal hypoglycemia results in a rebound morning hyperglycemia. Diabetic ketoacidosis (DKA) occurs from an acute insulin deficiency. In clients with diabetes, the nurse recognizes that exercise has blood glucose lowering effects, therefore inactivity and lack of exercise can contribute to hyperglycemia, not hypoglycemia. Additionally, increased food intake during exercise is recommended to prevent unexpected hypoglycemia. Illness and infection may precipitate the development of DKA, insulin deficiency, and hyperglycemia (not hypoglycemia). Inadequate insulin amount deprives cells of glucose and may lead to hyperglycemia.

9. The answer is 3

CORRECT OPTION: Due to the client's low blood glucose, the nurse's priority consideration is the risk for the client to develop **seizures**. The brain needs sufficient quantities of glucose, and seizures may occur in untreated hypoglycemia due to significant impairment in function of the central nervous system.

INCORRECT OPTIONS: Hypokalemia, osmotic diuresis, and hypovolemia are manifestations that may occur in clients with DKA when there is insulin deficiency and improper utilization of glucose.

10. The answer is 2, 3, and 5

CORRECT OPTIONS: The nurse's care plan to manage the client's low blood glucose should include **goals of achieve a normal blood glucose, reduce risk for injury due to low blood glucose, and promote self-care efforts to balance food, activity, and insulin.** To reverse low blood glucose and reduce injury (e.g., seizures, loss of consciousness, coma), immediate treatment for low blood glucose is essential. Promoting self-care efforts to balance food, activity, and insulin fosters active client management and can positively impact outcomes.

INCORRECT OPTIONS: To manage low blood glucose, the nurse does not include goals of replace electrolytes and restore fluid balance. These are goals related to conditions caused by insulin deficiency (e.g., DKA) that result in hypovolemia and electrolyte depletion. The client is a young, healthy athlete with a BMI of 21 kg/m². As a measure of obesity, the client's BMI indicates the client does not need to focus on losing weight.

11. The answer is 2, 3, 5, 7, and 8

CORRECT OPTIONS: A concentrated source of carbohydrates is needed to reverse low blood glucose of less than 70 mg/dL (39 mmol/L). Appropriate nursing actions include **administer 15 grams of carbohydrate** (e.g., 6 ounces regular soda, 4–6 ounces orange juice, or 1 tablespoon honey). The nurse should **obtain blood glucose 15 minutes after administering 15 grams of fast-acting carbohydrate. If blood glucose is < 70 mg/dL (3.9 mmol/L) after 15 grams of carbohydrate, the nurse should repeat 15 grams of fast-acting carbohydrate.** In acute care settings, it is also appropriate for the nurse to **administer 25–50 ml of 50% dextrose intravenous if the client is unconscious**. Additionally, for an unconscious client who cannot swallow or has no intravenous access, the nurse should **prepare 1 mg of glucagon intramuscular.** Glucagon will stimulate a hepatic response to make glucose quickly available.

INCORRECT OPTIONS: The nurse does not include actions of giving potassium chloride to correct electrolyte imbalance and administering continuous insulin drip as prescribed to treat low blood glucose. In clients who have DKA, a continuous insulin drip is needed to correct acute insulin deficiency, hyperglycemia, and ketosis. Potassium loss may occur from this process and should be replaced. The nurse should not give carbohydrates containing fat (e.g., candy bar or cookies) as the initial treatment for low blood glucose; response is delayed because the fat in these foods slows absorption of the glucose.

12. See explanation for answers

Assessment	Client Findings
Statements	"I understand my glucose can stay low for several hours after I finish soccer practice or a game."
	"I should always check my blood glucose more frequently when I exercise."
Vital Signs	Pulse 88 bpm, regular
	Respirations 28 and deep
Lab work	Blood glucose, 102 mg/dL (5.66 mmol/L)
Neurologic	Headache
	Dizziness when standing
	Coherent thoughts with smooth flow to speech
Respiratory	Fruity odor to breath

CORRECT OPTIONS: The client statements "**I understand my glucose can stay low several hours after I finish soccer practice or a game**" and "**I should always check my blood glucose more frequently when I exercise**" indicate understanding about the glucose-lowering effects of exercise. The nurse identifies normal client findings that indicate effective treatment for low blood glucose as a **regular pulse of 88, blood glucose 102 mg/dL (5.66 mmol/L), and coherent thoughts with smooth flow to speech.**

INCORRECT OPTIONS: In clients with diabetes, rapid, deep breathing can indicate a type of respirations called Kussmaul, which is associated with metabolic acidosis. Client findings of headache and dizziness when standing are symptoms that can occur with low blood glucose and may indicate the nursing actions have not been effective. Fruity odor to breath may be due to acetone, a byproduct of ketones that are produced when a client has DKA.

13. The answer is 2

The nurse is caring for clients in the outpatient clinic. Which phone call should the nurse return **first**?

Reworded Question: Which client should the nurse call back first?

Strategy: Think ABCs and expected vs. unexpected.

Needed Info: Need to meet client's needs. Physical stability is nurse's first concern. Most unstable client should be contacted first.

Category: Analysis/Safe and Effective Care Environment/Management of Care

(1) A client diagnosed with hepatitis A who states, "My arms and legs are itching."—caused by accumulation of bile salts under the skin; treat with calamine lotion and antihistamines

(2) A client with a cast on the right leg who states, "I have a funny feeling in my right leg."—CORRECT: may indicate neurovascular compromise; requires immediate assessment of circulation

(3) A client diagnosed with osteomyelitis of the spine who states, "I am so nauseous that I can't eat."—requires follow-up, but not highest priority

(4) A client diagnosed with rheumatoid arthritis who states, "I am having trouble sleeping."—requires assessment, but not a priority

14. The answer is 4

The nursing team consists of 1 RN, 2 LPN/LVNs, and 3 unlicensed assistive personnel (UAPs). The RN should care for which client?

Reworded Question: Which client is an appropriate assignment for the RN?

Strategy: Think about the skill level involved in each client's care.

Needed Info: Determine nursing care required to meet clients' needs; take into account time required, complexity of activities, acuity of client, and infection control issues. Consider knowledge and abilities of staff members and decide which staff person is best able to provide care. Give assignments to staff members (assign responsibility for total client care; avoid assigning only procedures). Provide additional help as needed.

Category: Planning/Safe and Effective Care Environment/Management of Care

(1) A client with a chest tube who is ambulating in the hallway—LPN/LVN can care for client

(2) A client with a colostomy who requires colostomy irrigation assistance—assign to the LPN/LVN

(3) A client with a right-sided stroke who requires assistance with bathing—assign to a UAP

(4) A client who is refusing medication to treat cancer of the colon—CORRECT: requires the assessment skills of the RN

15. The answer is 2

A 1-day-old client diagnosed with intrauterine growth restriction has a high-pitched, shrill cry and appears restless and irritable. The nurse also observes fist-sucking behavior. Based on this data, which action should the nurse take **first**?

Reworded Question: What do you do for a newborn experiencing withdrawal?

Strategy: Determine the outcome of each answer.

Needed Info: Drug withdrawal may manifest from 12 hours to 10 days after delivery. Symptoms: high-pitched cry, hyperreflexia, decreased sleep, diaphoresis, tachypnea, excessive mucus production, vomiting, uncoordinated sucking. Nursing care: assess muscle tone, irritability, vital signs; administer phenobarbital as prescribed; report symptoms of respiratory distress; reduce stimulation; provide adequate nutrition and fluids; monitor mother-newborn interactions.

Category: Implementation/Health Promotion and Maintenance

(1) Gently massage the client's back every 2 hours—may result in overstimulation of the client

(2) Tightly swaddle the client in a flexed position—CORRECT: promotes infant's comfort and security

(3) Schedule feeding times every 3–4 hours—small, frequent feedings are preferable

(4) Encourage eye contact with the client during feedings—may result in overstimulation of the client

16. The answer is 3

The client diagnosed with major depressive disorder who was admitted to the psychiatric unit for treatment and observation a week ago suddenly appears cheerful and motivated. The nurse should be aware of which possible cause of the change in behavior?

Reworded Question: What is the significance of sudden mood changes in a depressed client?

Strategy: Know the signs of impending suicide.

Needed Info: Assessment for suicidal ideation, suicidal gestures, suicidal threats, and actual suicidal attempt. Clients who have developed a suicide plan are more serious about following through, and are at grave risk. Clients emerging from severe depression have more energy with which to formulate and carry out a suicide plan (for which they had no energy before treatment). The nurse should determine risk for suicide; suspect suicidal ideation in depressed client; ask the client about thoughts of suicide; ask the client about the advantages and disadvantages of suicide to determine how the client sees the situation; evaluate client's access to a method of suicide; and support the client's reason to live.

Category: Analysis/Psychosocial Integrity

(1) The client is likely sleeping well because of the medication—sleeping well may improve overall mood, but nurse should first assess suicide risk due to sudden mood change

(2) The client has made new friends and has a support group—support on the nursing unit may improve overall mood, but nurse should first assess suicide risk due to sudden mood change

(3) The client may have finalized a suicide plan—CORRECT: as depressed clients improve, their risk for suicide becomes greater because they are able to mobilize more energy to plan and execute the suicide plan

(4) The client is no longer depressed due to treatment—sudden cheerful and energetic mood may indicate impending suicide, not resolution of depression

17. The answer is 3

The nurse is caring for a client who reports an off-white vaginal discharge with a curdlike appearance. The nurse observes the discharge and vulvular erythema. It would be **most** important for the nurse to ask which question?

Reworded Question: What is a predisposing factor to developing candidiasis?

Strategy: "Most important" indicates there may be more than one correct response.

Needed Info: *Candida albicans.* Symptoms: odorless, cheesy white discharge; itching, inflames vagina and perineum. Treatment: topical clotrimazole, nystatin.

Category: Assessment/Health Promotion and Maintenance

(1) "Do you have diabetes insipidus?"—diabetes mellitus, not diabetes insipidus, is a factor for the development of candidiasis

(2) "Are you sexually active?"—candidiasis not usually sexually transmitted; predisposing factors include glycosuria, pregnancy, and oral contraceptive use

(3) "What kind of birth control do you use?"—CORRECT: oral contraceptive use predisposes individuals to candidiasis

(4) "Do you take cough medicine?"—there's no relationship between cough medicine and candidiasis

18. The answer is 1

The nurse is caring for a client at 37 weeks' gestation who has a history of type 1 diabetes mellitus. The client states, "I am so thrilled that I will be breastfeeding my baby." Which response by the nurse is **best**?

Reworded Question: What are the insulin requirements of a client with a history of type 1 diabetes mellitus who breastfeeds an infant?

Strategy: Determine the outcome of each answer choice.

Needed Info: Nursing care of a pregnant client with a history of type 1 diabetes mellitus: reinforce need for careful monitoring throughout pregnancy; evaluate understanding of modifications in diet/insulin coverage. Teach client and significant other: diet (eat prescribed amount of food daily at same times); home glucose monitoring; insulin (purpose, dosage, administration, action, side effects, potential change in amount needed during pregnancy as fetus grows and immediately after delivery); no oral antidiabetic agents (teratogenic). Assist with stress reduction; fetal surveillance.

Category: Planning/Health Promotion and Maintenance

(1) "You will probably require less insulin while you breastfeed."—CORRECT: breastfeeding has an antidiabetogenic effect; requires less insulin

(2) "You will initially require more insulin after the baby is born."—insulin needs will decrease due to antidiabetogenic effect of breastfeeding and physiological changes during immediate postpartum period

(3) "You will be able to take an oral antidiabetic agent instead of insulin after the baby is born."—client has type 1 diabetes mellitus: insulin required

(4) "You will likely require the same dose of insulin that you require now."—during the third trimester, insulin requirements increase due to increased insulin resistance; breastfeeding after delivery has an antidiabetogenic effect, and the client will requires less insulin

19. The answer is 3

The nurse is caring for a client who had a thyroidectomy 6 hours ago for treatment of Graves disease. The nurse would be **most** concerned if which response was observed?

Reworded Question: What is a complication after a thyroidectomy?

Strategy: "Most concerned" indicates a complication.

Needed Info: Nursing care for Graves disease/hyperthyroidism: limit activities and provide frequent rest periods; advise light, cool clothing; avoid stimulants; use calm, unhurried approach; administer antithyroid medication, irradiation with I131 postoperatvely. Post-thyroidectomy care: low or semi-Fowler position; support head, neck, shoulders to prevent flexion or hyperextension of suture line; tracheostomy set at bedside; observe for complications—laryngeal nerve injury, thyroid storm, hemorrhage, respiratory obstruction, tetany (decreased calcium from parathyroid involvement), check Chvostek and Trousseau signs.

Category: Assessment/Physiological Integrity/Reduction of Risk Potential

(1) The client's vital signs include: blood pressure 138/82 mmHg, pulse 84 beats/minute, and respirations 16 breaths/minute—blood pressure not severely elevated; pulse and respirations within normal limits

(2) The client supports the head and neck to turn head to right—prevents stress on the incision

(3) The client spontaneously flexes the wrist when the blood pressure cuff is inflated during blood pressure measurement—CORRECT: carpal spasms indicate hypocalcemia

(4) The client becomes drowsy and reports a sore throat—expected outcome after surgery

20. See explanation for answers

Client is a 41-year-old primigravida at 34 weeks gestation. Client presented for a routine obstetric appointment today and reported increasing peripheral edema and daily headaches unresolved with the use of acetaminophen. The client's obstetrician evaluated the client. Findings included 2+ pretibial edema, a BP of 158/90, and weight gain of 11 lbs (4.98 kg) since previous office visit 2 weeks ago. Reflexes 3+ and brisk without clonus. Urine sample evaluated in provider's office revealed 2+ protein via dipstick. Client history significant for smoking 6 – 8 cigarettes daily, obesity with a pre-gravid body mass index (BMI) of 32. The client has consumed 2 servings of decaffeinated soda daily throughout pregnancy. Remainder of past medical history and obstetric history are unremarkable.

CORRECT OPTIONS: Risk factors for chromosomal abnormalities as well as pathophysiological pregnancy challenges are statistically increased in **women aged >35**. **Pre-gravid obesity** as well as **daily cigarette use** are known risk factors for the development of hypertension in pregnancy. The client is demonstrating current signs of pre-eclampsia with **daily headaches**, **peripheral edema**, **proteinuria**, **elevated blood pressure**, and **brisk reflexes**.

INCORRECT OPTION: Consumption of non-nutritive, sugar-laden beverages during pregnancy is not recommended, but are less concerning if they are decaffeinated.

21. The answer is 1, 2, 3, 4, 5, 6, 7, and 8

The client's age, physical findings and laboratory results are all indicative of a diagnosis of pre-eclampsia.

22. See explanation for answers

CORRECT OPTIONS: **Maternal hypertension**, whether pre-existing to the pregnancy or developing as the pregnancy progresses, **disrupts placental perfusion and causes endothelial dysfunction of the placenta**. With the resulting changes with blood flow capacity of the placenta, attachment to the uterine wall can be weakened and precipitate premature separation of the placenta, or **placental abruption**, before birth of the fetus has occurred.

INCORRECT OPTIONS: Placenta previa is the abnormal implantation of the placenta in the lower uterine segment such that it completely or partially covers the cervix, or is close enough to the cervix to cause bleeding when the cervix dilates or the lower uterine segment effaces. Placenta accreta is the unusual adherence of the placenta, penetrating slightly into the myometrium. While advanced maternal age can be a risk factor for the development of hypertension, advanced age alone has not been shown to increase the incidence of placental abruption. The use of IV oxytocin to stimulate or augment uterine contractions has not been shown to be a sole cause of placental abruption. Preterm gestation, as an individual characteristic, has not been demonstrated as a risk factor for placental abruption. Neither head compression nor umbilical cord compression has been shown to precipitate the premature separation of the placenta before birth.

23. See explanation for answers

FHR decreased with late decelerations: The most common symptoms of abruptio placentae are abrupt onset of focal uterine discomfort, vaginal bleeding, and fetal monitor indicators of fetal distress, including late deceleration and decreased FHR variability and rate. The nurse must plan potential interventions to address fetal compromise and detect and treat maternal hemorrhage. Due to the presence of fetal monitor indicators of distress, the nurse will **apply oxygen to the mother** to improve fetoplacental perfusion. INCORRECT OPTIONS: Applying anti-embolism stockings is not a priority concern. Trendelenburg position places pressure on the inferior vena cava and impedes maternal venous return, further decreasing blood flow to the fetus. The position of choice for the client as preparations are made for rapid delivery of the infant is left side lying.

Pink-tinged amniotic fluid: **Maternal vital signs must be monitored frequently** for signs of deteriorating hemodynamic status because pink-tinged amniotic fluid suggests bleeding. INCORRECT OPTIONS: Massive uterine hemorrhage may occur without overt and voluminous vaginal bleeding, as blood may be trapped between the wall of the uterus and the fetal sac. Massaging the uterus is performed after delivery to stimulate the fundus.

Focal uterine pain and rigidity: The **oxytocin infusion must be stopped immediately** to diminish uterine contractility. INCORRECT OPTIONS: The IV magnesium sulfate, with its smooth muscle relaxant effect, is infusing for management of the client's hypertension; discontinuing this medication will have no effect on the progression of the placental abruption. The client would be NPO, unable to take pain medication by mouth.

24. See explanation for answers

CORRECT OPTION: Indication for an emergency cesarean birth include both maternal and fetal issues. For this client, the placental abruption is causing **fetal compromise**. INCORRECT OPTIONS: There is no indication of cephalopelvic disproportion or malpresentation of the fetus.

CORRECT OPTION: **Notifying the blood bank is a priority** as excessive blood loss, hypovolemia, and thrombocytopenia can result from the placental abruption, depending upon the extent of placental detachment and the time that passes between placental detachment and birth. INCORRECT OPTIONS: While both the nursing supervisor and the NICU will be notified, the risk of hypovolemia and expected blood loss is of greatest concern. The blood bank must be notified.

CORRECT OPTION: The nurse caring for the client should anticipate going to the operating room with the client to provide information and **remain with and reassure the client until induction**. INCORRECT OPTIONS: Calling the operating room staff with a report of the client's condition is not the safest way to perform a hand-off of this client's care. The obstetrician or general surgeon performing the procedure will discuss the procedure with the family.

25. See explanation for answers

Improved: **Blood pressure**, **pulse**, **respirations**, and **uric acid** are all improved as a result of placental separation because the placenta is the root cause of pre-eclampsia. **Headache** likely improved due to decreased blood pressure and improved central nervous system (CNS) irritability, again related to placental separation.

No Change: The **hyperreflexia** is unchanged.

Declined: **Hematocrit** and **platelet count** have yet to improve following the cesarean birth and, in fact, have decreased further. This is related to the blood loss that likely accompanies the placental abruption and resulting coagulation cascade. Hemodilution from fluid volume replacement also can impact hematocrit at this time. All residual effects of CNS irritability related to pre-eclampsia, such as hyperreflexia, may take several days to several weeks to resolve.

26. The answer is 4

A client is admitted who reports severe pain in the right lower quadrant of the abdomen. Which action should the nurse take to assist the client with pain relief?

Reworded Question: What is an appropriate nonpharmacological method for pain relief?

Strategy: Determine the outcome of each answer choice.

Needed Info: Establish a 24-hour pain profile. Teach client about pain and its relief: explain quality and location of impending pain; slow, rhythmic, deep breathing promotes relaxation; effects of analgesics and benefits of preventative approach; splinting techniques to reduce pain. Reduce anxiety and fears. Provide comfort measures: proper positioning; cool, well-ventilated, quiet room; back massage; allow for rest.

Category: Implementation/Physiological Integrity/ Basic Care and Comfort

(1) Encourage rhythmic, shallow breathing—slow, rhythmic, deep breathing promotes relaxation

(2) Massage the lower right quadrant of the abdomen—if appendicitis is suspected, massage should never be performed as this action may cause the appendix to rupture

(3) Apply a warm heating pad to the client's abdomen—if pain is caused by appendicitis, increased circulation from heat may cause appendix to rupture

(4) Position client for comfort using pillows— CORRECT: non pharmacological method of pain relief

27. The answer is 2

The nurse is preparing a client for peritoneal dialysis. Which action should the nurse take **first**?

Reworded Question: What is the priority action for a client undergoing peritoneal dialysis?

Strategy: Determine if it is appropriate to assess or implement.

Needed Info: Peritoneal dialysis: takes place within the peritoneal cavity to remove excess fluids and waste products usually removed by the kidneys. Procedure: catheter surgically inserted into abdominal cavity; 1–2 liters of fluid infused into peritoneal space by gravity; fluid remains in cavity for about 20 minutes; fluid drained by gravity. Complications: peritonitis, abdominal pain, insufficient return of fluid. Nursing care before procedure: obtain baseline vital signs, breath sounds, weight, glucose, and electrolyte levels. During procedure: monitor vital signs, ongoing assessment for respiratory distress, pain, discomfort; use aseptic technique; check abdominal dressing around catheter for wetness.

Category: Implementation/Physiological Integrity/ Reduction of Risk Potential

(1) Assess access for a bruit and a thrill—used with hemodialysis through an access such as a fistula, graft, or shunt

(2) Warm the dialysate solution—CORRECT: solution should be warmed to body temperature in warmer or with heating pad; don't use microwave oven; cold dialysate increases discomfort

(3) Position client on the left side—client should be in supine or low Fowler position, and wearing a mask

(4) Insert an indwelling urinary catheter—unnecessary, client can void without a catheter

28. The answer is 3

The nurse is teaching an older adult client with right leg weakness how to use a cane. Which behavior by the client indicates that the teaching was effective?

Reworded Question: What is the appropriate technique used to ambulate with a cane?

Strategy: Determine the outcome of each answer choice.

Needed Info: Cane tip should have concentric rings (shock absorber for stability). Flex elbow 30 degrees and hold handle up; tip of cane should be 15 cm lateral to base of the 5th toe. Hold cane in hand opposite affected extremity; advance cane and affected leg; lean on cane when moving unaffected leg. To manage stairs, step up on unaffected (good) leg, place the cane and affected leg on step; reverse when going down ("up with the good, down with the bad"); same sequence used with crutches.

Category: Evaluation/Physiological Integrity/Basic Care and Comfort

(1) The client holds the cane with the right hand, moves the cane forward followed by the right leg, and then moves the left leg—should hold cane with the stronger (left) hand

(2) The client holds the cane with the right hand, moves the cane forward followed by the left leg, and then moves the right leg—should hold cane with the stronger (left) hand

(3) The client holds the cane with the left hand, moves the cane forward followed by the right leg, and then moves the left leg—CORRECT: the cane acts as a support and aids in weight-bearing for the weaker right leg

(4) The client holds the cane with the left hand, moves the cane forward followed by the left leg, and then moves the right leg—cane needs to be a support and aid in weight-bearing for the weaker right leg

29. The answer is 1

The nurse is helping an unlicensed assistive personnel (UAP) provide a bed bath to a comatose client who is incontinent. The nurse should intervene if which action is noted?

Reworded Question: Which is an incorrect action?

Strategy: "Should intervene" indicates that you are looking for something wrong.

Needed Info: Standard precautions used with all clients: primary strategy for preventing exposure to blood or body fluids. Gloves are worn when exposure to blood, body fluids, secretions, excretions, or contaminated articles is likely; remove and discard promptly after use; perform hand hygiene, before touching items and environmental surfaces to reduce the risk for pathogen transmission.

Category: Evaluation/Safe and Effective Care Environment/Safety and Infection Control

(1) The UAP answers the phone while wearing gloves—CORRECT: contaminated gloves should be removed and discarded, and then hand hygiene performed before answering the phone

(2) The UAP log-rolls the client to provide back care—appropriate action, maintains proper body alignment

(3) The UAP places an incontinence pad under the client—appropriate for a client with incontinence

(4) The UAP positions the client on the left side, with the head of bed elevated—appropriate position to prevent aspiration and protect the client's airway

30. The answer is 1

A client is brought to the emergency department for treatment after being found on the floor by a family member. X-rays reveal a displaced subcapital fracture of the left hip. When comparing the legs, the nurse would most likely make which observation?

Reworded Question: Which is a sign of a hip fracture?

Strategy: Think about each answer choice.

Needed Info: Symptoms of fracture: swelling, pallor, ecchymosis; loss of sensation to other body parts; deformity; pain, acute tenderness, or both; muscle spasms; loss of function, abnormal mobility; crepitus (grating sound on movement); shortening of affected limb; decreased or absent pulses distal to injury; affected extremity colder than contralateral part. Emergency nursing care: immobilize joint above and below fracture using splints before moving client; in open fracture, cover the wound with sterile dressings or cleanest material available, control bleeding by direct pressure; check temperature, color, sensation, capillary refill time distal to fracture; in the emergency department, manage pain.

Category: Assessment/Physiological Integrity/Physiological Adaptation

(1) The client's left leg is shorter than the right leg and externally rotated—CORRECT: affected leg externally rotates and shortens due to contraction of muscles attached above and below fracture site, fragments overlap by 1–2 inches (2.5–5 cm)

(2) The client's left leg is longer than the right leg and internally rotated—affected leg shortens and externally rotates

(3) The client's left leg is shorter than the right leg and adducted— affected leg shortens and externally rotates

(4) The client's left leg is longer than the right leg and is abducted—affected leg shortens and externally rotates

31. The answer is 2

The nurse is discharging a client from an inpatient alcohol treatment unit. Which statement by the client's family member indicates to the nurse that the family member is coping adaptively?

Reworded Question: What indicates that the client's family member is coping with the client's alcoholism?

Strategy: Think about what each statement means.

Needed Info: Nursing care for alcohol use disorder: safety; monitor for withdrawal; reality orientation; increase self-esteem and coping skills; balanced diet; abstinence from alcohol; identify problems related to drinking in family relationships, work, etc.; help client to acknowledge problem; confront denial with slow persistence; maintain relationship with client; establish control of problem drinking; provide support; Alcoholics Anonymous; disulfiram (drug sometimes used to maintain sobriety), based on behavioral therapy.

Category: Evaluation/Psychosocial Integrity

(1) "He will do well if I keep him engaged in his favorite activities."—the family member is accepting responsibility for the client's disorder and encouraging codependent behavior

(2) "My focus is learning how to live my life."—CORRECT: the family member is working to change codependent patterns

(3) "I am glad that our problems are behind us."—discharge from inpatient treatment is not the final step of treatment

(4) "I'll make sure that the children don't give him any problems."—family member is accepting responsibility for the client's disorder and promoting codependent behavior

32. The answer is 1

A client with a history of alcohol use disorder is brought to the emergency department in an agitated state. The client is vomiting and diaphoretic, and states that it has been 5 hours since the last drink. The nurse would expect to administer which medication?

Reworded Question: What is the best medication to treat acute alcohol withdrawal?

Strategy: Think about the action of each medication.

Needed Info: Alcohol sedates the central nervous system (CNS); rebound CNS effect during withdrawal. Early symptoms occur 4–6 hours after alcohol consumption. Symptoms: tremors; startles easily; insomnia; anxiety; anorexia; alcoholic hallucinosis (48 hours after last drink). Nursing care: administer sedation as needed, usually benzodiazepines; monitor vital signs, particularly pulse; institute seizure precautions; provide a quiet, well-lit environment; orient the client frequently; don't leave hallucinating, confused client alone; administer anticonvulsants as needed, thiamine IV or IM, and IV dextrose.

Category: Planning/Physiological Integrity/Pharmacological and Parenteral Therapies

(1) Chlordiazepoxide—CORRECT: antianxiety agent; used to treat symptoms of acute alcohol withdrawal; side effects (S/E): lethargy, hangover effect, agranulocytosis

(2) Disulfiram—used as a deterrent to compulsive drinking; contraindicated within 12 hours of alcohol consumption

(3) Methadone—opioid agonist; used to treat opioid withdrawal syndrome; S/E: respiratory depression, hypotension, dizziness, lightheadedness

(4) Naloxone—opioid antagonist used to reverse opioid-induced respiratory depression; S/E: ventricular fibrillation, seizures, pulmonary edema

33. The answer is 2

The nurse is caring for a client diagnosed with end-stage colon cancer. The spouse of the client says, "We have been married for so long. I am not sure how I can go on now." What is the **most** appropriate response by the nurse?

Reworded Question: What is the most therapeutic response to the spouse of the person diagnosed with end-stage colon cancer?

Strategy: Remember therapeutic communication.

Needed Info: The client in this interaction is the spouse of the client diagnosed with end-stage colon cancer; focus on the present; encourage verbalization of feelings; provide support.

Category: Implementation/Psychosocial Integrity

(1) "It sounds like your children will be there to help during your time of grieving."—dismisses client's concern; keep the focus on the client

(2) "I know this is difficult. Tell me more about what you are feeling now."—CORRECT: acknowledges the client's feelings and allows the client to express feelings

(3) "Think about the pain and suffering your spouse has endured lately."—gives advice and discourages verbalization of feelings

(4) "I will call the hospice nurse to discuss your spouse's condition with you."—passes the responsibility onto the hospice nurse; instead, the nurse should encourage the client to express feelings

34. The answer is 2

The nurse is teaching an older adult client how to use a standard walker. Which client behavior indicates that the nurse's teaching was effective?

Reworded Question: What is the correct technique when ambulating with a walker?

Strategy: Determine the outcome of each answer choice.

Needed Info: Elbows flexed at 20–30-degree angle when standing with hands on grips. Lift and move walker forward 8–10 inches (20–25 cm). With partial or non-weight-bearing, put weight on wrists and arms and step forward with affected leg, supporting self on arms, and follow with good leg. Nurse should stand behind client, hold onto a gait belt at waist as needed for balance. Sit down by grasping armrest on affected side, shift weight to good leg and hand, lower self into chair. Client should wear sturdy shoes.

Category: Evaluation/Physiological Integrity/Basic Care and Comfort

(1) The client slowly pushes the walker forward 12 inches (30 cm), then takes small steps forward while leaning on the walker—the client should not push the walker

(2) The client lifts the walker, moves it forward 10 inches (25 cm), and then takes several small steps forward—CORRECT: the client should pick up the walker, and then place it down on all legs

(3) The client supports weight on the walker while advancing it forward, then takes small steps while balancing on the walker—the client should not support weight on the walker while trying to move it

(4) The client slides the walker 18 inches (46 cm) forward, then takes small steps while holding onto the walker for balance—the client should pick up the walker, not slide it forward

35. The answer is 1

After receiving report, the nurse should see which client **first**?

Reworded Question: Who is the priority client?

Strategy: Think ABCs and "real" problems vs. "potential" problems.

Needed Info: Consider the following factors: chief complaint; age of client; medical history; potential for life-threatening event

Category: Analysis/Safe and Effective Care Environment/Management of Care

(1) A client in sickle-cell crisis experiencing an IV infiltration—CORRECT: IV fluids are critical for treating the clotting and pain associated with sickle cell crisis

(2) A client with leukemia receiving a red blood cell transfusion—there is no indication that this client is unstable or experiencing a transfusion reaction

(3) A client scheduled for an elective bronchoscopy—stable client

(4) A client reporting a leaking colostomy appliance—stable client

36. The answer is 2

The nurse is calculating the IV flow rate for a postoperative client. The client is to receive 3,000 mL of lactated Ringer solution IV infused over 24 hours. The IV administration set has a drop factor of 10 drops per milliliter. The nurse should regulate the client's IV administration set to deliver how many drops per minute?

Reworded Question: What is the IV flow rate?

Strategy: Remember the formula to calculate IV flow rate: Total volume × drop factor divided by the time in minutes. You will have a drop-down calculator on the computer to use while taking the NCLEX-RN® examination.

Needed Info: Lactated Ringer solution: electrolyte solution used to expand extracellular fluid volume, and reduce blood viscosity.

Category: Implementation/Physiological Integrity/Pharmacological and Parenteral Therapies

(1) 18—incorrect

(2) 21—CORRECT: $(3{,}000 \times 10)$ divided by (24×60) = 30,000 divided by 1,440 = 20.8 = 21

(3) 35—incorrect

(4) 40—incorrect

37. The answer is 1

A client diagnosed with emphysema becomes restless and confused. Which step should the nurse take next?

Reworded Question: What should the nurse do to raise the oxygen level of a client diagnosed with emphysema?

Strategy: Determine the outcome of each answer choice.

Needed Info: Emphysema: overinflation of alveoli resulting in destruction of alveoli walls; predisposing factors include smoking, chronic infections, environmental pollution. Teaching includes breathing exercises; stop smoking; avoid hot and cold air or allergens; instructions regarding medications; avoid crowds or close contact with persons who have colds or influenza; adequate rest and nutrition; oral hygiene; influenza vaccines; observe sputum for indications of infection.

Category: Implementation/Physiological Integrity/Reduction of Risk Potential

(1) Encourage pursed-lip breathing—CORRECT: pursed-lip breathing helps the client control the rate and depth of breathing

(2) Measure the client's temperature—confusion is most likely caused by poor oxygenation

(3) Assess the client's potassium level—confusion is most likely caused by poor oxygenation, not electrolyte imbalance

(4) Increase the oxygen flow rate to 5 L/minute—the client should receive low-flow oxygen to prevent carbon dioxide narcosis

38. The answer is 2

The nurse is caring for a client one day after an abdominal-perineal resection for rectal cancer. The nurse should question which prescription?

Reworded Question: Which is an incorrect prescription?

Strategy: Determine the outcome of each answer choice.

Needed Info: Stoma skin care: effect on skin depends on composition, quality, consistency of drainage, location of stoma, frequency of appliance adhesive removal. Principles of skin protection: use skin sealant under tape; use skin barrier to protect skin around stoma; cleanse skin gently and pat dry, do not rub; change appliance immediately when seal breaks.

Category: Analysis/Physiological Integrity/Basic Care and Comfort

(1) Remove nasogastric tube if audible bowel sounds—audible bowel sounds usually indicate the return of peristalsis. The health care provider will also prescribe a clear liquid diet, and then advance the diet as tolerated

(2) Irrigate the colostomy every 8 hours for 2 days—CORRECT: colostomy irrigation should not be performed immediately after surgery when the colostomy is not yet functioning; the colostomy commonly begins to function 3–6 days after surgery

(3) Cover the stoma site with petrolatum gauze—petrolatum gauze may be used to cover the stoma and keep the stoma moist if there is not a pouch in place

(4) Administer meperidine 50 mg IM for postoperative pain—opioid analgesic that can effectively relieve postoperative pain

39. The answer is 4

The nurse is caring for a client 4 hours after intracranial surgery. Which action should the nurse take immediately?

Reworded Question: What is a priority after intracranial surgery?

Strategy: Determine the outcome of each answer choice.

Needed Info: Monitor vital signs hourly. Elevate the head of bed 30 to 45 degrees (as prescribed) to promote venous return from brain, and prevent increased intracranial pressure. Avoid neck flexion and head rotation. Reduce environmental stimuli. Prevent Valsalva maneuver by teaching the client to exhale when turning or moving in bed. Administer stool softeners. Restrict fluids to 1200–1500 mL/day. Administer medications: an osmotic diuretic, corticosteroid, and anticonvulsant.

Category: Implementation/Physiological Integrity/Reduction of Risk Potential

(1) Instruct the client to deep breathe, cough, and expectorate into a tissue—coughing should be avoided because it increases intracranial pressure

(2) Position the client in a left lateral position with the neck flexed—the head should be maintained in a neutral position to promote venous return and reduce the risk for increased intracranial pressure

(3) Perform passive range-of-motion exercises every 2 hours—position changes required during range-of-motion exercise can increase intracranial pressure

(4) Use a turning sheet under the client's head to midthigh to reposition client in bed—CORRECT: Using a turning sheet under the client's head to midthigh helps move the client as a unit maintaining body alignment, and reducing the risk for increased intracranial pressure

40. The answer is 2

A pediatric client with a congenital heart defect is admitted with a diagnosis of heart failure. Digoxin 0.12 mg by mouth daily is prescribed for the client. The bottle contains 0.05 mg of digoxin in 1 mL of solution. Which amount of digoxin should the nurse administer to the client?

Reworded Question: How much of the medication should the nurse give?

Strategy: Remember how to calculate dosages. Be careful and don't make math errors. You will have a drop-down calculator on the computer to use while taking the NCLEX-RN® examination.

Needed Info: Formula: dose on hand over 1 mL = dose desired over x.

Category: Implementation/Physiological Integrity/ Pharmacological and Parenteral Therapies

(1) 1.2 mL—inaccurate

(2) 2.4 mL—CORRECT: 0.05 mg/1 mL = 0.12 mg/x mL, $0.05x = 0.12$, $x = 2.4$ mL

(3) 3.5 mL—inaccurate

(4) 4.2 mL—inaccurate

41. The answer is 3

The nurse is caring for a client with cervical cancer. The nurse notes that the radium implant has become dislodged. Which action should the nurse take **first**?

Reworded Question: What is the best action when a radium implant becomes dislodged?

Strategy: Think about the outcome of each answer choice.

Needed Info: Limit radioactive exposure: assign client to private room; place "Caution: Radioactive Material" sign on door; wear dosimeter film badge at all times when interacting with client (measures amount of exposure); rotate staff caring for client; organize tasks so limited time is spent in client's room; limit visitors; encourage client to do own care; provide shield in room. Client care: use antiemetics for nausea; consider body image; provide comfort measures; provide good nutrition.

Category: Implementation/Safe and Effective Care Environment/Safety and Infection Control

(1) Grasp the implant with a sterile hemostat and carefully reinsert it into the client—the implant should be picked up with long-handled forceps, not a hemostat, and deposited into a lead container in the room, not reinserted into the client

(2) Wrap the implant in a blanket and place it behind a lead shield until reimplantation—the implant should be picked up with long-handled forceps and put into a lead container in the room for disposal

(3) Ensure the implant is picked up with long-handled forceps and placed in a lead container—CORRECT: the priority is to secure the implant to prevent unwanted and dangerous radiation exposure; the implant should be picked up with long-handled forceps and then placed in a lead container; this equipment should be kept in the room of any client receiving this therapy so that it is readily available; institutional guidelines and procedures for managing dislodgement should be followed; radiology is usually involved as soon as dislodgement occurs

(4) Obtain a dosimeter reading on the client and report it to the health care provider—the priority is to secure the implant and place it into a lead container

42. See explanation for answers

1030: Client reports worsening cough, headache, and new onset shortness of breath since last clinic visit. Started antibiotic therapy at home but reports "not feeling well" the last 2 days and inability to take anything by mouth, including antibiotics. Client is alert and oriented × 3. Lungs sounds are clear to left lung fields but coarse crackles noted to the right lung base. S1 and S2 heart sounds heard, no murmur or gallop noted. Skin is warm to the touch and appears flushed, capillary refill >3 seconds.

CORRECT OPTIONS: The nurse will be concerned about **worsening cough, headache, new onset shortness of breath, and coarse crackles at the right lung base** in a client with an upper respiratory infection (URI). These symptoms indicate that the client's condition is worsening. **Inability to take anything by mouth** is a red flag; the client would be unable to take the full course of the antibiotic which can cause the development of resistant bacteria. **Flushed, warm skin** is seen in early sepsis due to vasodilation. **Capillary refill >3 seconds** indicates impaired tissue perfusion.

INCORRECT OPTIONS: After a diagnosis of a URI, the client will be started on empiric antibiotic therapy while cultures are pending. Alert and oriented × 3 means the client is able to accurately state name, location, and time. Intact orientation indicates that the client has adequate cerebral perfusion. Distinct heart sounds are a positive finding and indicate normal pumping action of the heart.

43. The answer is 1 and 3

CORRECT OPTIONS: The client is exhibiting symptoms of worsening infection. **Pneumonia** can occur due to a URI if the infectious agent travels lower in the airway. Spread of the infection into the bloodstream can cause sepsis and **septic shock**.

INCORRECT OPTIONS: At this time, the client is not having symptoms of a urinary tract infection (UTI), airway obstruction, or anaphylaxis. Additionally, UTI and anaphylaxis are not common complications of a URI.

44. See explanation for answers

CORRECT OPTIONS: The profound vasodilation that occurs with sepsis, if untreated, can cause severe hypotension that is not responsive to fluid administration. If this occurs, the condition has progressed to septic shock; inadequate tissue perfusion and acute organ failure can result. Crucial indicators of impaired perfusion include **decreased urine output**, **change in level of consciousness**, and **decreased oxygenation**.

INCORRECT OPTIONS: Hematocrit, temperature, and creatinine do not give insight on perfusion within the body. Hematocrit is the volume of erythrocytes present in blood. Temperature is a parameter to measure to confirm infection. Creatinine is a lab monitored for renal function.

45. See explanation for answers

Respiratory: Titrating **supplemental oxygen to maintain SpO$_2$ greater than 92%** is a crucial intervention. INCORRECT OPTIONS: Nasotracheal suctioning can be a helpful intervention for clients unable to clear their own airways, but no data indicates that this is a problem for this client. A V/Q scan gives detailed insight into lung function but takes time; it does not help the client right now.

Cardiovascular: A crucial measure to increase BP in sepsis is fluid resuscitation; therefore, it would be appropriate to **administer an IV fluid bolus**. INCORRECT OPTIONS: An echocardiogram is an ultrasound showing the heart's chambers, adequacy of valve function, and motion of the myocardial wall. There is no data that indicates the heart's structure is abnormal. Elevating the head of bed (HOB) is a common intervention to assist with respiratory concerns but may actually worsen blood pressure in this client.

Genitourinary: **Inserting an indwelling urinary catheter** can help with accurate monitoring of intake and output (I&O). Perfusion of the kidneys is likely impaired in this client, and tracking the I&O can help assess the effectiveness of interventions. INCORRECT OPTIONS: Urine specific gravity is a laboratory test that measures the kidneys' ability to concentrate urine; it is unnecessary at this time. Setting up a toileting schedule is not an appropriate intervention for this client; this intervention is often used in clients who are confused and may forget to use the bathroom.

46. The answer is 1

CORRECT OPTION: Immediate, one-hour management for sepsis includes: **obtain blood and sputum cultures**, measure serum lactate, administer broad-spectrum antibiotics, and rapidly infuse crystalloid fluids for hypotension.

INCORRECT OPTIONS: Administration of a broad-spectrum antibiotic prior to cultures will interfere with the results. It's crucial to identify the causative organism and begin antimicrobial therapy promptly, because mortality rates rise when antibiotic therapy is delayed. Acetaminophen will treat the client's fever but is not the most important intervention. Inserting an indwelling urinary catheter will be necessary to track I&O but is not the first action to take.

47. See explanation for answers

Improved: Normalization or improvement of blood pressure is evidence that adequate fluid administration has improved the client's circulatory status. **Minimum hourly urine output of 30 m L** indicates adequate kidney perfusion and is another parameter to judge response to fluid resuscitation. **Decreasing rate and depth of respirations** indicates resolution of metabolic acidosis. Additionally, **pulse oximetry > 90%** is within normal limits.

No Change: The client continues to have coarse crackles to bilateral lung bases, which can occur related to fluid shifting that occurs with the inflammatory process.

48. The answer is 2

The nurse is caring for clients in the emergency department of an acute care facility. Four clients have been admitted in the last 20 minutes. Which admission should the nurse see **first**?

Reworded Question: Who is the priority client?

Strategy: Think ABCs.

Needed Info: Factors to consider: chief complaint; age of client; medical history; potential for life-threatening event.

Category: Planning/Safe and Effective Care Environment/Management of Care

(1) A client with chest pain unrelieved by nitroglycerin—an airway issue takes priority

(2) A client with third-degree burns to the face—CORRECT: face, neck, chest, or abdominal burns can cause severe edema that restricts the airway; airway issues take priority

(3) A client with a fractured left hip—airway issue takes priority

(4) A client reporting epigastric pain—airway issue takes priority

49. The answer is 2

The nurse is caring for clients on the pediatric unit. A client with second- and third-degree burns on the right thigh is being admitted. The nurse should assign the new client to which roommate?

Reworded Question: Who is the appropriate roommate for a client with burns?

Strategy: Think about the transmission of diseases.

Needed Info: Burns: increase the risk for infection; contact precautions to prevent spread of pathogens transmitted by direct contact or contact with items in the client's environment, such as *Clostridium difficile* and methicillin-resistant *Staphylococcus aureus*; airborne and contact precautions required until chickenpox lesions become dry and crusted.

Category: Implementation/Safe and Effective Care Environment/Safety and Infection Control

(1) A client with chickenpox—infectious disease that requires airborne and contact precautions

(2) A client with asthma—CORRECT: lowest risk of cross-contamination because client with asthma is not infectious

(3) A client who developed acute diarrhea after antibiotic—requires contact precautions because the client may have *Clostridium difficile* diarrhea

(4) A client with methicillin-resistant *Staphylococcus aureus*—a resistant organism that requires contact precautions

50. The answer is 4

The nurse is teaching a client about elastic stocking use. Which statement by the client indicates to the nurse that teaching was successful?

Reworded Question: Which is a correct statement about elastic stocking use?

Strategy: Determine the outcome of each answer choice.

Needed Info: Maintain pressure on muscles of the lower extremities. Don't use if there are any skin lesions or gangrenous areas. Remove and reapply at least twice per day. Stockings should be kept clean and dry.

Category: Evaluation/Physiological Integrity/Basic Care and Comfort

(1) "I will wear the stockings until I'm told to remove them."—the client should remove elastic stockings daily for bathing and to inspect extremities

(2) "I should wear the stockings even when I am asleep."—elastic stockings promote venous return and are not necessary during prolonged periods of sleep; client can elevate leg on pillow while sleeping to promote venous return

(3) "Every 4 hours I should remove the stockings for a half-hour."—stockings should be worn when client is out of bed to promote venous return

(4) "I'll put on the stockings before I get out of bed in the morning."—CORRECT: elastic stockings promote venous return by applying external pressure on veins; should be applied in the morning because this is the time of day that the legs are usually the least swollen

51. The answer is 2

A client is ordered 1,000 mL of 5% dextrose in half normal saline solution IV to infuse over 8 hours. The IV administration set tubing delivers 15 drops per milliliter. The nurse should regulate the flow rate so it delivers how many drops of fluid per minute?

Reworded Question: What is the correct IV flow rate?

Strategy: Use the correct formula and be careful not to make math errors. You will have a drop-down calculator on the computer to use while taking the NCLEX-RN® examination.

Needed Info: Formula: total volume × drip factor divided by the total time in minutes.

Category: Planning/Physiological Integrity/Pharmacological and Parenteral Therapies

(1) 15—incorrect
(2) 31—CORRECT: (1,000 × 15) divided by (8 × 60)
(3) 45—incorrect
(4) 60—incorrect

52. The answer is 3

A client is to receive 3,000 mL of normal saline solution IV infused over 24 hours. The IV administration set tubing delivers 15 drops per milliliter. The nurse should regulate the flow rate so that the client receives how many drops of fluid per minute?

Reworded Question: How should the nurse regulate the IV flow rate?

Strategy: Use the formula and avoid making math errors. You will have a drop-down calculator on the computer to use while taking the NCLEX-RN® examination.

Needed Info: Formula: total volume × the drop factor divided by the total time in minutes

Category: Planning/Physiological Integrity/Pharmacological and Parenteral Therapies

(1) 21—inaccurate
(2) 28—inaccurate
(3) 31—CORRECT: (3,000 × 15) divided by (24 × 60)
(4) 42—inaccurate

53. The answer is 3

The nurse is supervising the care of a client receiving parenteral nutrition through a single-lumen central venous access device (CVAD). The nurse would be **most** concerned if which step in client care was observed?

Reworded Question: Which is an incorrect action?

Strategy: "Most concerned" indicates that you are looking for an incorrect intervention.

Needed Info: Parenteral nutrition: method of supplying nutrients to the body by the IV route. Nursing care: change IV tubing and filters every 24 hours, transparent semipermeable dressing changed every 5–7 days, gauze dressing changed every 2 days, dressing changed immediately if soiled, loosened, or dislodged; initial rate of infusion 50 mL/hr and gradually increased (100–125 mL/hr) as client's fluid and electrolyte tolerance permits; increased rate of infusion causes hyperosmolar state (headache, nausea, fever, chills, malaise); slowed rate of infusion results in "rebound" hypoglycemia caused by delayed pancreatic reaction to change in insulin requirements.

Category: Evaluation/Physiological Integrity/Pharmacological and Parenteral Therapies

(1) The client receives insulin through the single-lumen CVAD—insulin compatible with parenteral solution
(2) A mask is placed on the client during the site dressing change—this decreases the risk of site contamination from respiratory droplets; nurse also wears mask during dressing changes

(3) The client's dressing is changed daily using sterile technique—CORRECT: transparent semipermeable dressing changed every 5–7 days, gauze dressing is changed every 2 days, and both are immediately changed if soiled, dislodged, or integrity compromised

(4) The client is weighed 2–3 times per week in the morning—weighing the client helps assess fluid balance

54. The answer is 2

The nurse is caring for clients in the outpatient clinic. A client reports weakness and numbness in the legs. The client's vital signs include: blood pressure 120/60 mmHg, pulse 86 beats/minute, and respiratory rate 20 breaths/minute. The client denies any pain but appears anxious to the nurse. It would be **most** important for the nurse to ask which question?

Reworded Question: What is a possible cause of Guillain-Barré syndrome (GBS)?

Strategy: Determine the relationship between the answers and GBS.

Needed Info: GBS Plan/Implementation: intervention is symptomatic; steroids in acute phase; plasmapheresis; aggressive respiratory care; prevent hazards of immobility; maintain adequate nutrition; physical therapy; pain-reducing measures; eye care; prevention of complications (urinary tract infection, aspiration); psychosocial support.

Category: Assessment/Physiological Integrity/Physiological Adaptation

(1) "Have you recently fallen or suffered a physical injury?"—client has symptoms consistent with GBS; not injury-related

(2) "Have you recently had a viral infection, such as a cold?"—CORRECT: A viral infection or immunizations commonly precede GBS

(3) "Have you recently taken any over-the-counter medication?"—no association with symptoms; appropriate question for health history

(4) "Have you experienced any headaches over the past week?"—headache is not a typical symptom of GBS

55. The answer is 4

A client diagnosed with anorexia nervosa is admitted to the hospital. Which statement by the client requires immediate follow-up by the nurse?

Reworded Question: Which problem has the highest priority for this client?

Strategy: Remember Maslow's hierarchy of needs.

Needed Info: Anorexia nervosa: a disorder characterized by restrictive eating resulting in emaciation, disturbance in body image, and an intense fear of being obese. Physical needs must be met first to maintain the client in stable condition. Adequate fluid and electrolyte balance are difficult to maintain.

Category: Planning/Psychosocial Integrity

(1) "My gums bled this morning."—vitamin deficiencies may cause bleeding gums, but not the highest priority

(2) "I'm getting fatter every day."—body image disturbance occurs in clients diagnosed with anorexia nervosa, but such psychosocial needs do not take priority

(3) "Nobody likes me, I'm so ugly."—chronic low self-esteem commonly occurs with anorexia nervosa; this psychosocial need does not take priority

(4) "I feel dizzy and weak today."—CORRECT: fluid volume deficit takes highest priority; dehydration, a common occurrence with anorexia nervosa, could lead to irreversible kidney damage and vital sign instability

56. The answer is 4

A client is admitted to the hospital for treatment of *Pneumocystis jiroveci* pneumonia and Kaposi's sarcoma secondary to human immunodeficiency virus (HIV). The client informs the nurse about a personal decision to become an organ donor. Which response by the nurse is **best**?

Reworded Question: Can this client be an organ donor?

Strategy: Think about each answer choice.

Needed Info: Criteria for organ and tissue donation: no history of significant disease process in the organ or tissue to be donated; no untreated sepsis; brain death of donor; no history of extracranial malignancy; relative hemodynamic stability; blood group compatibility; newborn donors must be full-term; only absolute restriction for organ donation is documented HIV disease. Family members can give consent. Nurse can discuss organ donation with other death-related topics (funeral home to be used, autopsy request).

Category: Implementation/Physiological Integrity/ Physiological Adaptation

(1) "What does your family think about your decision?"—client has the right to make the decision

(2) "You will help many people by donating your organs."—clients with documented HIV are prohibited from donating organs

(3) "Would you like to speak to an organ donor coordinator?"—passes responsibility for the discussion to the organ donor coordinator

(4) "Your illness prevents you from becoming an organ donor."—CORRECT: clients with documented HIV are prohibited from donating organs

57. The answer is 3

The nurse is caring for a client 5 hours after a pancreatectomy for cancer of the pancreas. The nurse observes minimal drainage from the nasogastric (NG) tube. It is **most** important for the nurse to take which action?

Reworded Question: Which is the best action when an NG tube is not draining?

Strategy: Determine whether it is appropriate to assess or implement.

Needed Info: Insertion of NG tube: measure distance from tip of nose to earlobe, plus distance from earlobe to bottom of xyphoid process. Mark distance on tube with tape and lubricate end of tube. Insert tube through

nose to stomach. Offer sips of water and advance tube gently. Observe for respiratory distress. Secure with hypoallergenic tape or a securement device. Verify tube position initially and before feeding. Aspirate for gastric contents, assess appearance, and check pH.

Category: Assessment/Physiological Integrity/Basic Care and Comfort

(1) Notify health care provider—should assess first

(2) Monitor vital signs every 15 minutes—does not address lack of drainage

(3) Assess the NG tube for kinking—CORRECT: assess prior to implementing; maintain tubing in a dependent position to promote drainage

(4) Replace the NG tube immediately—assess before implementing; think "least invasive first"

58. The answer is 1

The nurse is caring for a client who was involved in a motor vehicle accident one day ago. The client has a double-lumen tracheostomy tube with a cuff. Which action should the nurse perform?

Reworded Question: Which is a correct action when caring for a tracheostomy?

Strategy: Determine the outcome of each answer choice. Pay close attention to absolute words (e.g., "all").

Needed Info: Cuffed tracheostomy tube permits mechanical ventilation and seals off lower airways. Inject air with a syringe into one-way valve in pilot line to secure the tracheostomy in place. Nursing responsibilities: perform trachesotomy care, change client's position frequently, provide humidification and hydration, suction the tracheostomy as needed.

Category: Implementation/Physiological Integrity/ Basic Care and Comfort

(1) Change tracheostomy dressing every 8 hours and as needed—CORRECT: doing so prevents infection and moisture-associated skin breakdown

(2) Change the tracheostomy ties every 48 hours— change tracheostomy ties when needed

(3) Maintain the inner cannula in place at all times—keep the inner cannula of the tracheostomy in place at all times, except when cleaning

(4) Push the outer cannula back in if it accidentally dislodges—do not push the dislodged tracheostomy back in the stoma; maintain a patent airway and contact the health care provider

59. The answer is 1

The nurse is assisting the health care provider with removal of a chest tube. Which instruction should the nurse give to the client before chest tube removal?

Reworded Question: What should the client do during chest tube removal?

Strategy: Determine the outcome of each answer choice.

Needed Info: Pneumothorax: air in pleural space causes collapse of lung. Chest tubes: attached to a three-chamber chest drainage system to restore negative pressure in pleural space. Removal: chest tube is clamped, client performs Valsalva maneuver; petroleum gauze dressing applied over the exit site and sealed with tape.

Category: Implementation/Physiological Integrity/Reduction of Risk Potential

(1) "Exhale and bear down."—CORRECT: Valsalva maneuver (exhaling and bearing down) increases intrathoracic pressure to prevent air from entering the chest during tube removal

(2) "Hold your breath for 5 seconds."—unnecessary

(3) "Inhale and exhale rapidly."—unsafe manuever

(4) "Cough as hard as you can."—unnecessary

60. The answer is 4

The nurse is preparing discharge teaching for a client with a new colostomy. The nurse knows teaching was successful when the client chooses which menu option?

Reworded Question: What is the appropriate diet for a client with a colostomy?

Strategy: Recall the type of diet required and then select the menu that is appropriate.

Needed Info: Diet: a low-residue diet for 4–6 weeks postoperatively, avoiding gas-forming, odor-producing, and excessively laxative-producing or constipating foods.

Category: Evaluation/Physiological Integrity/Basic Care and Comfort

(1) Sausage, sauerkraut, baked potato, and fresh fruit—sausage and sauerkraut are gas-producing and should be avoided with a new colostomy

(2) Cheese omelet with bran muffin and fresh pineapple—bran muffin and fresh fruit are high-fiber (residue)

(3) Pork chop, mashed potatoes, turnips, and salad—turnips are odor-causing and salad is high-residue

(4) Baked chicken, boiled potato, cooked carrots, and yogurt—CORRECT: provides balanced nutrition, high-protein, low-residue, low-fat, and non-irritating foods

61. The answer is 2

The nurse is teaching a client how to breastfeed her newborn. The nurse knows that teaching has been successful if the client makes which statement?

Reworded Question: What indicates that a newborn is receiving adequate nutrition when breastfeeding?

Strategy: Think about each statement. Is it true?

Needed Info: Breastfeeding is recommended for the first 6–12 months of life; human milk is considered ideal food. Colostrum is secreted at first; clear and colorless; contains protective antibodies; high in protein and minerals. Milk is secreted after 2–4 days; milky white appearance; contains more fat and lactose than colostrum.

Category: Evaluation/Health Promotion and Maintenance

(1) "My baby's weight should equal the birth weight in 5 to 7 days."—breastfed infants should surpass birth weight in 10–14 days

(2) "My baby should have at least 6 to 8 wet diapers per day."—CORRECT: indicates newborn adequately hydrated and ingesting adequate nutrition

(3) "My baby will sleep at least 6 hours between feedings."—newborns feed approximately every 2–3 hours during the day and every 4 hours at night

(4) "My baby will feed for about 10 minutes per feeding."—should feed for about 15–20 minutes per breast

62. The answer is 2

A client is admitted to the telemetry unit for evaluation of reported chest pain. Eight hours after admission, the client's cardiac monitor shows ventricular fibrillation. The health care provider defibrillates the client. The nurse understands that the purpose of defibrillation is to accomplish which goal?

Reworded Question: Why is a client defibrillated?

Strategy: Think about each answer choice.

Needed Info: Defibrillation: delivers an electrical current to the heart that depolarizes myocardial cells. When the cells repolarize, the sinoatrial (SA) node commonly recaptures its role as the heart's pacemaker.

Category: Analysis/Physiological Integrity/Physiological Adaptation

(1) Increase cardiac contractility, preload, and cardiac output—inaccurate, not a function of defibrillation

(2) Depolarize cells allowing SA node to recapture pacing role—CORRECT: electrical current delivered to the heart depolarizes myocardial cells allowing the SA node to recapture its pacing role

(3) Reduce the degree of cardiac ischemia and acidosis—inaccurate

(4) Provide electrical energy for depleted myocardial cells—inaccurate

63. The answer is 3

A client is brought to the emergency department reporting chest pain. The nurse assesses the client. Which symptom would be **most** characteristic of an acute myocardial infarction (MI)?

Reworded Question: What type of pain is characteristic of an MI?

Strategy: Think about the cause of each type of pain.

Needed Info: MI signs and symptoms: chest pain radiating to neck, jaw, shoulder, back, or left arm; unrelieved by nitroglycerin. Also apprehension, diaphoresis, palpitations, shortness of breath.

Category: Assessment/Physiological Integrity /Physiological Adaptation

(1) Intermittent, localized epigastric pain—indicates GI disorder

(2) Sharp, localized, unilateral chest pain—symptom of possible pneumothorax

(3) Severe substernal pain radiating down the left arm—CORRECT: pain may be crushing; radiate; unrelated to emotion or exercise

(4) Sharp, burning chest pain moving from place to place—may be caused by anxiety

64. The answer is 3

A client is admitted with diagnoses of deep vein thrombosis (DVT) and pulmonary embolism. A continuous heparin infusion is prescribed. Five days after receiving the infusion continuously, which finding **most** concerns the nurse?

Reworded Question: Which is most concerning after receiving heparin continuously for 5 days?

Strategy: Prioritize using the ABCs.

Needed Info: Heparin: anticoagulant. Adverse effects: hemorrhage, heparin-induced thrombocytopenia (HIT). HIT suspected if platelet count drops below 150,000/mm^3 (150 × 10^9/L) or if platelet count drops more than 50% from baseline. Incidence of HIT: as many as 3% of clients receiving heparin therapy. Treatment: discontinuation of heparin therapy. Direct or indirect thrombin inhibitor may be prescribed to maintain anticoagulation.

Category: Planning/Physiological Integrity/Pharmacological and Parenteral Therapies

(1) Potassium level increases from 4 to 5 mEq/L (4 to 5 mmol/L)—hyperkalmia is an adverse effect of heparin therapy, but a potassium level of 5 mEq/L (5 mmol/L) is still within normal limits

(2) The client states, "I just found out that I'm pregnant."—heparin does not cross the placenta but should only be used when potential benefits outweigh potential risks; should notify health care provider of client's report of pregnancy but not highest priority

(3) Platelet count drops to 135,000/mm^3 (135 × 10^9/L)—CORRECT: indicative of HIT; priority is to discontinue heparin therapy

(4) Aspartate aminotransferase (AST) level 20 U/L (0.33μkat/L)—within normal limits

65. The answer is 2

A client returns to the clinic 2 weeks after hospital discharge. The client is taking warfarin sodium 2 mg PO daily. Which statement by the client to the nurse indicates that further teaching is necessary?

Reworded Question: What is contraindicated for warfarin?

Strategy: Think about what each statement means and how it relates to warfarin.

Needed Info: Warfarin sodium: anticoagulant. Major adverse effect: hemorrhage. Prothrombin time (PT) or international normalized ration (INR) used to monitor effectiveness; PT usually maintained at 1.5–2 times normal, goal INR is typically 2–3. Antidote: vitamin

K. Nursing responsibilities: check for bleeding gums, bruises, nosebleeds, petechiae, melena, tarry stools, hematuria. Use electric razor, soft toothbrush; maintain consistent dietary intake of vitamin K once PT/INR levels are therapeutic.

Category: Evaluation/Physiological Integrity/Pharmacological and Parenteral Therapies

(1) "I take an antihistamine before bedtime."—no contraindication

(2) "I take aspirin whenever I have a headache."—CORRECT: inhibits platelet aggregation; increases the risk for bleeding; avoid use with warfarin

(3) "I put on sunscreen whenever I go outside."—does not require an intervention

(4) "I take an antacid if my stomach gets upset."—does not require an intervention

66. The answer is 3

To enhance the percutaneous absorption of nitroglycerin ointment, it would be **most** important for the nurse to select a site with which characteristic?

Reworded Question: What is the best site for nitroglycerin ointment?

Strategy: Think about each site.

Needed Info: Nitroglycerin: used in treatment of angina pectoris to reduce ischemia and relieve pain by decreasing myocardial oxygen consumption; dilates veins and arteries. Adverse effects: throbbing headache, flushing, hypotension, tachycardia. Nursing responsibilities: teach appropriate administration, storage, expected pain relief, adverse effects, when to seek emergency care. Ointment applied to skin; sites rotated to avoid skin irritation. Prolonged effect up to 24 hours.

Category: Implementation/Physiological Integrity/Pharmacological and Parenteral Therapies

(1) Muscular—most important is that the site be non hairy since hair interferes with absorption

(2) Near the heart—most important is that the site be non hairy since hair interferes with absorption

(3) Non hairy—CORRECT: hair interferes with absorption, a skin site free of hair helps ensure drug absorption

(4) Bony prominence—most important is that the site be non hairy since hair interferes with absorption

67. The answer is 4

A client newly diagnosed with major neurocognitive disorder (NCD) due to Alzheimer's disease is admitted to the unit. Which action by the nurse is **best**?

Reworded Question: What is the best assessment?

Strategy: Determine whether to assess or implement.

Needed Info: Alzheimer's disease: chronic, progressive, degenerative neurocognitive disorder, resulting in cerebral atrophy. Signs and symptoms: changes in memory, confusion, disorientation, change in personality; most common after age 65. Nursing responsibilities: reorient as needed; speak slowly; place a clock and calendar in room; place bed in low position with side rails up (all side rails raised is a restraint).

Category: Assessment/Psychosocial Integrity

(1) Place the client in a semi-private room away from the nurses' station—for purposes of safety, should be in a room near nurses' station; needs frequent assessment

(2) Ask family members to wait in the waiting room during the admission process—familiar people decrease confusion in an unfamiliar environment

(3) Assign a different nurse daily to care for client—consistency is important

(4) Ask the client to state the current date—CORRECT: assessment is the first step in planning care

68. The answer is 2

The nurse in the postpartum unit is caring for a client who delivered her first child the previous day. While assessing the client, the nurse notes multiple varicosities on the client's lower extremities. Which action should the nurse perform?

Reworded Question: What is the best way to prevent thrombophlebitis?

Strategy: Think about what causes thrombophlebitis.

Needed Info: High risk of developing thrombophlebitis during pregnancy and immediate postpartum period. Thrombophlebitis: inflammation of vein associated with formation of a thrombus or blood clot. Other risk factors: prolonged immobility, use of oral contraceptives, sepsis, smoking, dehydration, and heart failure. Signs and symptoms: pain in the calf, localized edema of one extremity. Homan sign (pain in calf when foot is dorsiflexed) is not a reliable indicator of DVT. Prevention: early and frequent ambulation. Treatment: bed rest and elevation of extremity, anticoagulant (heparin).

Category: Planning/Health Promotion and Maintenance

(1) Teach the client to rest in bed when the baby sleeps—not preventive; bed rest can cause thrombophlebitis

(2) Encourage early and frequent ambulation—CORRECT: facilitates emptying of blood vessels in lower extremities

(3) Apply warm soaks for 20 minutes every 4 hours—not a preventive measure but an intervention used to treat; must be prescribed by health care provider

(4) Perform passive range-of-motion (ROM) exercises 3 times daily—early ambulation more effective; passive ROM exercises retain joint function, maintain circulation; passive exercises: no assistance from client

69. The answer is 1, 2, 4, and 6

CORRECT OPTIONS: The nurse will be concerned about a **low arterial pH**, an **elevated pCO_2**, a **low pO_2**, and an **elevated WBC count**. In a client with COPD, infection can often induce an exacerbation of symptoms.

INCORRECT OPTIONS: The HCO_3 and hematocrit are normal findings that indicate adequate kidney function and concentration of red blood cells, respectively.

70. See explanation for answers

Hypercapnia: The client has an **acidic pH**; this is due to the **buildup of CO_2**, which is an acid, in the client's bloodstream. This causes hypercapnia. The client could be **lethargic** due to a buildup of CO_2.

Hypoxemia: The **low pO_2** is consistent with hypoxemia. The client could also be **lethargic** due to low oxygenation; altered level of consciousness is seen with changes in acid-base balance or poor oxygenation/perfusion to the brain.

71. See explanation for answers

CORRECT OPTIONS: **Buildup of acidic CO_2** in the client's bloodstream will cause pH to become acidic. To determine if the acidosis is respiratory or metabolic, the nurse will evaluate the **pCO_2**. The alveoli control of the amount of CO_2, and if this value is high, then the **cause of the acidosis is respiratory**. Tip: high pCO_2 and low pH = respiratory acidosis.

INCORRECT OPTIONS: Metabolic acidosis would be indicated by a low pH and a low bicarbonate (HCO_3) level, but normal or even low pCO_2. Metabolic and respiratory alkalosis are evidenced by an elevated pH. In metabolic alkalosis, the HCO_3 level is elevated. In respiratory alkalosis, the pCO_2 level is low. WBC levels do not affect the arterial blood pH.

72. See explanation for answers

Wheezes to bilateral lung fields: Wheezes are caused by the squeezing of air through narrowed pathways. This indicates constriction of the lung tissue. **LABAs** dilate the bronchioles. A **CT scan of the chest** will help to visualize exactly what is happening in the airway.

pO_2 60 mmHg (7.98 kPa): Low oxygen levels in clients can be improved by **raising the HOB** to open the airway. Additionally, **continuously monitoring pulse oximetry** is a noninvasive technique that will alert the nurse of changes in oxygenation.

pCO_2 65 mmHg (8.64 kPa): Elevated CO_2 is seen in clients with COPD because they have difficulty fully exhaling, and expired CO_2 is "trapped." **Pursed-lip breathing** is a technique that prolongs expiration as clients exhale through pursed lips. INCORRECT OPTION: Administering sodium bicarbonate would not improve CO_2 levels, the source of the acidosis.

Copious amounts of thick, tan sputum: Clients experiencing a COPD exacerbation often see changes in sputum amount and consistency. **Expectorants** reduce viscosity of secretions so they are more easily expectorated. INCORRECT OPTION: Checking gag reflex is an intervention that would be used to determine if a client is able to protect the airway. This intervention is not appropriate for this client.

73. The answer is 2, 3, and 6

CORRECT OPTIONS: Administering **salmeterol prior to fluticasone** allows bronchodilation prior to steroid absorption within the airway. Because salmeterol is a LABA, administration may stimulate other symptoms of sympathetic nervous system activation, such as tremors or **tachycardia**. The **inhaled medications should not be abruptly discontinued** as this could cause sudden bronchoconstriction.

INCORRECT OPTIONS: Gargling and rinsing the mouth is necessary after inhalation of fluticasone, not salmeterol. Salmeterol causes bronchodilation but does not thin secretions. The nurse will instruct the client to hold the breath for about 10 seconds after inhaling the medications, to keep the medication in the lungs.

74. See explanation for answers

Assessment	Assessment Findings
Neurologic	Client awake and alert . Oriented × 3.
Cardiovascular	S1 and S2 heart sounds heard, no murmur or gallop noted. HR 98 bpm and BP 120/76 mmHg.
Respiratory	Client denies shortness of breath at rest. Auscultation of lung sounds reveals wheezes bilaterally, RR 20 bpm. Pulse oximetry 92% on oxygen per 50% venturi mask.

CORRECT OPTIONS: The client is **no longer lethargic** and has notable **improvements to HR, BP, shortness of breath, and pulse oximetry** since implementation of interventions. The decreased HR and BP indicate that the client's body is no longer as stressed by the COPD exacerbation as it was on admission. Improvement of pulse oximetry indicates oxygen and inhaler therapy are effective, which likely has improved perfusion to the brain.

INCORRECT OPTIONS: There was no change to the client's orientation, heart sounds, lung sounds, or RR since admission.

75. The answer is 2

The nurse is caring for a client who sustained a left femur fracture in a bicycle accident. A cast is applied. The nurse knows that which exercise would be **most** beneficial for this client?

Reworded Question: What exercise is best for a client in a cast?

Strategy: Picture the client as described. Imagine client performing each type of exercise. Also think about the key words "most beneficial."

Needed Info: Fracture: break in continuity of bone. Complications: hemorrhage (bone vascular), shock, fat embolism (long bones), sepsis, peripheral nerve damage, delayed union, nonunion. Treatment: reduction (closed or open), immobilization (cast, traction, splints, internal and external fixation). Cast allows early mobility. Nursing responsibilities: teach isometric exercises.

Category: Planning/Physiological Integrity/Reduction of Risk Potential

(1) Passive exercise of the affected limb—nurse moves extremity; unable to perform with cast in place

(2) Quadriceps setting of the affected limb—CORRECT: isometric exercise: contraction of muscle without movement of joint; maintains strength in the affected limb

(3) Active range-of-motion exercises of unaffected limb—not best, doesn't strengthen affected limb

(4) Passive exercise of the upper extremities—need strengthening exercises, not passive exercises

76. The answer is 3

A client is to receive 35 mg/hr of intravenous aminophylline. The nurse mixes 350 mg of aminophylline in 500 mL dextrose 5% in water. At which rate should the nurse infuse this solution?

Reworded Question: What is the IV flow rate?

Strategy: Set up a ratio and solve for x. If you miss this, review your nursing math. You will have a drop-down calculator on the computer to use while taking the NCLEX-RN® examination.

Needed Info: Formula: med on hand over volume on hand = desired med over x. Solve for x.

Category: Implementation/Physiological Integrity/Pharmacological and Parenteral Therapies

(1) 20 mL/hr—incorrect

(2) 35 mL/hr—incorrect

(3) 50 mL/hr—CORRECT: 350 mg/500 mL = 35 mg/x, $350x = 17{,}500$, $x = 50$

(4) 70 mL/hr—incorrect

77. The answer is 2

The nurse is inserting an IV catheter into a client's left arm. Suddenly the client exclaims, "It feels like an electric shock is going all the way down my arm and into my hand!" Which action will the nurse take **first**?

Reworded Question: What should the nurse do if a nerve is struck during IV catheter insertion?

Strategy: Determine the outcome of each answer. Is it appropriate?

Needed Info: When choosing location to insert a peripheral IV catheter, consider the condition of the vein, type of fluid and medications to be infused, duration of therapy, and client's age, size, and status.

Category: Implementation/Physiological Integrity/Reduction of Risk Potential

(1) Instruct the client to take slow, deep breaths—incorrect action; will cause harm to the client if IV catheter is left in place

(2) Remove the catheter from the client's left arm—CORRECT: electric shock sensation indicates catheter tip is touching a nerve; remove IV catheter immediately to prevent permanent nerve injury; can also occur during routine venipuncture

(3) Tell the client this is a common response to IV catheter insertion—it does sometimes happen; important to remove IV catheter immediately

(4) Withdraw the catheter slightly and then push it forward—action can cause nerve damage

78. The answer is 1

The nurse is caring for a group of clients. The nurse knows that it is **most** important for which client to receive their scheduled medication on time?

Reworded Question: Which medication, if given late, might cause harm to the client?

Strategy: Think about each answer.

Needed Info: Myasthenia gravis is deficiency of acetylcholine at myoneural junction; symptoms include muscular weakness produced by repeated movements that soon disappears following rest, diplopia, ptosis, impaired speech, and dysphagia

Category: Analysis/Physiological Integrity/Pharmacological and Parenteral Therapies

(1) A client diagnosed with myasthenia gravis receiving pyridostigmine bromide—CORRECT: Pyridostigmine bromide is a cholinesterase inhibitor which increases acetylcholine concentration at the neuromuscular junction; early administration can precipitate a cholinergic crisis; late administration can precipitate myasthenic crisis

(2) A client diagnosed with bipolar disorder receiving lithium carbonate—Lithium carbonate is a mood stabilizer; targeted initial blood level = 1–1.5 mEq/L (1–1.5 mmol/L); targeted maintenance blood level = 0.8–1.2 mEq/L (0.8–1.2 mmol/L)

(3) A client diagnosed with tuberculosis receiving isoniazid—Isoniazid is given in a single daily dose; side effects include hepatitis, peripheral neuritis, rash, and fever

(4) A client diagnosed with Parkinson's disease receiving levodopa—Levodopa is thought to restore dopamine levels in extrapyramidal centers; sudden withdrawal can cause parkinsonian crisis; priority is to administer pyridostigmine bromide

79. The answer is 3

A school-age client is admitted to the hospital for evaluation for a kidney transplant. During the initial assessment, the nurse learns that the client received hemodialysis for 3 years due to stage 5 kidney disease. The nurse knows that the illness can interfere with this client's achievement of which stage of personality development?

Reworded Question: Which developmental stage is altered in a client due to this chronic disease?

Strategy: Picture the client described in the question. Think about the activities and interests of a school-age child. This helps eliminate incorrect answer choices. A school-age child may be thinking about homework and doing chores at home.

Needed Info: Eric Erikson developed a theory of the stages of personality development that progressed in predictable stages from birth to death. Other stages: autonomy versus shame and doubt (task of 1–3 yrs); initiative versus guilt (task of 3–6 yrs).

Category: Analysis/Health Promotion and Maintenance

(1) Intimacy—young adult: 19–40 yrs; achieving sexual and loving relationship with another; alternative: isolation

(2) Trust—infancy; results from consistent care by a loving caretaker; teaches that basic needs will be met; alternative: mistrust

(3) Industry—CORRECT: 6–12 yrs; aspires to be the best; learns social skills, how to finish tasks; sensitive about school expectations; may be impaired due to absences from school, growth retardation, and emotional difficulties; alternative: inferiority

(4) Identity—adolescence; peer groups important; used to define identity, establish body image, form new relationships; alternative: role confusion

80. The answer is 4

The nurse is assessing a client with a history of Addison disease who has received steroid therapy for several years. The nurse could expect the client to exhibit which changes in appearance?

Reworded Question: What changes are seen in a client after taking steroids long-term?

Strategy: All the options in an answer choice must be correct for the option to be right.

Needed Info: Meds: cortisone and hydrocortisone usually given in divided doses: Two-thirds in morning and one-third in late afternoon with food to decrease GI irritation. Teach client to report signs and symptoms of excessive drug therapy (rapid weight gain, face, fluid retention).

Category: Assessment/Physiological Integrity/Physiological Adaptation

(1) Buffalo hump, girdle-obesity, gaunt facial appearance—hump and girdle-obesity true; gaunt face seen with lack of steroids

(2) Skin tanning, mucous membrane discoloration, weight loss—tanning and weight loss seen with lack of steroids; mucous membrane discoloration not seen

(3) Emaciation, nervousness, breast engorgement, hirsutism—emaciation and breast engorgement are not related to steroids; however, steroids may cause nervousness and anxiety and hirsutism (excessive growth of hair) can result from excess cortisol

(4) Truncal obesity, purple striations on the skin, moon face—CORRECT: effects of excess glucocorticoids

81. The answer is 3

The nurse is caring for a client who reports being beaten and sexually assaulted by a friend. Which action will the nurse take **first**?

Reworded Question: What is the initial nursing action to take with a client who reports being a victim of sexual assault?

Strategy: Discriminate between what is appropriate and inappropriate nursing behavior.

Needed Info: Nursing care for crime victims must address both physical and emotional needs. The nurse must be cautious not to disturb or eliminate any evidence until the victim has been examined by a health care provider. The nurse must document all evidence found during the nursing assessment. After the client has been examined and a course of action determined, the nurse can begin to address the expressed needs of the client, such as contacting legal counsel or the chaplain.

Category: Implementation/Psychosocial Integrity

(1) Encourage the client to notify the family's legal counsel—not the first action the nurse should take with this client

(2) Request a consult with a psychiatric health care provider—not the first action that should be taken with this client (physical needs [assessing for injuries] take priority over psychosocial needs)

(3) Remain with the client during the physical examination—CORRECT: provide consistent emotional and physical support for the client; priority is for client to be examined for physical injuries

(4) Clean and dress wounds before the physical examination—contraindicated; eradicates potential evidence

82. The answer is 4

The nurse is preparing discharge instructions for a client who underwent cataract surgery with lens implantation. Which point should the nurse include in the discharge teaching?

Reworded Question: What's important for the client to know after cataract surgery to avoid complications?

Strategy: Think about each answer and how it relates to cataract surgery.

Needed Info: Cataract: change in the transparency of crystalline lens of eye. Causes: aging, trauma, congenital, systemic disease. Signs and symptoms: blurred vision, decrease in color perception, photophobia.

Treated by removal of lens under local anesthesia with sedation. Intraocular lens implantation, eyeglasses, or contact lenses after surgery. Complications: glaucoma, infection, bleeding, retinal detachment.

Category: Planning/Physiological Integrity/Physiological Adaptation

(1) Importance of reporting a scratchy feeling in the eye—a scratchy feeling in the eye may be expected for a few days after surgery

(2) Lie on the side of the affected eye the night after surgery—the client should avoid lying on the side of the affected eye the night after surgery

(3) Wipe eye with a single gesture from outer canthus inward—if needed, the client should wipe the closed eye with a clean tissue using a single gesture from the inner canthus outward

(4) Avoid lifting objects that weigh more than 15 lb (6.8 kg)—CORRECT: to avoid increasing intraocular pressure, the client should avoid lifting, pushing, or pulling objects that weigh more than 15 lb (6.8kg)

83. The answer is 1

A client is preparing to take a 1-day-old infant home from the hospital. The nurse discusses the test for phenylketonuria (PKU) with the client. The nurse's teaching should be based on an understanding that the test is **most** reliable in which circumstance?

Reworded Question: When is the PKU test most reliable?

Strategy: Focus on the key words in the question. Think about what you know about the PKU test.

Needed Info: PKU: genetic disorder caused by a deficiency in liver enzyme phenylalanine hydroxylase. Body can't metabolize essential amino acid phenylalanine, allows phenyl acids to accumulate in the blood. If not recognized, resultant high levels of phenylketone in the brain cause intellectual disability. Guthrie test: screening for PKU. Treatment: dietary restriction of foods containing phenylalanine. Blood levels of phenylalanine monitored to evaluate the effectiveness of the dietary restrictions.

Category: Analysis/Health Promotion and Maintenance

(1) After a source of protein has been ingested—CORRECT: recommended to be performed before newborns leave hospital; if initial blood sample is obtained within first 24 hrs, recommended to be repeated at 3 weeks

(2) After the meconium has been excreted—no relationship; dark-green, tarry stool passed within first 48 hrs of birth

(3) After the danger of hyperbilirubinemia has passed—no relationship; excessive accumulation of bilirubin in blood; signs and symptoms: jaundice (yellow discoloration of skin); common finding in newborn; not cause for concern

(4) After the effects of delivery have subsided—no relationship to PKU testing

84. The answer is 2

The nurse is caring for a client who receives a balanced complete formula through an enteral feeding tube. The nurse knows that the **most** common complication of an enteral tube feeding is which of the following?

Reworded Question: What is a common complication of a tube feeding?

Strategy: Focus on the words "most common," which indicate there may be more than one correct answer. And in this situation, there is—(4) is a complication, but it is not as common.

Needed Info: Enteral tube feedings are used for clients who are unable to tolerate feeding by the oral route but who have a functioning GI tract. May be given by intermittent or continuous infusion. Elevate head of bed 30–45 degrees. Give at room temperature. Check for placement before feeding. Don't hang solution for more than 6 hrs. Flush tubing with 30 mL water every 4 hrs. Change feeding set every 24 hrs. Balanced complete formula contains intact protein.

Category: Evaluation/Physiological Integrity/Basic Care and Comfort

(1) Edema—not frequently seen; if present, health care provider may change to a low-sodium formula

(2) Diarrhea—CORRECT: formula intolerance or rate intolerance; give slowly; other symptoms of intolerance: nausea, vomiting, aspiration, glycosuria, diaphoresis

(3) Hypokalemia—normal potassium 3.5–5 mEq/L (3.5–5 mmol/L); hypokalemia may occur secondary to prolonged diarrhea, but not all clients with diarrhea will develop hypokalemia; common causes of hypokalemia: diuretics, diarrhea, GI drainage

(4) Vomiting—can happen with rapid rate increase; administer slowly

85. The answer is 1

A client is brought to the emergency department bleeding profusely from a stab wound in the left chest area. Vital signs are: blood pressure 80/50 mmHg, pulse 110 beats/minute, and respiratory rate 28 breaths/minute. The nurse should expect which potential problem?

Reworded Question: What type of shock is described?

Strategy: Form a mental image of the person described.

Needed Info: Symptoms of hypovolemic shock: tachycardia, reduced urine output, irritability. Treatment: oxygen therapy, IV fluids to restore volume, vasopressors (if hypotension persists despite adequate fluid resuscitation). Nursing responsibilities: secure airway, monitor vital signs, insert large bore IV catheter, arterial blood gas analysis, central venous pressure measurements, insert indwelling urinary catheter, hourly intake and output measurement, position flat with legs elevated, keep warm.

Category: Planning/Physiological Integrity/Physiological Adaptation

(1) Hypovolemic shock—CORRECT: loss of circulating volume

(2) Cardiogenic shock—decrease in cardiac output; cause: cardiac dysfunction, myocardial infarction, or heart failure

(3) Neurogenic shock—increase in vascular bed; cause: spinal anesthesia, spinal cord injury

(4) Septic shock—decreased cardiac output, hypotension; cause: gram-positive or gram–negative bacteria

86. The answer is 3

A client is admitted to the hospital for surgical repair of a detached retina in the right eye. In planning care for this client postoperatively, the nurse should encourage the client to undertake which action?

Reworded Question: What should you do after surgery for a detached retina?

Strategy: Picture the client as described.

Needed Info: Detached retina: separation of retina from pigmented epithelium. Signs and symptoms: curtain falling across field of vision, black spots, flashes of light, sudden onset. Treatment: surgical repair (photocoagulation, diathermy, cryosurgery, scleral buckling). Complications: infection, redetachment, increased intraocular pressure, development of cataracts. Nursing responsibilities post-op: check eye patch for drainage, position with detached area dependent; no rapid eye movement (reading, sewing); no coughing, vomiting, sneezing.

Category: Planning/Physiological Integrity/Reduction of Risk Potential

(1) Perform self-care activities—activity restrictions depend on location and size of tear

(2) Maintain patches over both eyes—only affected eye covered

(3) Limit movement of both eyes—CORRECT: eye movements increase intraocular pressure

(4) Refrain from excessive talking—no restriction

87. See explanation for answers

CORRECT OPTIONS: The client is at very high risk for falls, and **could sustain a fracture or head injury** as a result. The client is taking three medications which lower the blood pressure: losartan, an angiotensin II receptor blocker (ARB); carvedilol, a beta blocker; and hydrochlorothiazide, a thiazide diuretic. The combination of these medications and the initiation of an increased dosage can cause severe orthostatic hypotension. The nurse will need to **monitor for postural hypotension** when taking the blood pressure. It will be very important to **teach the client to change position slowly** when getting up from a lying or sitting position to standing. Because the client has diabetes, the client must be made aware that sympathetic nervous symptoms of hypoglycemia are masked when taking a beta blocker, and the **blood glucose must be checked more regularly**.

INCORRECT OPTIONS: The client is "off balance," not confused or voicing any other symptoms of UTI, such as urinary frequency or urgency. The client and spouse have been managing the client's care at home and there is no indication the client's condition warrants placement in an assisted living facility. The physician will not need to be notified until the client has been assessed and more data is gathered. The client's blood pressure has been monitored over a period of time, and readings have been consistent. Most of the client's medications need to be taken with food, with the exception of the sulfonylurea, which needs to be taken 30 minutes prior to breakfast. Taking carvedilol with food can decrease the incidence of orthostatic hypotension. The client should never skip a dose of medication, but should notify the home health nurse or physician regarding adverse effects. The client will not need to limit fluids while taking a diuretic unless instructed by the physician. The client with hypertension will continue to limit sodium intake to avoid fluid retention.

88. The answer is 3

An infant is brought to the pediatrician's office for a well-baby visit. During the examination, congenital subluxation of the left hip is suspected. The nurse would expect to see which symptom?

Reworded Question: What will you see with congenital hip dislocation?

Strategy: Form a mental image of the deformity.

Needed Info: Subluxation: most common type of congenital hip dislocation. Head of femur remains in contact with acetabulum but is partially displaced. Diagnosed in infant less than 4 weeks old. Signs/symptoms: unlevel gluteal folds, limited abduction of hip, shortened femur affected side, Ortolani's sign (click). Treatment: abduction splint, hip spica cast, Bryant's traction, open reduction.

Category: Assessment/Health Promotion and Maintenance

(1) Lengthening of the limb on affected side—inaccurate

(2) Deformities of the foot and ankle—inaccurate

(3) Asymmetry of the gluteal and thigh folds—CORRECT: restricted movement on affected side

(4) Plantar flexion of the foot—seen with clubfoot

89. The answer is 3

After 2 weeks of receiving lithium therapy, a client in the psychiatric unit becomes depressed. Which evaluation of the client's behavior by the nurse would be **most** accurate?

Reworded Question: Is the depression normal, or something to be concerned about?

Strategy: Think about each answer and how it relates to lithium therapy.

Needed Info: Lithium is used to control manic episodes of bipolar psychosis; nursing care includes monitoring blood levels 2–3 times a week when started and monthly while on maintenance. Need fluid intake of 2,500–3,000 mL/day and adequate salt intake. Side effects include dizziness, hand tremors, impaired vision.

Category: Evaluation/Psychosocial Integrity

(1) The treatment plan is not effective; the client requires a larger dose of lithium—not accurate

(2) This is an abnormal response to lithium therapy; the client should stop the lithium immediately—normal response

(3) This is a normal response to lithium therapy; the client should be monitored for suicidal behavior—CORRECT: delay of 1–3 weeks before mood-stabilizing benefits of medication seen

(4) The treatment plan is not effective; the client requires an antidepressant—normal response

90. The answer is 4

The nurse is supervising care at an adult day-care center. Four meal choices are available to the residents. The nurse should ensure that a resident on a low-cholesterol diet receives which meal?

Reworded Question: What should a client on a low-cholesterol diet eat?

Strategy: Think about each answer.

Needed Info: Low-cholesterol diet should reduce total fat to 20–25% of total calories and reduce the ingestion of saturated fat. Carbohydrates (especially complex carbohydrates) should be 55–60% of calories. High-cholesterol foods: eggs, dairy products, meat, poultry.

Category: Implementation/Physiological Integrity/Basic Care and Comfort

(1) Egg custard and boiled liver—high amounts of cholesterol

(2) Fried chicken and potatoes—avoid fried foods

(3) Hamburger and French fries—avoid fried foods

(4) Grilled salmon and green beans—CORRECT: fish instead of meat, increase vegetables

91. See explanation for answers

Condition Most Likely Experiencing	
Atrial fibrillation.	☑

CORRECT OPTION: The client is displaying symptoms of **atrial fibrillation** which include rapid, irregular heart rate and feelings of a "racing" heartbeat. Atrial fibrillation is the loss of organized atrial electrical activity within the heart. It usually occurs in a client with underlying heart disease, such as coronary artery disease (CAD), and hypertension. It often develops acutely with stress. Atrial fibrillation is readily treated with medical or electrical cardioversion.

INCORRECT OPTIONS: The client is not having any classic symptoms of myocardial infarction (MI), such as shortness of breath or chest pain. Pneumonia would not cause a racing heartbeat or feeling faint. Ventricular tachycardia (VT) is a lethal dysrhythmia. Clients experiencing VT are usually hemodynamically unstable or unresponsive; neither is true of this client.

Actions to Take	
12 lead electrocardiogram (EKG).	☑
Prepare for diltiazem continuous IV infusion.	☑

CORRECT OPTIONS: In a client reporting symptoms of dysrhythmia, the first step is to **obtain an EKG** to verify the rhythm. Once the rhythm is known, the client may require treatment, especially if symptomatic. The priority treatment goal of atrial fibrillation is ventricular rate control. A controlled atrial fibrillation is defined as a ventricular rate less than 100 beats per minute. A calcium channel blocker (e.g., **diltiazem**) is one of the most common antidysrhythmic classes of medications used to treat atrial fibrillation.

INCORRECT OPTIONS: Incentive spirometry is a tool used to help prevent atelectasis, most notably in post-operative clients. An exercise-induced cardiac stress test is utilized for clients who have CAD symptoms to determine EKG changes when the heart is stressed. Immediate cardioversion is indicated when the ventricular rate exceeds 150 beats per minute and the client becomes hemodynamically unstable. This client, however, is fully responsive and blood pressure is within normal limits. None of these actions is appropriate to take.

Parameters to Monitor	
Neurological status.	☑
Heart rate.	☑

CORRECT OPTIONS: Prevention of complications is crucial to treating atrial fibrillation. It is very important to monitor the client's **neurologic status**. Clients with atrial fibrillation are more likely to develop clots within the atria, which can embolize and travel to the brain, causing a stroke. **Heart rate** less than 100 beats/minute is a parameter indicating the effectiveness of treatment. If ventricular rates are controlled, the client can live with this dysrhythmia comfortably.

INCORRECT OPTIONS: Serum troponin is crucial to draw in clients reporting symptoms of an MI but does not change in response to a dysrhythmia. A chest x-ray is helpful to obtain a snapshot visual of the heart and lungs but will not show changes with dysrhythmia. Capillary refill indicates peripheral perfusion but is not a priority assessment needed to determine if the client's dysrhythmia is responding to treatment.

92. The answer is 3

The nurse is teaching a primigravid client how to measure the frequency of uterine contractions. The nurse should explain to the client that the frequency of uterine contractions is determined by which approach?

Reworded Question: How do you determine the frequency of uterine contractions?

Strategy: Think about each answer.

Needed Info: There must be at least 3 contractions to establish frequency.

Category: Implementation/Health Promotion and Maintenance

(1) By timing from the beginning of one contraction to the end of the next contraction—not accurate

(2) By timing from the beginning of one contraction to the end of the same contraction—defines duration

(3) By the number of contractions that occur within a given period of time—CORRECT

(4) By the strength of the contraction at the peak of the contraction—describes intensity

93. The answer is 2

The nurse is teaching a woman who is receiving estrogen replacement therapy. Which statement by the nurse indicates that the nurse is aware of the possible complications of estrogen therapy?

Reworded Question: What complications are seen with the use of estrogen therapy?

Strategy: Think about each answer and the effects of estrogen therapy.

Needed Info: Estrogen therapy predisposes to cancer of reproductive organs. Other side effects are skin rashes, pruritus, breast soreness, headaches, nausea, vomiting, eye irritation with contact lenses, depression, and thromboembolic disorders. Used cautiously with family history of breast or genital tract cancer.

Category: Implementation/Health Promotion and Maintenance

(1) "Take an analgesic before you take estrogen, because estrogen may cause discomfort."—not accurate; may cause nausea, weight gain, lethargy

(2) "Make sure you keep your clinic appointments, especially your gynecologic checkup."—CORRECT: requires a checkup at 6 months; endometrial and breast cancer risk increased

(3) "Increase your fluid intake, because estrogen promotes diuresis and weight loss."—causes fluid retention and edema; monitor weight; restrict sodium intake

(4) "You need to increase roughage in your diet to avoid constipation."—not a complication of estrogen therapy

94. The answer is 3

Several days after being admitted for depression, a client is observed sitting alone in the clients' dining room. The nurse notes that the client has not finished the meal. Which action is **most** appropriate?

Reworded Question: How would you meet this client's needs?

Strategy: Determine the outcome of each answer. Is it desired?

Needed Info: Symptoms of depression: withdrawn, regressive behavior, psychomotor retardation.

Category: Planning/Psychosocial Integrity

(1) Allow the client to eat alone until more comfortable eating with other clients—social isolation, reinforces depression

(2) Ask the client's family to bring in some of the client's favorite foods—assumes client did not finish the meal because the client did not like the food that was provided

(3) Order small, frequent meals and sit with the client during meals in the dining room—CORRECT: diminished appetite, prevents social isolation

(4) Do not focus on eating behaviors; appetite will improve over time—does not meet nutritional needs

95. The answer is 3

A client receives 10 units of isophane insulin subcutaneously every morning at 0800. At 1600, the nurse observes that the client is diaphoretic and slightly confused. The nurse takes which action **first**?

Reworded Question: What is the cause of these symptoms? What is the first thing you should do?

Strategy: "First" indicates that this is a priority question.

Needed Info: Isophane insulin: intermediate-acting preparation: onset 1–2 hrs, peak 4–12 hrs, duration 16 hrs. Signs and symptoms (S/S) hypoglycemia: confusion, tremors, tachycardia, cool clammy skin, diaphoresis, headache, hunger. Treatment: if conscious, liquids containing sugar; dextrose 50% IV if unconscious; client education.

Category: Planning/Physiological Integrity/Pharmacological and Parenteral Therapies

(1) Obtain the client's vital signs—not first action; should recognize S/S hypoglycemia

(2) Check urine for glucose and ketones—indicates only hyperglycemia, no information about hypoglycemia; should recognize S/S hypoglycemia

(3) Give 6 oz (180 mL) of skim milk—CORRECT: S/S of hypoglycemia; give 15–20 grams of glucose or simple carbohydrates; recheck blood glucose level in 15 minutes and repeat, if needed

(4) Contact the health care provider—not first action; contact health care provider if hypoglycemia does not improve

96. The answer is 2

Prior to the client undergoing a scheduled intravenous pyelogram (IVP), the nurse reviews the client's health history. It would be **most** important for the nurse to obtain the answer to which question?

Reworded Question: What do you need to know before an IVP?

Strategy: Think about each answer and how it relates to an IVP.

Needed Info: IVP: radiopaque dye containing iodine is injected into the body, filtered through the kidneys, and excreted by the urinary tract. Visualizes kidneys, ureters, and bladder. Preparation: nothing by mouth after midnight, cathartics evening before test. Injection of dye causes flushing of face, nausea, salty taste in mouth.

Category: Assessment/Physiological Integrity/Reduction in Risk Potential

(1) Does the client have any difficulty voiding?—not most important

(2) Does the client have any allergies to shellfish or iodine?—CORRECT: anaphylactic reaction; itching, hives, wheezing; treatment: antihistamine, oxygen, epinephrine, vasopressor

(3) Does the client have a history of constipation?—not essential information

(4) Does the client have a history of frequent headaches?—not most important

97. The answer is 1

Parents bring their child to the primary health care provider for suspected chickenpox. The nurse knows the rash characteristic of chickenpox can be described as which of the following?

Reworded Question: What does the rash from chickenpox look like?

Strategy: Form a mental image of client with characteristic rash.

Needed Info: Chickenpox transmission: direct contact, respiratory droplets; requires airborne precautions and contact precautions until lesions are dry and crusted. Incubation period: 14–16 days. Treatment: Acyclovir, diphenhydramine hydrochloride, calamine lotion for itching, good skin care to prevent secondary infection, bathe daily, change clothes and linens, at home isolate until vesicles have dried (usually 1 week after onset), short fingernails, avoid use of aspirin due to Reye's syndrome.

Category: Assessment/Health Promotion and Maintenance

(1) Maculopapular—CORRECT: prodromal stage: slight fever, malaise, anorexia, maculopapular rash; becomes vesicular: fluid-filled vesicles form crusts, communicable 1–2 days before eruption of lesions (during prodromal stage) up to 6 days after first vesicles appear and crusts form

(2) Small, irregular red spots with minute bluish-white centers—Koplik spots: prodromal stage of measles, first seen on buccal mucosa 2 days before rash

(3) Round or oval erythematous scaling patches—psoriasis: treatment: exposure to sunlight and ultraviolet light, topical corticosteroids, coal-tar derivatives

(4) Petechiae—pinpoint, nonraised, perfectly round purplish red spots caused by intradermal or submucosal hemorrhage, seen in severe sepsis with disseminated intravascular coagulation (DIC), Rocky Mountain spotted fever, and subacute bacterial endocarditis (SBE)

98. The answer is 3

The nurse is caring for a client admitted for a possible herniated intervertebral disk. The health care provider prescribed ibuprofen and cyclobenzaprine hydrochloride to be given as needed for pain. Several hours after admission, the client reports pain. Which action will the nurse take **first**?

Reworded Question: What should you do first?

Strategy: Set priorities. Compare the answers to the steps in the nursing process.

Needed Info: Herniated disk: knifelike pain aggravated by sneezing, coughing, straining.

Category: Planning/Physiological Integrity/Pharmacological and Parenteral Therapies

(1) Give the client ibuprofen to promptly manage the pain—implementation; not first step

(2) Ask the health care provider which medication to give first—the NCLEX is testing your ability to critically think and prioritize; there is important information that you can gather

(3) Gather more information from the client about the pain—CORRECT: assess; first step in nursing process

(4) Allow the client some time to rest to see if the pain subsides—implementation; not first step

99. The answer is 3

During visiting hours the nurse finds a visitor unconscious on the floor of a client's room. Which of the following nursing assessment findings indicates the the need for cardiopulmonary rescusitation (CPR)?

Reworded Question: What are the signs of cardiopulmonary arrest?

Strategy: Think about the steps you would take to evaluate an unconscious client.

Needed Info: Cardiopulmonary arrest: no normal breathing and no pulse identifies cardiac arrest. CPR: (1) determine unresponsiveness, (2) activate emergency response system (shout for help), (3) determine breathlessness (look for no breathing or only gasping) and pulselessness (no pulse within 5–10 sec?), (4) begin CPR (cycles of 30 compressions and 2 breaths).

Category: Assessment/Physiological Integrity/Physiological Adaptation

(1) Shallow respirations and thready pulse—Not indicator for CPR

(2) Rapid respirations and slow, weak pulse—not indicator for CPR

(3) Gasping respiration and pulselessness—CORRECT: No breathing or only gasping and no pulse identifies cardiac arrest and the need for CPR

(4) Pupillary changes and rapid pulse—not indicator for CPR

100. The answer is 4

A client is transferred to a long-term care facility after a stroke. The client has right-sided paralysis and dysphagia. The nurse observes an unlicensed assistive personnel (UAP) preparing the client to eat lunch.

Which situation would require an intervention by the nurse?

Reworded Question: Which option is wrong?

Strategy: This is a negative question. Make sure you know if you are looking for a correct situation or a problematic situation.

Needed Info: Dysphagia: difficulty swallowing. Provide head support if needed, position the client upright, feed the client slowly in small amounts, place food in the unaffected side of mouth. Maintain client in an upright position for 30–45 minutes after eating. Provide oral care after eating.

Category: Evaluation/Physiological Integrity/Reduction of Risk Potential

(1) The client remains in bed in the high Fowler position—correct positioning to prevent aspiration, or the client may sit in chair

(2) The client's head and neck are positioned slightly forward—correct positioning; helps client chew and swallow

(3) UAP places food in the back of the mouth on the unaffected side—helps client handle food

(4) UAP adds tap water to the pudding to help the client swallow—CORRECT: requires intervention, soft or semisoft foods are more easily swallowed; liquids increase the risk for aspiration

101. The answer is 3

A parent with 4 children calls the clinic for advice on how to care for the oldest child, who has developed chickenpox. Which statement by the parent indicates a need for further teaching?

Reworded Question: What teaching is necessary for parent of child with chickenpox?

Strategy: Be careful! This is a negative question. You are looking for an incorrect statement.

Needed Info: Teaching: calamine lotion for itching, good skin care to prevent secondary infection, bathe daily, change clothes and linens, isolate until vesicles

have dried (usually 1 week after onset), short fingernails, avoid use of aspirin due to Reye's syndrome.

Category: Evaluation/Safe and Effective Care Environment/Safety and Infection Control

(1) "I should keep my child home from school until the vesicles are crusted."—correct information; chickenpox transmitted by direct contact with droplets of infected person; communicable period: 1–2 days before rash until vesicles crusted (scabbed), then child may interact with siblings and others

(2) "I can use calamine lotion if needed."—correct information, used to treat itching

(3) "I should remove the crusts so the skin can heal."—CORRECT: indicates need for further teaching; good skin care important; crusts usually not removed, can cause scarring

(4) "I can use mittens if scratching becomes a problem."—rash itches; mittens used to prevent scratching

102. The answer is 4

The nurse is teaching a woman who comes to the clinic at 32 weeks' gestation with a diagnosis of pregnancy-induced hypertension (PIH). Which statement by the client indicates to the nurse that further teaching is required?

Reworded Question: What is not accurate about the care of a woman with PIH?

Strategy: This is a negative question. It can be reworded to say, "All of the following are true *EXCEPT*."

Needed Info: PIH, preeclampsia: development of hypertension with proteinuria or edema (dependent or facial) or both after 20 weeks' gestation. Risk factors: previous history of PIH, parity (first-time mothers), age (younger than 20 or older than 35), underweight or overweight, geographic location (southern or western U.S.), multifetal gestation, hydatidiform mole, kidney disease, hypertension, and diabetes mellitus. Prevention: early prenatal care, identify high risk clients, recognize signs/symptoms early; bed rest lying on left side, daily weights. Treatment: urine checks for proteinuria; diet (increased protein and decreased sodium). Can develop into eclampsia (convulsions or coma).

Category: Evaluation/Health Promotion and Maintenance

(1) "Lying in bed on my left side is likely to increase my urinary output."—true; bed rest promotes good perfusion of blood to uterus; decreases blood pressure and promotes diuresis

(2) "If the bed rest works, I may lose a pound or two in the next few days."—true; causes diuresis; results in reduction of retained fluids; instruct to monitor weight daily and notify health care provider if notices abrupt increase even after resting in bed for 12 hrs

(3) "I should be sure to maintain a diet that has a good amount of protein."—true; replaces protein lost in urine; increases plasma colloid osmotic pressure; avoid salty foods; avoid alcohol; drink 8 glasses of water daily; eat foods high in roughage

(4) "I will have to keep my room darkened and not watch much television."—CORRECT: incorrect information, not necessary; diversional activities helpful

103. The answer is 2

The nurse evaluates the care provided to a client hospitalized for treatment of adrenal crisis. Which change would indicate to the nurse that the client is responding favorably to medical and nursing treatment?

Reworded Question: What shows a positive response to treatment for adrenal crisis?

Strategy: Think about each answer.

Needed Info: In adrenal crisis, the required adrenal hormones exceed the supply available. Usually precipitated by stress, surgery, trauma, or infection. Signs/symptoms (S/S): hypotension, cool pale skin, increased urinary output, dehydration.

Category: Evaluation/Physiological Integrity/Physiological Adaptation

(1) The client's urinary output has increased—indicates continuing lack of hormones; will decrease with treatment

(2) The client's blood pressure has increased—CORRECT: hypotension S/S of adrenal insufficiency; without treatment sodium level falls, resulting in volume depletion and hypotension; potassium level rises, resulting in cardiac dysrhythmias

(3) The client has experienced weight loss—indicates continuing loss of water and continuing lack of hormones

(4) The client's peripheral edema has decreased—edema not seen with adrenal crisis

104. The answer is 4

After completing an assessment, the nurse determines that a client is exhibiting early symptoms of a dystonic reaction related to the use of an antipsychotic medication. Which action by the nurse would be **most** appropriate?

Reworded Question: What is the first thing you do for a client with a dystonic reaction?

Strategy: Set priorities. Remember Maslow's hierarchy of needs.

Needed Info: Dystonic reaction: muscle tightness in throat, neck, tongue, mouth, eyes, neck, and back; difficulty talking and swallowing. Treatment: IM or IV diphenhydramine hydrochloride or benztropine mesylate.

Category: Implementation/Psychosocial Integrity

(1) Reality-test with the client and assure the client that physical symptoms are not real—real symptoms, not delusions

(2) Teach the client about common side effects of antipsychotic medications—physical needs are highest priority

(3) Explain to the client that there is no treatment that will relieve these symptoms—diphenhydramine hydrochloride used IM or IV

(4) Notify the primary health care provider to obtain a prescription for IM diphenhydramine—CORRECT: emergency situation, can occlude airway

105. The answer is 1

A client underwent vagotomy with antrectomy for treatment of a duodenal ulcer. Postoperatively, the client develops dumping syndrome. Which statement by the client indicates to the nurse that further dietary teaching is necessary?

Reworded Question: What is contraindicated for the client with dumping syndrome?

Strategy: Be careful! You are looking for incorrect information.

Needed Info: Antrectomy: surgery to reduce acid-secreting portions of stomach. Delays or eliminates gastric phase of digestion. Dumping syndrome occurs in clients after a gastric resection. It occurs after eating and is related to the reduced capacity of the stomach.

Undigested food is dumped into the jejunum, resulting in distention, cramping, pain, diarrhea 15–30 min after eating. Subsides in 6–12 months. S/S 5–30 min after eating: vertigo, tachycardia, syncope, diarrhea, nausea. Treatment: octreotide acetate to slow gastric emptying; antispasmodics; high-protein, high-fat, low-carbohydrate, dry diet. Eat in semirecumbent position, lying down after eating.

Category: Evaluation/Physiological Integrity/Basic Care and Comfort

(1) "I should eat bread with each meal."—CORRECT: incorrect information; should decrease intake of carbohydrates

(2) "I should eat smaller meals more frequently."—true; 5–6 small meals per day

(3) "I should lie down after eating."—true; delays gastric emptying time

(4) "I should avoid drinking fluids with my meals."—true; no fluids 1 hr before, with, or 1 hr after meal

106.   See explanation for answers

Troponin is a biomarker that is highly specific to myocyte damage. The laboratory test will increase within 4–6 hours of onset of myocardial infarction (MI) symptoms, peak within 24 hours, and return to baseline over the several days following the incident. CORRECT ANSWERS: The nurse expects the troponin level will **decrease** and return to normal if **perfusion is adequately restored**, regardless of cellular damage that has already occurred. INCORRECT ANSWERS: If the troponin continues to increase, this means that blockage of blood flow within the coronary circulation is actively occurring and has not been treated. The results show that symptoms have subsided, so ischemia is no longer under way. Regardless of cellular damage that has already occurred, troponin level will decline. The troponin will not fluctuate.

107. The answer is 3

The nurse is caring for a client diagnosed with bipolar disorder. The client paces endlessly in the halls and makes hostile comments to other clients. The client resists the nurse's attempts to move the client to a room in the unit. Which action by the nurse is **most** important?

Reworded Question: What is priority for the client who is experiencing mania?

Strategy: "Most important" indicates priority.

Needed Info: Bipolar disorder is a chronic mood syndrome that causes mania, hypomania, and depression; during mania, client is hyperactive, anxious, and unable to meet physical needs; also see flight of ideas, inappropriate dress, and a lack of inhibitions.

Category: Planning/Psychosocial Integrity

(1) Offer the client fluids every hour—appropriate action; at risk for cardiac collapse due to dehydration; first give medication to decrease hyperactivity

(2) Inform the client about unit rules—inappropriate timing; may increase hostility and agitation; administer medication, reduce environmental stimuli

(3) Administer haloperidol IM—CORRECT: decrease hyperactive behavior so client can take fluids and food

(4) Encourage the client to rest—important; first decrease hyperactive behavior

108. The answer is 3

The nurse is caring for an Rh-negative client who has delivered an Rh-positive child. The mother states, "The doctor told me about Rho GAM, but I'm still a little confused." Which response by the nurse is **most** appropriate?

Reworded Question: What is RhoGAM and why is it used?

Strategy: Remember what you know about RhoGAM.

Needed Info: RhoGAM: given to unsensitized Rh-negative (Rh−) mother after delivery or abortion of an Rh-positive (Rh+) infant or fetus to prevent development of sensitization. Rh− mother produces antibodies in response to the Rh+ RBCs of fetus. If occurs during pregnancy, fetus is affected. If occurs during delivery, later pregnancies may be affected. An indirect Coombs test is performed on the mother during pregnancy, and a direct Coombs test is done on cord blood after delivery. If both are negative and the neonate is Rh+, the mother is given RhoGAM to prevent sensitization. RhoGAM is usually given to unsensitized mothers within 72 hrs of delivery, but may be effective when given 3–4 weeks after delivery. To be effective, RhoGAM must be given after the first delivery and repeated after each subsequent delivery. RhoGAM is ineffective against Rh+ antibodies that are already present in the maternal circulation. The administration of RhoGAM at 26–28 weeks' gestation is also recommended.

Category: Implementation/Health Promotion and Maintenance

(1) "RhoGAM is given to your child to prevent the development of antibodies."—not given to neonate

(2) "RhoGAM is given to your child to supply the necessary antibodies."—not given to neonate

(3) "RhoGAM is given to you to prevent the formation of antibodies."—CORRECT: prevents maternal circulation from developing antibodies

(4) "Rho GAM is given to you to encourage the production of antibodies."—not accurate; given to discourage antibody production

109. The answer is 3

The nurse is teaching a client diagnosed with osteoarthritis. The client asks how to effectively decrease pain and stiffness in the joints before beginning the daily routine. Which instruction should the nurse give the client?

Reworded Question: What should the client with osteoarthritis do first thing in the morning?

Strategy: Which answer would reduce an osteoarthritic client's pain?

Needed Info: Osteoarthritis results in articular cartilage loss with formations of bony outgrowths (osteophytes) at the joint margins. Causes include:

hematologic disorders (e.g., hemophilia), inflammation, joint instability, mechanical stress (e.g., sports), medications (e.g., colchicine, corticosteroids), neurologic disorders (e.g., pain and loss of reflexes from diabetic neuropathy), skeletal deformities (e.g., hip dislocation), trauma (fractures). Treatment: acetaminophen, nonsteroidal anti-inflammatory drugs (NSAIDs), intraarticular corticosteroids.

Category: Implementation/Physiological Integrity/ Basic Care and Comfort

(1) "Perform isometric exercises for at least 10 minutes."—done to preserve muscle strength; tighten muscle, hold for few seconds, then relax without moving joint

(2) "Do range-of-motion exercises then apply ointment to your joints."—done after ointment applied; range-of-motion exercises do not reduce pain

(3) "Take a warm bath, and then rest for a few minutes."—CORRECT: heat reduces pain, spasms, stiffness in joints; ice may be helpful for acute inflammation

(4) "Perform stretching exercises for all muscle groups."—would be painful

110. The answer is 2

The nurse is caring for a client receiving paroxetine. It is **most** important for the nurse to report which of the following to the health care provider?

Reworded Question: What is a potential medication interaction?

Strategy: "Most important" indicates priority.

Needed Info: Paroxetine is a selective serotinin reuptake inhibitor (SSRI) used to treat depression, panic disorder, obsessive-compulsive disorder, anxiety; side effects include palpitations, bradycardia, nausea and vomiting, and decreased appetite.

Category: Evaluation/Physiological Integrity/Pharmacological and Parenteral Therapies

(1) The client reports no change in appetite—medication causes anorexia; monitor weight and nutritional intake; report continued weight loss

(2) The client reports recently being started on digoxin—CORRECT: medication may decrease effectiveness of digoxin

(3) The client reports applying sunscreen to go outdoors—appropriate action; prevents photosensitivity reactions

(4) The client reports driving the car to work—driving is acceptable after determining client's response to medication

111. The answer is 1

A pediatric client is seen in a clinic for treatment of attention-deficit/hyperactivity disorder (ADHD). Medication has been prescribed for the client along with family counseling. The nurse is teaching the parents about the medication and discussing parenting strategies. Which statement by the parents indicates that further teaching is necessary?

Reworded Question: What information is wrong for child with ADHD?

Strategy: Be careful! You are looking for incorrect information.

Needed Info: ADHD: developmentally inappropriate inattention, impulsivity, hyperactivity. Treatment: medication (methylphenidate hydrochloride), family counseling, remedial education, environmental manipulation (decrease external stimuli), psychotherapy.

Category: Evaluation/Psychosocial Integrity

(1) "We will give the medication at night so it doesn't decrease appetite."—CORRECT: incorrect information; stimulants (methylphenidate hydrochloride) used; side effects: insomnia, palpitations, growth suppression, nervousness, decreased appetite; give 6 hrs before bedtime

(2) "We will provide a regular routine for sleeping, eating, working, and playing."—true

(3) "We will establish firm but reasonable limits on behavior."—true

(4) "We will reduce distractions and external stimuli to help concentration."—true

K 477

112.   The answer is 2, 3, 5, 6, 8, and 9

CORRECT OPTIONS: This client's lab work indicates worsening iron deficiency anemia as evidenced by decreasing Hgb, Hct, RBC, and serum ferritin levels. The client's condition is exacerbated due to inability to tolerate the prescribed iron supplement (ferrous sulfate). Due to decreased oxygen-carrying capacity related to decreased hemoglobin, the client may develop severe fatigue, **dizziness, exercise intolerance**, **shortness of breath**, **pagophagia** (craving ice or cold foods), **brittle fingernails**, and **stomatitis**.

INCORRECT OPTIONS: Weight gain and increased urine output are not caused by iron deficiency anemia. Yellow sclera is associated with jaundice or liver disease. In some cases, the client may develop pearly white to bluish sclera.

113. The answer is 1

The nurse is teaching a client undergoing a paracentesis for treatment of cirrhosis. The client asks about positioning for the procedure. Which description from the nurse would be **most** appropriate?

Reworded Question: What is the correct position for a paracentesis?

Strategy: Visualize the procedure.

Needed Info: Paracentesis: removal of fluid from abdominal or peritoneal cavity. Can be used for diagnostic purposes, to remove ascitic fluid for symptomatic relief, to prepare for peritoneal dialysis. Preparation: have client void, measure vital signs, weigh client, measure abdominal girth. During procedure: check vital signs every 15 min. Measure and document amount of drainage (2–3 L can be removed), characteristics. After procedure: apply pressure dressing, check for leakage. Bed rest until vital signs stable. Complications: hypovolemia and shock. Cirrhosis: degenerative liver disease; tissue is replaced by scar tissue. Causes: alcoholism, hepatic inflammation or necrosis, chronic biliary obstruction. Signs/symptoms: ascites, lower leg edema, jaundice, esophageal varices, hemorrhoids, bleeding tendencies, pruritus, dark urine, clay-colored stools. Nursing responsibilities: high-protein (unless ascites, edema, or signs of impending hepatic coma are present), high-carbohydrate, low-sodium diet; good skin care; promote rest; reduce exposure to infection.

Category: Analysis/Physiological Integrity /Reduction of Risk Potential

(1) Sitting with the lower extremities well supported—CORRECT: Fowler position or sitting on side of bed with feet on stool; easy access to abdominal area; allows intestines to float to prevent laceration

(2) Side-lying with a pillow between the knees—not accurate

(3) Prone with the head turned to the left side—not accurate

(4) Dorsal-recumbent with a pillow at the back of the head—not accurate

114. The answer is 2

A client is calling the suicide prevention hotline to report a personal suicide plan. Which question should the nurse ask **first**?

Reworded Question: What is most important to know about a client who has threatened suicide?

Strategy: "First" indicates priority.

Needed Info: Signs of suicide: symptoms of depression, client gives away possessions, gets finances in order, has a means, makes direct or indirect statements, leaves notes, has increased energy. Predisposing factors: male over age 50, age 15–19, poor social attachments, client with previous attempts, client with auditory hallucinations, overwhelming precipitating events (terminal disease, death or loss of loved one, failure at school or job).

Category: Assessment/Psychosocial Integrity

(1) "What has happened to cause you to want to end your life?"—does not determine immediate need for safety

(2) "Tell me the details of the plan that you developed to kill yourself?"—CORRECT: lets you prioritize interventions to assure safety

(3) "When did you start to feel as though you wanted to die?"—does not determine immediate need for safety

(4) "Do you want me to prevent you from killing yourself?"—yes/no question, closed

115. The answer is 4

A client is admitted for treatment of hypovolemic shock. The health care provider prescribes normal saline solution IV to infuse at 125 mL/hr and central venous pressure (CVP) readings every 4 hours. Sixteen hours after admission, the client's CVP reading is less than 2 mmHg. Which evaluation of the client's fluid status by the nurse would be **most** accurate?

Reworded Question: What does this CVP reading indicate?

Strategy: Consider each answer and remember normal CVP reading values.

Needed Info: CVP: central venous line placed in superior vena cava. To obtain a reading: client placed supine, 0 on manometer placed at level of right atrium (midaxillary line at 4th intercostal space), turn stopcock to allow manometer to fill with fluid, turn to allow fluid to go into client. Fluid will fluctuate with respirations. When stabilized, take reading at highest level of fluctuation. Normal: 2–8 mmHg (3–11 cm H_2O). Elevated: hypervolemia, heart failure, pericarditis. Low: hypovolemia.

Category: Evaluation/Physiological Integrity/Reduction of Risk Potential

(1) The client has received enough fluid—inaccurate, CVP remains low

(2) The client's fluid status remains unaltered—nothing to compare to

(3) The client has received too much fluid—inaccurate, CVP remains low

(4) The client requires additional IV fluid—CORRECT: normal 2–8 mmHg (3–11 cm H_2O); indicates hypovolemia

116. The answer is 1

A client hospitalized for treatment of delusions tells the nurse, "I'm head of the hospital system working undercover to gather information on client abuse." Which statement by the nurse to the client is **best** initially?

Reworded Question: How would you handle a client with delusions?

Strategy: Know when further assessment is needed and what the appropriate communication techniques are to use with delusional clients.

Needed Info: The initial approach to delusions is to clarify meanings. After clarification, the delusions should not be discussed as this could reinforce them. Arguing with a client about delusions may also reinforce them. Delusions that entail injury or death should be addressed immediately and client protections put into place.

Category: Assessment/Psychosocial Integrity

(1) "Tell me what you mean about being head of the hospital system and gathering client abuse information."—CORRECT: initial approach is to further assess by clarifying the meaning of the delusion to the client

(2) "I think you should share this story with the other clients at dinnertime and see what they say."—could cause disruption among other clients and embarrass the client

(3) "You are not the head of the hospital system; you are an accountant under treatment for a mental disorder."—arguing with client about delusion is ineffective, inappropriate, and may strengthen the client's belief in it

(4) "It worries me when you say these things; it means you are not responding to the medication."—nurse is communicating disappointment to the client and treating the delusion as though it were a behavior under the client's control

117. The answer is 1

The nurse is caring for a client in labor. The nurse palpates a firm, round form in the uterine fundus, small parts on the client's right side, and a long, smooth, curved section on the left side. Based on these findings, the nurse should anticipate auscultating the fetal heart in which of the following locations?

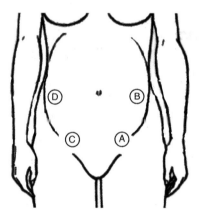

Reworded Question: If a fetus is left occiput anterior (LOA), where should the nurse listen for the fetal heart tone?

Strategy: Examine the diagram carefully. Know the client's right from left.

Needed Info: Fetal reference point: vertex presentation—dependent upon degree of flexion of fetal head on chest; full flexion/occiput (O), full extension chin (M), moderate extension (military) brow (B). Breech presentation—sacrum (S). Shoulder presentation—scapula (Sc). Maternal pelvis is designated per her right/left and anterior/posterior/transverse. Position = relationship of fetal reference point to mother's pelvis; expressed as standard 3-letter abbreviation: LOA (left occiput anterior) (most common), LOP (left occiput posterior), ROA (right occiput anterior), ROP (right occiput posterior), LOT (left occiput transverse), ROT (right occiput transverse).

Category: Planning/Health Promotion and Maintenance

(1) A—CORRECT: point of maximum intensity for fetal heart with fetus in LOA position

(2) B—PMI location for fetus in LOP position

(3) C—PMI location for fetus in ROA position

(4) D—PMI location for fetus in ROP position

118. The answer is 1

A client admitted with a diagnosis of pneumonia is receiving gentamicin. For this client, which laboratory values would be **most** important for the nurse to monitor?

Reworded Question: What are the adverse effects of gentamicin?

Strategy: Use the process of elimination, noting the key words "most important," which indicate that more than one answer choice may be correct. Also, every part of the answer choice must be correct in order to select the answer.

Needed Info: Gentamicin is a broad-spectrum antibiotic used to treat bacterial infections, particularly those caused by gram-negative bacteria. Adverse effects: neuromuscular blockage, encephalopathy, seizures, ototoxic to the eighth cranial nerve (tinnitus, vertigo, hearing loss), nephrotoxicity; less commonly, may cause

anemia and hypokalemia. Blood should be drawn for peak and trough level.

Category: Implementation/ Physiological Integrity/ Reduction of Risk Potential

(1) Blood urea nitrogen and creatinine—CORRECT: gentamicin is nephrotoxic; proteinuria, oliguria, hematuria, increased blood urea nitrogen, decreased creatinine clearance

(2) Hemoglobin and hematocrit—gentamicin can cause anemia, but is less common

(3) Sodium and potassium—hypokalemia is an infrequent problem with gentamicin therapy

(4) Prothrombin time and bleeding time—prothrombin time not affected; thrombocytopenia is a risk with gentamicin therapy

119. The answer is 2

The nurse is preparing a client newly diagnosed with Addison disease for discharge. Which statement by the client indicates a need for further instruction from the nurse?

Reworded Question: Which instruction about Addison's disease does the client not understand?

Strategy: Use the process of elimination, noting the key words "need for further instruction." Be careful: you are looking for an answer choice that contains incorrect information. If you had trouble with this question, review client teaching for Addison disease.

Needed Info: Addison disease is the most common form of adrenal hypofunction. It occurs when more than 90 percent of the adrenal gland is destroyed. Early diagnosis and adequate hydrocortisone replacement therapy indicate a good prognosis. Acute adrenal insufficiency, or adrenal crisis, is a medical emergency requiring immediate treatment. Corticosteroid replacement is the primary lifelong treatment for clients with primary or secondary adrenal hypofunction. An adrenal crisis usually subsides quickly with proper treatment, and subsequent oral maintenance doses of hydrocortisone preserve stability.

Category: Analysis/Physiological Integrity/Reduction of Risk Potential

(1) "I understand that I will need lifelong cortisone therapy."—indicates the client understands the discharge teaching; clients with Addison disease require lifelong cortisone replacement therapy

(2) "When stressed, I will need to decrease my medication."—CORRECT: indicates the client does not understand discharge teaching and requires further instructions; during times of stress, clients with Addison disease need to *increa*se the medication dosage, not decrease it

(3) "I must take precautions to prevent injuring myself."—indicates the client understands the discharge teaching; clients with Addison disease should be warned that infection, injury, or profuse sweating in hot weather (leading to sodium loss) may precipitate a crisis

(4) "I should always carry a medical identification card."—indicates the client understands the discharge teaching; clients with Addison disease should always carry a medical identification card and wear a bracelet stating the name and dosage of the steroid the client takes

120. The answer is 2 and 4

The nurse is assessing a client newly diagnosed with initial-stage chronic glomerulonephritis. Which finding should the nurse expect to see? **(Select all that apply.)**

Reworded Question: What are the signs and symptoms of initial-stage chronic glomerulonephritis?

Strategy: Focus on the key words "Select all that apply." There may be only 1 correct answer, more than 1 correct answer, or all of the answer choices may be correct. Think about the signs and symptoms of initial-stage chronic glomerulonephritis as opposed to late-stage findings.

Needed Info: Chronic glomerulonephritis is a slowly progressive, noninfectious disease characterized by inflammation of the renal glomeruli. By the time it produces symptoms, it is usually irreversible and eventually results in kidney failure. Symptoms of the initial stage are nephrotic syndrome, hypertension, proteinuria, and hematuria. Late-stage findings include azotemia, nausea, vomiting, pruritus, dyspnea, malaise, fatigue, mild to severe anemia, and severe hypertension.

Category: Assessment/Physiological Integrity/Physiological Adaptation

(1) Hypotension—initial-stage findings include hypertension; late-stage symptoms include severe hypertension

(2) Proteinuria—CORRECT: this is an initial-stage finding

(3) Severe anemia—this is a late-stage finding

(4) Hematuria—CORRECT: this is an initial-stage finding

(5) Azotemia—this is a late-stage finding

(6) Nausea—this is a late-stage finding

121. The answer is 2

The nurse is caring for a client who underwent a lumbar spinal fusion for a herniated intervertebral disk. To promote comfort and minimize complications, the nurse tells the client to **avoid** which activity?

Reworded Question: What should the client avoid after having undergone a lumbar spinal fusion?

Strategy: Note the key word "avoid" in the question stem. Focus on the surgical procedure and recall that activity and positioning should not cause discomfort or unnecessary strain on the lower back.

Needed Info: To avoid complications and promote comfort after spinal fusion, the client should be advised to bend at the knees when lifting (never at the waist); lie down when tired and sleep on the side with a pillow between the knees. Lying on the stomach causes strain on the back; use a firm mattress to reduce tension on the spine. Choose a firm, hardback chair for sitting, no longer than 20 minutes at a time.

Category: Implementation/Physiological Integrity/ Basic Care and Comfort

(1) Bending the knees when lying on one side—will decrease the strain on the shoulders, neck, and arms

(2) Sitting for longer than 20 minutes at a time—CORRECT: puts strain on the back; it is better to walk around or lie down to rest

(3) Using an extra firm mattress—reduces tension on the spine

(4) Sitting in a hardback chair—provides support for the back

122. The answer is 4

The nurse is preparing a client for surgery. When obtaining informed consent, the nurse should **initially** take what action?

Reworded Question: What are the elements of informed consent, and what are the nurse's responsibilities?

Strategy: Think about the elements of informed consent and the responsibilities of the health care provider and nurse. "Initially" indicates there may be more than one correct response.

Needed Info: Informed consent is more than simply getting a client to sign a written consent form. It is a process of communication between a client and health care provider that results in the client's authorization or agreement to undergo a specific medical intervention. The client should have an opportunity to ask questions to better understand the treatment or procedure and make an informed decision to proceed or refuse.

Category: Assessment/Safe and Effective Care Environment/Management of Care

(1) Explain the risks, benefits, and alternatives to the procedure—this is the responsibility of the health care provider performing the procedure, not the nurse

(2) Tell the client that a signature is needed for all surgeries—although this is true, it does not determine the client's ability to give informed consent

(3) Witness the client's signature on the informed consent form—this is true; however, the nurse should first assess the client's knowledge of the procedure

(4) Assess whether client understands procedure enough to give consent—CORRECT: informed consent means the client understands and comprehends the risks, benefits, and alternatives of the planned procedure.

123. **See explanation for answers**

CORRECT OPTIONS: This client is at risk for the development of post-operative **pneumonia** primarily due to **shallow breathing** and **decreased ambulation**, which lead to atelectasis and stagnation of respiratory secretions. Stagnant secretions may lead to inflammation and infection in the lungs. Post-operative pneumonia is a complication of abdominal surgery because pain may cause a decrease in movement, deep breathing, use of incentive spirometer, and ambulation. This client's shortness of breath, coarse rhonchi, and thick respiratory secretions are all symptoms associated with decreased ventilation.

INCORRECT OPTIONS: There is no increased risk of pneumothorax in this client who has had abdominal surgery. The client has active bowel sounds and is tolerating liquids, which indicates the client has not developed an ileus. The elevation of pulse and blood pressure are more likely due to pain, not pneumonia. The urinary catheter and PCA pump are related to the routine post-operative care for this client, but do not increase the risk for pneumonia.

124. The answer is 3

The nurse is preparing to administer heparin sodium to a client diagnosed with thrombophlebitis. The nurse should ensure that which agent is available if the client develops a significant bleeding problem?

Reworded Question: What is the antidote for heparin sodium?

Strategy: Focus on the name of the medication administered and remember that the antidote for heparin sodium is protamine sulfate. Review antidotes for commonly administered medications.

Needed Info: Heparin sodium is indicated for prophylaxis and treatment of venous thromboembolism and atrial fibrillation with embolization. Heparin prevents clot formation. Its antidote is protamine sulfate.

Category: Planning/Safe and Effective Care Environment/Management of Care

(1) Phytonadione—antidote for warfarin

(2) Fresh frozen plasma—reverses bleeding associated with warfarin therapy

(3) Protamine sulfate—CORRECT: antidote for heparin sodium

(4) Reteplase—a thrombolytic agent that breaks up blood clots; it is not an antidote

125. The answer is 3

The nurse finds a client sitting on the bathroom floor. The nurse assesses the client, obtains assistance, and assists the client back to bed. The nurse notifies the health care provider and completes an incident report. Which is the **most** appropriate nursing action?

Reworded Question: What is the nurse's responsibility related to incident reporting?

Strategy: Use the process of elimination.

Needed Info: Incident reports are confidential and privileged information. They should not be placed in a client's medical record, copied, or referenced in the medical record. The person who witnesses the incident should complete the report. An objective entry of the incident should be documented in the client's medical record.

Category: Implementation/Safe and Effective Care Environment/Management of Care

(1) Document in medical record that incident report was filed—reference to incident reports should not be documented in a client's medical record

(2) Make a copy of the incident report for the nurse manager—incident reports should never be copied

(3) Document the incident in the client's medical record—CORRECT: objective details of the incident should be documented in the client's medical record

(4) Place the incident report in the client's medical record—incident reports should not be placed in a client's medical record but routed to the hospital's risk management or legal department

126. The answer is 3

The nurse is performing an initial post-operative assessment on a client who has a chest tube attached to a water seal drainage system. The nurse should immediately intervene for which observation?

Reworded Question: Which observation of chest tube and water seal drainage system requires immediate attention?

Strategy: Use the process of elimination. Three of the answer choices need no intervention.

Needed Info: A chest tube with water seal drainage allows air and fluid to be removed from the intrapleural space. The water seal drainage to which the chest tube is connected prevents backflow into the pleural space. The chest tube is attached to a valve mechanism designed to allow air or fluid to drain out of, but not into, the chest cavity. There should be no dependent loops or kinks in the tube, and the tube should be unclamped, including during transport and ambulation, unless prescribed by the health care provider. The fluid level in the water seal chamber should be at 2 cm.

Category: Assessment/Safe and Effective Care Environment/Management of Care

(1) There are no dependent loops in the chest tube—no need to intervene because this is correct

(2) The chest tube remains unclamped—no need to intervene; chest tube should be unclamped

(3) Water seal drainage system is above the client's chest—CORRECT: water seal drainage system should be *be*low the client's chest to facilitate removal of air or fluid

(4) Fluid level in the water seal is at 2 cm—no need to intervene; this is the correct fluid level

127. The answer is 2

The nurse is caring for a client diagnosed with terminal cancer in the client's home. The nurse knows that which of the following ethical principles **best** supports keeping client and family care consistent with the nurse's professional code of ethics?

Reworded Question: Keeping client and family care consistent with the nurse's professional code of ethics is the definition of which principle?

Strategy: Think about the definition of each principle. Review ethical principles if you had trouble with this question.

Needed Info: A nurse should be able to identify ethical issues that affect client care. If ethical issues arise, the nurse must be able to handle them according to ethical principles.

Category: Analysis/Safe and Effective Care Environment/Management of Care

(1) Virtues—refers to compassion, trustworthiness, integrity, and veracity

(2) Fidelity—CORRECT: refers to keeping faithful to ethical principles and the American Nurses Association Code of Ethics for Nurses

(3) Beneficence—refers to a nurse's duty to do what is in the best interest of the client

(4) Justice—refers to a fair, equitable, and appropriate treatment

128. The answer is 4

Prior to administering a tuberculin (Mantoux) skin test, the nurse in an outpatient clinic is educating a client suspected of having tuberculosis (TB). The nurse determines that the client understands the teaching when the client gives which response?

Reworded Question: What is the purpose of the Mantoux skin test?

Strategy: Use the process of elimination.

Needed Info: A Mantoux skin test is performed to see if a client has ever had TB. It is done by putting a small amount of TB protein under the top layer of skin on the inner forearm. If a client has ever been exposed to the bacteria, the skin will react to the antigens by developing a firm red bump at the site within 2 days. A TB skin test cannot tell how long a person has been infected with TB or if the infection is inactive or active and can be passed to others.

Category: Assessment/Safe and Effective Care Environment/Safety and Infection Control

(1) "I know the test will tell me how long I've been infected with TB."—tuberculin test cannot tell how long a client has been infected with TB

(2) "This test will tell me if I can spread TB to other people."—tuberculin test cannot differentiate between an active TB infection and a dormant TB infection

(3) "I will need to come back and have a nurse look at the site in a week."—site of the skin test must be read within 48–72 hours

(4) "The test will tell us if I've ever been infected with the TB bacteria."—CORRECT: tuberculin skin test is done to see if a client has ever been infected with TB

129. The answer is 2

A client diagnosed with metastatic breast cancer is admitted with neutropenic fever. The client informs the nurse of the personal decision to not receive cardiopulmonary resuscitation. The nurse explains that this information can be outlined in an advance directive.

The nurse understands that which regulation addresses the client's right to identify treatment desires in advance?

Reworded Question: What ensures that clients are informed of their right to create advance directives?

Strategy: Knowledge regarding each of these choices is required to answer this question. If you had difficulty with this question, review the Patient's Bill of Rights, the Patient Self-Determination Act, the Health Insurance Portability and Accountability Act (HIPAA), and the Americans with Disabilities Act to be sure you understand the objective of each.

Needed Info: The Patient Self-Determination Act outlines the requirements for informing clients they have right to refuse medical treatment and to specify their wishes for treatment through advance directives.

Category: Analysis/Safe and Effective Care Environment/Management of Care

(1) Patient's Bill of Rights—does not address advance directives

(2) Patient Self-Determination Act—CORRECT: ensures that clients are informed of their right to refuse medical treatment and (in advance directives) to specify their wishes for treatment

(3) Health Insurance Portability and Accountability Act—does not address advance directives

(4) Americans with Disabilities Act—does not address advance directives

130. The answer is 1

A non-English-speaking client is being discharged after having a central venous access device (CVAD) inserted. Which description **best** describes the nurse's role in advocating for the client?

Reworded Question: Which answer best characterizes advocacy?

Strategy: Think about the definition of nurse advocacy. Focus on the key word "best," which may indicate there is more than one correct response. Consider each

answer and select the action that is most representative of a nurse advocating for her client.

Needed Info: Advocacy: the act of promoting a client's rights and interests.

Category: Implementation/Safe and Effective Care Environment/Management of Care

(1) The nurse uses a translator to help provide discharge instructions—CORRECT: using a translator is the best example of an act of advocacy that promotes the client's rights and interests

(2) The nurse provides the client with written discharge instructions—providing written instructions may benefit the client, but is not the best example of advocacy (simply providing written discharge instructions does not validate the client's understanding)

(3) The nurse ensures the client has transportation home upon discharge—asking if the client has a ride home is appropriate, but not the best example of advocacy

(4) The nurse provides discharge instructions in a private room—providing discharge instructions in a way that maintains privacy is important, but not the best example of advocacy

131. The answer is 2

A nurse is caring for a client with a new colostomy. Which activity **best** describes the nurse's role as an advocate for the client?

Reworded Question: Which task best advocates for the client?

Strategy: Focus on the key word "best." This indicates there may be more than one correct response. Consider each option and select the action that best advocates for the client.

Needed Info: Nurse advocacy is based on the premise that a nurse acts to protect the best interests of the client, as well as to protect a client's right to make decisions. Nurse advocacy includes empowering a client through education.

Category: Implementation/Safe and Effective Care Environment/Management of Care

(1) Ensuring the skin is dry before re-adhering the pouch—proper procedure, but does not provide client with education needed to care for the ostomy

(2) Teaching the client how to care for the ostomy pouch—CORRECT: best represents nurse's role as client advocate; educating about self-care empowers the client to self-advocate

(3) Providing the client's family member with a list of foods to avoid—may be important to client in terms of dietary choices, but does not teach client directly how to manage the ostomy

(4) Explaining that adjustment to an ostomy takes time—likely useful to client, but does not teach client directly how to manage ostomy

132. The answer is 1, 2, 4, and 5

A client was admitted to a rehabilitation center after hip replacement surgery. During an episode of confusion, the client became a danger to self and required vest restraint application. The nurse knows that which implementation is also considered a form of restraint? **(Select all that apply.)**

Reworded Question: What are examples of restraints?

Strategy: Consider each response.

Needed Info: Know the definition of medical restraints and be able to provide examples.

Category: Analysis/Safe and Effective Care Environment/Safety and Infection Control

(1) Administering haloperidol to a combative client—CORRECT: a medication administered to control a client's behavior is considered a chemical restraint

(2) Raising all of the side rails on the client's hospital bed—CORRECT: a mechanical restraint

(3) Assigning unlicensed assistive personnel (UAP) to sit with client—nonrestraint effort to protect the client

(4) Fastening a bed sheet tightly across the client's chest—CORRECT: a mechanical restraint

(5) Clipping a tray across the front of the client's wheelchair—CORRECT: trays that clip across the front of a wheelchair so that the client can't fall out easily are a form of mechanical restraint

133. The answer is 3 and 4

A client has an unsteady gait and requires assistance with ambulation. The nurse decides to use a gait belt. Which step should the nurse take when using a gait belt? **(Select all that apply.)**

Reworded Question: Which of the following are correct when using a gait belt?

Strategy: Focus on the key words "Select all that apply." There may be only 1 correct answer, more than 1 answer may be correct, or all of the answer choices may be correct. Think about elements of proper gait belt use, and use the process of elimination to rule out the incorrect responses.

Needed Info: Know proper technique for gait belt use.

Category: Implementation/Safe and Effective Care Environment/Safety and Infection Control

(1) Secure the gait belt loosely around the client's waist—the gait belt should fit snugly, with room for the nurse's fingers between the belt and client

(2) Twist the upper body when positioning the client—the nurse should keep the back straight to practice proper body mechanics and prevent injury

(3) Remove gait belt from the client immediately after use—CORRECT: gait belts should be removed after use

(4) Place the gait belt over the client's clothes with the clip in front—CORRECT: allows for easier adjustment

(5) Walk in front of the client who is wearing the gait belt—the nurse should stand behind and to the side of the client during ambulation; the nurse should remain very close to the client and not keep the client at an arm's length

134. The answer is 3

A pediatric client with acute otitis media has been prescribed ofloxacin ear drops. The nurse knows that which statement by the parent demonstrates an understanding of how to properly administer the ear drops?

Reworded Question: What is the proper way to administer ear drops?

Strategy: Consider each of the statements. Using the process of elimination, select the statement that best reflects the technique that should be used to administer ear drops to a pediatric client.

Needed Info: Ear drop medication technique: warm the drops to body temperature to prevent pain and dizziness; lie the client down with affected ear facing up; place drops on the wall of the ear canal to allow air to escape and the medication to flow into the ear; give the medication as prescribed.

Category: Implementation/Physiological Integrity/Pharmacological and Parenteral Therapies

(1) "I can stop giving the ear drops as soon as my child's fever is gone."—medication should be administered as prescribed and should not be discontinued based on the presence or absence of a fever

(2) "I should give the drops directly on the eardrum to help get rid of the infection quickly."—ear drops should not be administered directly on the eardrum

(3) "I should warm the ear drops before giving them by wrapping the bottle in my hand."—CORRECT: temperature should be between 95–98.6° F (35–37° C) for administration

(4) "I should have my child lie flat while I administer the ear drops."—client should assume a side-lying position with the affected ear facing upwards

135. The answer is 1

A client recently diagnosed with hypertension has been taking furosemide 40 mg PO twice daily. During a clinic appointment, the client reports new onset muscle weakness and abdominal cramping. Blood samples are drawn for laboratory analysis. The nurse knows which result is the best explanation for the symptoms experienced by the client?

Reworded Question: What is the most likely reason for the client's symptoms?

Strategy: Consider the adverse effects of furosemide. What effects does the medication have on potassium levels? What symptoms might be seen with this adverse effect?

Needed Info: Furosemide is a diuretic that can lead to electrolyte imbalances. The normal range for potassium is 3.5 to 5 mEq/L (3.5 to 5 mmol/L). Symptoms associated with hypokalemia include abdominal cramping and muscle weakness.

Category: Analysis/Physiological Integrity/Reduction of Risk Potential

(1) Potassium 3 mEq/L (3 mmol/L)—CORRECT: a potassium level of 3 mEq/L (3 mmol/L) falls below normal range; may be associated with symptoms such as abdominal cramping and muscle weakness

(2) Creatinine 1.2 mg/dL (106.1 μmol/L)—this falls within normal range; it is not the correct response

(3) Fasting glucose 105 mg/dL 5.8 mmol/L)—this falls within normal range; it is not the correct response

(4) Total calcium 10 mg/dL (2.5 mmol/L)—this falls within normal range; it is not the correct response

136. See explanation for answers

Condition Most Likely Experiencing	
Asthma attack.	☑

CORRECT OPTION: The client is most likely experiencing an **asthma attack**, characterized primarily by wheezing, coughing, dyspnea, and hyperventilation. Airflow obstruction occurs and expiration can be prolonged after exposure to a risk factor or allergen. The client has a history of asthma, reports recent poor control with rescue medication, and is not taking the controller medicine, an inhaled glucocorticoid.

INCORRECT OPTIONS: Pneumonia is acute infection of the lung tissue, typically characterized by cough, fever, chills, pleuritic chest pain, and coarse crackles in the affected area; this client denies chest pain and is afebrile. Heart failure may have symptoms of peripheral edema, fatigue, and dyspnea due to pulmonary overload. Pulmonary embolism (PE), a thrombus in the pulmonary arteries, is a complication from peripheral venous thromboembolism (VTE). Primary risk factors for VTE include venous stasis, blood hypercoagulability, or endothelial damage; these do not appear the client history.

Actions to Take	
Give short acting beta-2-adrenergic agonist (SABA) medication.	☑
Speak calmly and guide client in methods to control breathing.	☑

CORRECT OPTIONS: To relieve airway constriction and hypoxemia, the nurse will give **short acting beta-2-adrenergic agonist (SABA) medication**. SABA medications are the most effective for alleviating acute bronchospasm and promoting bronchodilation in mild to moderate asthma attacks. It is important for the nurse to relieve client anxiety and fear during an acute attack. The **nurse should calmly talk and guide the client in using breathing methods** that slow the respiratory rate and control breathing.

INCORRECT OPTIONS: The nurse does not elevate the legs above the heart; this is helpful for improving circulation and reducing edema. The nurse should position the client comfortably, in semi-Fowler to high Fowler to maximize chest expansion, or sitting forward to maximize diaphragmatic movement. Hypoxemia is managed by giving oxygen (target pulse oximetry of > 93%) by nasal cannula or mask. Flow rates greater than 5 L/minute can dry and irritate nasal and pharyngeal mucosa. Chest physiotherapy with postural drainage is effective when the client has difficulty clearing excessive bronchial secretions, as in chronic obstructive pulmonary disease and cystic fibrosis.

Parameters to Monitor	
Lungs sounds.	☑
Pulse oximetry.	☑

CORRECT OPTIONS: To determine the client's progress, the nurse should monitor the client's respiratory status, including **lung sounds**, and vital signs, including **pulse oximetry**. These findings provide information about the client's respiratory function and response to treatment actions. A sudden absence of wheezing could indicate deterioration in the client's condition.

INCORRECT OPTIONS: The nurse does not monitor orthostatic blood pressure. Orthostatic blood pressure readings are taken to assess for a type of hypotension occurring when the client changes position from supine to sitting or standing. Skin temperature provides information about an increase or decrease in blood circulating through the dermis; it is not a parameter to monitor in an acute asthma attack. Serum hemoglobin measures oxygen carrying capacity of red blood cells. Changes in hemoglobin and other red blood cell indices are useful in determining causes of anemia. Potentially more useful parameters to monitor in evaluating the client's response to treatment include serial peak expiratory flow rate (PEFR) results, oximetry, and arterial blood gases.

137. The answer is 4

Which pediatric client should the nurse provide assessment and intervention for **first**?

Reworded Question: Which client requires immediate intervention?

Strategy: Think ABCs and airway.

Needed Info: Understand the ABCs framework of prioritizing airway, breathing, and circulation in order of importance. Always assess the client before checking alarms.

Category: Assessment/Safe and Effective Care Environment/Management of Care

(1) A client who has suddenly developed hives on the trunk—no indication that the client with hives is in immediate distress; requires an assessment but is not the priority

(2) A stable client who is receiving mechanical ventilation—no indication that an alarm is sounding; client requires an assessment but not immediately

(3) A client who reports mild difficulty breathing after femur fracture repair—no indication of *immediate* distress; requires an assessment to determine whether fat embolism syndrome, pulmonary embolism, or atelectasis may be present but is not the priority; this client should be seen second

(4) A client whose apnea monitor sounds with an oxygen saturation level of 82%—CORRECT: an abnormally low oxygen saturation level must be assessed immediately and an intervention initiated; it may be simple repositioning, suctioning, or readjusting the probe, but apnea alarms should not be ignored

138. The answer is 2

The nurse is assigning rooms for a group of clients. The nurse knows that which client requires an airborne infection isolation room?

Reworded Question: Which pathogen is spread by airborne droplet nuclei or small particles that remain infectious over time and distance?

Strategy: Think about the transmission of pathogens.

Needed Info: Transmission-based precautions help to limit the spread of pathogens. Airborne precautions prevent the spread of infectious agents that remain infectious over time and distance. Droplet precautions are for pathogens spread by direct or indirect contact with respiratory droplets when a client coughs, sneezes, or talks. These pathogens travel short distances (less than 3 feet). Contact precautions are required for pathogens spread by direct or indirect contact with the client or the client's environment.

Category: Implementation/Safe and Effective Care Environment/Safety and Infection Control

(1) A client with *Pneumocystis jiroveci* pneumonia— *Pneumocystis jiroveci* pneumonia requires standard precautions; no special room placment needed

(2) A client with suspected rubeola—CORRECT: rubeola is a highly contagious infection that's spread through droplets that remain infectious over long distances when suspended in air; requires airborne precautions with client placement in an airborne infection isolation room

(3) A client with meningococcal pneumonia—meningococcal pneumonia requires droplet precautions; a single-client room is sufficient

(4) A client with suspected seasonal influenza— seasonal influenza requires droplet precautions; a single-client room is sufficient

139. The answer is 2

In the event of a fire, the nurse should take which action **first**?

Reworded Question: Which should the nurse do *first* in the event of a fire?

Strategy: Think about what you know about the steps involved in fire safety in a hospital setting.

Needed Info: If a fire occurs, the first step is to get clients out of immediate danger (rescue and remove). Then, activate the alarm, confine the floor (close doors and windows, turn off oxygen and electric equipment), and extinguish the fire with an appropriate extinguisher.

Category: Implementation/Safe and Effective Care Management/Safety and Infection Control

(1) Leave the building—the nurse should not leave the building without attempting to remove clients from danger

(2) Attempt to get clients out of immediate danger—CORRECT: this is the first step the nurse should take in the event of fire

(3) Work to contain the fire—the first thing the nurse should do is attempt to get clients out of immediate danger

(4) Extinguish the fire with a fire extinguisher—not the first step

140. The answer is 2

The nurse is conversing with a client about a prescribed blood transfusion. It is clear to the nurse that the client does not understand the risks involved with the transfusion. Which intervention **best** supports the nurse's responsibility in the informed consent process?

Reworded Question: What is the nurse's responsibility in the informed consent process?

Strategy: Think about the process of informed consent and whose responsibility it is to obtain informed consent.

Needed Info: The health care provider prescribing the procedure is responsible for explaining the risks, benefits, and alternatives to the client. The nurse may witness the signing of the consent form but should only sign if confident that the client does indeed understand and wants the procedure. The nurse should also be familiar with the ethics of decision making for any client.

Category: Implementation/Safe and Effective Care Environment/Management of Care

(1) Tell client that blood transfusion carries few risks—telling the client that blood transfusion carries few risks leaves the client without the information required to make an informed decision

(2) Inform prescribing health care provider that client needs further explanation of associated risks—CORRECT: the nurse should advocate for the client and inform the health care provider who prescribed

the procedure that the client needs further information

(3) Have another health care professional witness the client's signature on the informed consent form—the nurse should not have someone else witness the client's signature on the consent form, especially if the nurse knows that the client does not fully understand the risks involved

(4) Describe alternative treatments to blood transfusion—it's the health care provider's role to describe alternative treatments

141. The answer is 3

The nurse is caring for a celebrity who may have sustained a career-changing injury. When asked by coworkers about the status of the client, the nurse refuses to discuss the client's condition. Which ethical principle **best** support the nurse's action?

Reworded Question: Which ethical principle should the nurse use when asked about a client by other staff not caring for the client?

Strategy: Think about ethical practice and the Code of Ethics for Nurses.

Needed Info: Understand the ethical principles that determine what is right and wrong when caring for clients. You should be able to define and review outcomes and interventions to promote ethical practice. Justice, nonmaleficence, fidelity, confidentiality, and accountability are some of the ethical principles that a nurse should understand and practice.

Category: Implementation/Safe and Effective Care Environment/Management of Care

(1) Justice—providing fair and appropriate treatment

(2) Beneficence—doing what is in the best interest of the client

(3) Confidentiality—CORRECT: maintaining the client's privacy and supporting what the nurse's role is by not talking to coworkers about the client

(4) Accountability—being responsible for one's actions

PART THREE
THE PRACTICE TEST

142.   See explanation for answers

Highest Risk Condition
Ischemic stroke. ☑

CORRECT OPTION: This client has multiple risk factors for **ischemic stroke**. For clients older than 55 years, the risk of stroke more than doubles each decade. Other risk factors include diagnoses of diabetes mellitus, obesity, hypertension, and migraine headaches. This client also smokes tobacco, which increases the risk of ischemic stroke dramatically. Most importantly, the client has had a confirmed TIA, as well as symptoms suggestive of previous TIA, which is considered a warning of an impending stroke.

INCORRECT OPTIONS: The client's lab work does not support a diagnosis of kidney failure, and the client's symptoms are not consistent with the conditions of cerebral aneurysm or pulmonary embolism.

Treatments Anticipated for Condition
Prescriptions for a statin and aspirin. ☑
Smoking cessation program. ☑

CORRECT OPTIONS: The client will need to be placed on a **statin and low-dose aspirin**. Platelet-inhibiting medications like aspirin decrease the incidence of cerebral infarction for clients who had experienced a TIA. Statin medications are recommended to reduce both coronary events and ischemic strokes, especially for clients with high cholesterol in which low HDL cholesterol accompanies high LDL cholesterol levels. Excessive cholesterol increases plaque formation and consequent narrowing of the carotid arteries. The client should also **stop smoking immediately**. Smoking doubles the risk of stroke and is a leading risk factor for stroke mortality.

INCORRECT OPTIONS: A sulfonylurea would be added in order to decrease blood glucose levels. However, the client's fasting glucose and hemoglobin A_{1c} levels do not indicate a need to alter the client's diabetes medication. Recombinant t-PA is given when a client is experiencing acute stroke symptoms and hemorrhagic stroke is ruled out. It is not given preventively for TIA. Typically, carotid endarterectomy is not performed until carotid occlusion is severe (70–99%) for clients with few risk factors and moderate (50–69%) for clients with multiple risk factors. The client's care may include planned endovascular surgery, but medical management would be initiated first based on the ultrasound results.

Parameters to Monitor	
Cholesterol and triglyceride levels.	☑
Neurologic status.	☑

CORRECT OPTIONS: The client will require a great deal of education about ways to modify risk factors. By taking statin medications, the client should have a **decrease in total cholesterol and triglyceride levels**, as well as a decrease in LDL. The nurse will also need to ensure the family is aware of neurologic signs and symptoms of acute stroke. The client remains at high risk for stroke; therefore, **ongoing assessment of the neurologic system** is imperative.

INCORRECT OPTIONS: Maintaining the blood glucose within normal parameters is important to reduce stroke mortality, but the most important parameters to monitor for this client are the neurologic status and cholesterol levels. The client's weight and BMI are high, but there is no comparative data indicating weight gain or loss or lose weight with diabetes treatment and exercise. Pulmonary functions tests are important to monitor considering the client's smoking history but would not be the priority parameter to monitor for ischemic stroke.

143. The answer is 1, 3, 4, and 5

The charge nurse is preparing assignments on a medical unit. For this shift, there are several LPN/LVNs, several RNs, and one unlicensed assistive personnel (UAP). Which assignment by the charge nurse is appropriate? **(Select all that apply.)**

Reworded Question: Which tasks are within the scope of practice for the RN, the LPN/LVN, and the UAP?

Strategy: Eliminate the choices that are outside the scope of practice for the professional assigned to the task.

Needed Info: Think through which tasks can be appropriately delegated to trained personnel. You also should review the principles of delegation, the Nurse Practice Act, and know what it means to supervise those who have been assigned tasks.

Category: Analysis/Safe and Effective Care Environment/Management of Care

(1) The UAP is assigned to bathe all clients that cannot self-bathe—CORRECT: bathing clients is within the scope of practice for a UAP

(2) An LPN/LVN is assigned initial assessment on a newly-admitted client—LPN/LVNs can collect client data, but not perform an initial assessment

(3) An LPN/LVN is assigned clients needing prescribed oral medications and vital sign measurements—CORRECT: LPN/LVNs are permitted to administer oral medications and obtain vital signs

(4) The RNs are assigned clients that require IVP medication administration—CORRECT: It is in the RN scope of practice to administer IVP medications

(5) LPN/LVN assigned indwelling urinary catheter insertion—CORRECT: inserting an indwelling urinary catheter is within the scope of practice of an LPN/LVN

144. The answer is 4

The nurse is educating new nursing staff members about client safety on the pediatric unit. Which comment by a new staff member **best** demonstrates that teaching has been successful?

Reworded Question: Which statement is correct about pediatric client safety practices in and out of the hospital setting?

Strategy: Think prevention and safety with children.

Needed Info: Begin by reviewing pediatric growth and development, including age-related safety regulations for each age group. Review prevention strategies for children, including car seat safety, poisoning, falls, and injury prevention.

Category: Evaluation/Safe and Effective Care Environment/Safety and Infection Control

(1) "A toddler may be transported to the car by wheelchair when discharged, and then the parents are responsible for how the child is transported home in the family car."—a toddler should not be discharged to parents if they do not have an appropriate car seat

(2) "School-aged children do not require booster seats if they weigh less than 80 lb (36.3 kg), and they do not require bicycle helmets if they weigh more than 80 lb (36.3 kg)."—school-aged children weighing less than 80 lb (36.3 kg) should remain in an appropriate booster seat or car restraint until they reach 57 in (145 cm) and weigh more than 80 lb (36.3 kg); all clients should wear bicycle helmets

(3) "Medications can be left at the bedside for pediatric clients, so the parents can dispense them when needed."—medications should not be left at the bedside of any client

(4) "Medications and cleaning supplies must be stored in a locked, child-proof cabinet at all times."—CORRECT: all medications and cleaning supplies must be stored in a locked, child-proof cabinet

145. The answer is 2

The nurse is calling a client after discharge to follow-up regarding care of the newborn. The client reports that the newborn's eyes look yellow. Which is the **most** appropriate response by the nurse?

Reworded Question: What are the causes of newborn jaundice after discharge from the hospital?

Strategy: Think breastfeeding and hydration. The phrase "most appropriate" indicates that more than one answer may be correct.

Needed Info: You should have a basic understanding of newborn feeding and care, breastfeeding issues for the new mother, and the significance of jaundice in the newborn. Clients who breastfeed need to maintain good hydration and pay attention to how much milk they are producing for their newborn. You should understand the risks of dehydration for the newborn and jaundice if it remains a long-term issue.

Category: Assessment/Physiological Integrity/Reduction of Risk Potential

(1) "How often are you nursing your baby?"—this should be the second question after finding out how the baby is being fed

(2) "Are you breastfeeding or bottle feeding?"—CORRECT: it is important to know how the baby is being fed; breastfed newborns may have jaundice for a few days due to lack of milk production or inadequate feeding; bottle-fed newborns who are taking the appropriate amount of formula tend to not be as jaundiced after discharge; determining how the newborn is fed is important to assess the risk for dehydration

(3) "Do you know your baby's last bilirubin level?"—the mother may or may not know the bilirubin level at discharge, but this is not the most important question; the most important information is about the way the newborn is being fed

(4) "Has your baby been seen by the pediatrician?"—the next pediatrician appointment is important but not before finding out how the newborn eats and the hydration state of the newborn

146. The answer is 1

The nurse is assessing a client who begins to have a grand mal seizure for the first time. Which action does the nurse take **first**?

Reworded Question: What is the nurse's first response to a client having a seizure?

Strategy: Think ABCs and priority—this suggests that all the answers may be correct; however, one takes precedence.

Needed Info: Seizures can be life-threatening if the client's airway becomes obstructed. Know the types of seizures, treatments, and the emergency care of a client who seizes. Understanding the causes of seizures can assist you in planning for the follow-up care of a client who has a seizure. First-time seizures often require a neurological workup, including a CT scan or MRI of the brain. A seizing client must be protected from aspiration and choking by placing the client on the side or turning the head.

Category: Implementation/Physiological Integrity/Physiological Adaptation

(1) Protect client's airway—CORRECT: the priority is to protect the client's airway and prevent aspiration by turning the head or positioning the client on the side

(2) Restrain the client—attempts to restrain can cause injury; it is better to move objects away, lower the client to the floor, or protect the client from hitting the side rails if in bed

(3) Record the duration of the seizure—you must record the duration of the seizure, but timing can be done while you protect the airway; airway always takes priority

(4) Notify the health care provider—you must notify the health care provider of the seizure activity, but don't leave the client during a seizure to do so; call for help and protect the airway

147. The answer is 1

A new staff nurse working on the intensive care unit is concerned about the client's status. The client's blood pressure, heart rate, and oxygen saturation level have progressively decreased. The nurse discusses the client's condition with the charge nurse. The charge nurse says "Don't worry, the client always does that." Which action should the nurse take?

Reworded Question: What is the *most* appropriate action for the nurse to take?

Strategy: Determine the outcome of each answer choice.

Needed Info: The nurse caring for the client has the ultimate responsibility and ethical obligation to act on behalf of the client. If the new nurse is concerned for the client's status, and the charge nurse is not inducing actions that support the appropriate provision of care, the new nurse must escalate concerns up the chain of command to ensure client safety.

Category: Implementation/Safe and Effective Care Environment/Management of Care

(1) Call the nursing supervisor for assistance—CORRECT: the nurse should escalate up the chain of command to advocate for the client

(2) Wait and see how the client progresses—this is incorrect because the client is exhibiting serious symptoms

(3) Take the advice of the experienced nurse—this is incorrect because the nurse must trust their own clinical judgment even if it conflicts with an experienced nurse

(4) Discuss this with other nurses on the unit—this might be an appropriate strategy, but a supervisor can provide more immediate assistance

148. The answer is 3

The nurse on a surgical unit has just received hand-off report for assigned clients. Which of the following clients should the nurse see **first**?

Reworded Question: Which client is least stable?

Strategy: Think ABCs.

Needed Info: The most unstable client should be seen first. The most urgent client needs should be attended to first.

Category: Analysis/Safe and Effective Care Environment/Management of Care

(1) A client awaiting discharge after surgical repair of an arm fracture—client remains stable

(2) A client using a continuous passive motion machine after knee replacement surgery—client is stable and not the first priority

(3) A client who developed new oxygen requirements and wheezing after abdominal surgery—CORRECT: a new oxygen requirement could indicate a complication of the surgery

(4) A client whose blood pressure is elevated one day after hip replacement surgery—you would want to address the blood pressure elevation, but it is not as urgent as the client recovering from abdominal surgery

149. The answer is 2

The nurse is working on a unit that is equipped with bar-code technology. Which method by the nurse is **best** when using this technology?

Reworded Question: What is a best practice for nurses who work with medication administration bar-code technology?

Strategy: Consider the outcome of each answer.

Needed Info: Electronic medication administration programs, such as scanners that use bar-coding, encourage safer practices and promote the reduction of errors in the medication administration process. However, a machine does not take the place of nursing clinical judgment. Appropriate nursing judgment and practices are paramount.

Category: Analysis/Safe and Effective Care Environment/Management of Care

(1) Rely solely on bar-code technology for safer medication administration practices—although bar-code

technology promotes safer medication administration practices, they do not replace nursing judgement

(2) Rely on nursing judgement, decision-making, and bar-code technology—CORRECT: computers do not take the place of nursing judgment

(3) Never give a medication that bar-code technology identifies as "incorrect medication."—this is not true; computerized systems can be inaccurate; the nurse should confirm the medication prescription, the medication, and the client, and then make the decision to administer or not based on nursing judgment

(4) Override bar-code technology when it identifies "incorrect medication" and administer it—this may be true in certain situations, but there is insufficient information in this case

150. The answer is 4

The nurse is working at a skilled nursing facility. The nurse witnesses a client getting up from a sitting position on the floor. When the nurse asks the client what happened, the client responds, "I fell." Which documentation should the nurse record in the incident report?

Reworded Question: How does a nurse report an event?

Strategy: Determine the outcome of each answer choice.

Needed Info: As a measure of tracking and preventing future events, the nurse is required to report events or injuries that are not expected with the typical provision of care. When reporting, the nurse should state events factually and objectively.

Category: Implementation/Safe and Effective Care Environment/Safety and Infection Control

(1) Client fell on the floor and there was no injury noted—not an appropriate answer because the nurse did not witness the client fall

(2) Client fell on floor and landed in a sitting position on the floor—not an appropriate answer because the nurse did not witness the client fall

(3) Client found on flood but was able to get up without assistance. Client most likely slipped or tripped—nurse's conjecture about cause of fall should not be documented

(4) Client found on floor and reported, "I fell." Assessment findings reveal no injury; primary health care provider notified—CORRECT: this is the best answer that states the facts objectively

PART FOUR

THE LICENSURE PROCESS

[CHAPTER 12]

APPLICATION, REGISTRATION, AND SCHEDULING

The process of obtaining an American nursing license requires a definite sequence of actions by the candidate. Because this may be your first experience with the RN licensure process, and because there are no established test dates, you may have difficulty knowing exactly how to complete the paperwork and go through the process. This chapter will give you a checklist to follow when planning to take the NCLEX-RN® exam. This is a general list, so you must individualize it according to the requirements for the state or province in which you wish to become licensed. We will outline the questions that you need to ask and the steps you need to take to complete the licensure process.

How to Apply for the NCLEX-RN® Exam

During your last semester of nursing school, you will be given the following applications:

(1)   Application for licensure that goes to your state board of nursing/regulatory body

(2)   Application for the NCLEX-RN® exam that goes to Pearson VUE

On a predetermined date, you will submit the completed forms and the required licensure fees to your nursing school.

Application Fees

- The NCLEX-RN® exam fee is $200 ($360 CAD). Additional licensure fees are determined by each state nursing board. Refer to your state board of nursing's web site to determine your state's fee.

- You are responsible for submitting the completed test application and the $200 fee to Pearson VUE. All applications will be processed by phone or online.

The Registration Process

```
A   →  APPLY
P      to Board of Licensure  ──────────┐
P                                        ↓
L                            Licensure application  ──────┐
I                            COMPLETE?                     │
C   →  REGISTER                                            │
A      with Pearson VUE  ──────────────┐                  │
N      for exam                         │                  │
T      $200 NCLEX-RN® exam fee          ↓                  │
S                            Acknowledgment email          │
 ←──────────────────────────  sent to applicant            │
                                        ↓                   │
                             Pearson VUE receives  ←────────┘
                             eligibility status from Board
                                        ↓
                             Pearson VUE emails
 ←──────────────────────────  Authorization to Test (ATT)
                                to applicant
    →  SCHEDULE
       testing appointment
       with test center using ATT
```

Applicant must APPLY, REGISTER, and SCHEDULE

Registration

You can register for the NCLEX-RN® exam with Pearson VUE using either of the following two methods:

(1) *Internet registration:* To register online, go to **nclex.com** (the NCLEX® candidate website). Payment is by credit, debit, or prepaid card (using Visa, MasterCard, or American Express only).

(2) *Telephone registration:* Call VUE NCLEX Candidate Services at 1-866-496-2539 (1-866-49-NCLEX). To register by phone, you must pay using a Visa, MasterCard, or American Express credit or debit card. Even if you register by phone, you must provide an email address to receive communications from Pearson VUE about your registration.

Pearson VUE does not accept registrations submitted by mail.

Some states require that the testing application form and fee be sent along with the licensure application and fee.

For more information, visit **nclex.com/prepare.page** and download the most recent *NCLEX-RN® Examination Candidate Bulletin.* For questions regarding registering to take the NCLEX® exam, your Authorization to Test (ATT), a lost ATT, acceptable forms of identification, or comments about the test center, visit the NCLEX® candidate website (**nclex.com**) or contact:

NCLEX® Candidate Services
1-866-496-2539 (1-866-49-NCLEX)
https://www.ncsbn.org/exam-contacts.htm

NCLEX-RN® Examination Program
Pearson Professional Testing
5601 Green Valley Drive
Bloomington, MN 55437-1099
pvamericascustomerservice@pearson.com

How Do You Know Your Application Has Been Received?

You will receive an acknowledgment from your state board stating that all of your information has been received.

Potential Problems with Licensure Application

Some states require that your permanent transcript be mailed with your application.

Here is a checklist to help avoid problems with your application:

- Have you met all requirements for graduation? Do you have any electives still outstanding?
- Has your nursing school received a permanent transcript for any credits that you transferred from another institution?
- Do you owe any fines or have any unpaid parking tickets? (This can delay the release of your permanent transcript. Check at your nursing school office, just to be sure.)

- Some states require that a statement be sent from your nursing school stating that you have met all requirements for graduation.
- Did you change your mind about the state in which you want to apply for licensure? If so, you must apply to a new state—and forfeit the original application fee.

What If You Want to Apply for Licensure in a Different State?

If you plan to apply for licensure in a different state from the one in which you are attending nursing school, contact the state board of nursing in the state in which you wish to become licensed.

Here's a checklist for obtaining a license in another state:

- Contact the state board of nursing of that state and find out what their requirements are for licensure.
- Find out what their fees are.
- Request a new candidate application for licensure.

After you pass the NCLEX-RN® exam, you will receive your nursing license from the state in which you applied for licensure regardless of where you took your exam. For example, if you applied for licensure in Michigan, you can take the test in Florida, if you wish. You would then receive a license to practice as an RN in Michigan because that is where you applied for licensure.

When Can You Schedule Your NCLEX-RN® Exam?

Pearson VUE will send you a document entitled "Authorization to Test" (ATT). The ATT will be sent to you via email at the email address you provided when you registered. You will be unable to schedule your test date until you receive this form.

On the ATT is your assigned candidate number; you will need to refer to this when scheduling your exam. Your ATT is valid for a time determined by the individual state board of nursing/regulatory body, and you must test before your ATT expires. If you don't, you will need to reapply to take the exam and pay the testing fees again. With your ATT, you will receive a list of test centers. You can schedule your NCLEX-RN® exam using the following procedures:

- Log on to the NCLEX® Candidate Website at **nclex.com**
- Call NCLEX® Candidate Services

    United States and Canada: 1-866-496-2539 (1-866-49-NCLEX) (toll-free)

    Asia Pacific Region: +852-3077-4923 (pay number)

    Europe, Middle East, Africa: +44-161-855-7445 (pay number)

    India: 91-120-439-7837 (pay number)

    All other countries not listed above: 1-952-905-7403 (pay number)

Candidates with hearing impairments who use a Telecommunications Device for the Deaf (TDD) can call the U.S.A. Relay Service at 1-800-627-3529 (toll-free) or the Canada & International Inbound relay service at 1-605-224-1837 (pay number).

Those with special testing requests, such as persons with disabilities, must call the NCLEX-RN®
Program Coordinator at NCLEX® Candidate Services at one of the numbers listed above. If you require
special accommodations, you cannot schedule your exam through the NCLEX® Candidate Website.

There is a space on the ATT for you to record the date and time of your scheduled exam. You will also
receive confirmation of your scheduled date and time.

Potential Rescheduling Problems

- You must test prior to the expiration date of your ATT. If you miss your appointment, you
  forfeit your testing fees and must reapply to both the state board of nursing/regulatory body and
  Pearson VUE.
- If you wish to change your appointment, you must notify Pearson VUE during business hours, at
  least 24 hours prior to your scheduled appointment. Call one of the numbers listed above or go
  the NCLEX® candidate website (**nclex.com**). If your test date is on Saturday, Sunday, or Monday,
  make sure to call on or before Friday.

Do not call the test site directly or leave a message if you are unable to take your test on the scheduled
date. You must follow the procedure outlined here.

When Will You Take the Exam?

The earliest date on which you can take the NCLEX-RN® exam varies depending on your state, but the
majority of students test approximately 45 days after the date of their graduation. Variables include:
when you submit the applications and fees, the length of time the ATT is valid, personal factors
(weddings, births, vacations), and job requirements. Each state determines the requirements for graduate nurses, licensure pending. If you are working as a graduate nurse, you must be knowledgeable about
the rules in your state.

Taking the Exam

What Happens on the Day of My NCLEX-RN® Exam?

Arrive at the test center at least 30 minutes before your scheduled test time. Wear layered clothing—the
rooms may be cool in the morning but can warm up as the day progresses.

Here's a checklist of things to bring on the day of the exam:

- Your Authorization to Test (ATT). (Although your ATT is no longer required for admission to
  your exam, you may wish to refer to it.)
- One form of unexpired, government-issued, signed identification that includes a picture. If you
  have changed your hair color, lost weight, or grown a beard, have a new picture ID made before
  Test Day. The name on your ID must match exactly the name on your ATT. Acceptable forms of
  identification include driver's license, state/territorial/provincial identification, passport, and U.S.
  military ID.

- A snack and something to drink.
- Do not bring any study materials to the test center.

Check-in procedure:

- Present a valid, acceptable form of ID.
- Provide your digital signature, take a palm vein scan, and have your photograph taken.
- Agree to the Candidate Statement via digital signature.
- Seal all electronic devices in a plastic bag provided by the test center.
- Place all other personal belongings in secure storage outside the testing room. This includes watches, large jewelry, scarfs and hats, lip balm, food and drink, and medical devices.

Earplugs are available on request. Request them, in case you find yourself distracted by background noise.

You will be provided an erasable note board for scratch work.

Where Will I Take My Test?

You will be in a room separate from the rest of the test center. Many testing sites consist of a room with 10–15 computers placed around the outside walls. Each computer sits on a full-size desk, with an adjustable chair for you to sit on. There are dividers between desks, but you will be able to see the person sitting next to you. There is a picture window from which the proctor will observe each person testing. There are also video cameras and sound sensors mounted on the walls to monitor each candidate.

What Will the Computer Screen Look Like?

The number of the question you are answering is located in the lower-right side of your computer screen. In the upper-right corner is a digital clock that counts down from 5:00:00—representing the 5 hours you have to complete the short tutorial that begins the exam, the exam itself, and all breaks.

If the question is a traditional four-option, text-based, multiple choice question, the question stem is located in the top half of the screen and the four answer choices are located in the lower half of the screen (Figure 12.1). Radio buttons are in front of each answer choice.

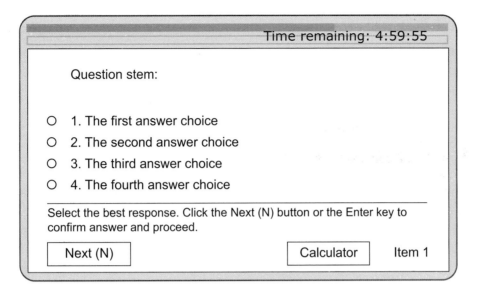

Figure 12.1

You will notice that there are two buttons at the bottom of the computer screen. You use the Next (N) button to confirm your answer selection and move to the next question. Click the Calculator button to display a drop-down calculator that can be used to perform computations.

If the question is an alternate format question that may have more than one correct answer, you will see the phrase "Select all that apply" between the stem of the question and five to nine answer choices. A small box is in front of each answer choice. The Next (N) button and Calculator button are at the bottom of the computer screen.

If the question is a hot spot alternate format question, the screen will contain a graphic or a picture. The Next (N) button and Calculator button are at the bottom of the computer screen.

If the question is a fill-in-the-blank alternate format question, a text box will be under the question. The Next (N) button and Calculator button are at the bottom of the computer screen.

If the question is a drag-and-drop/ordered response alternate format question, the unordered options will be under the question and to the left. The space for the ordered response will be to the right of the unordered options. The Next (N) button and Calculator button are at the bottom of the screen.

If the question is a chart/exhibit alternate format question, it will include the following prompt after the question stem: "Click on the Exhibit button below for additional client information." The Exhibit button is located in the bottom of the computer screen between the Next (N) button and the Calculator button. Click on the Exhibit button to display a pop-up box containing 3 tabs. Click on each of the tabs to display information needed to answer the question.

If the question is an audio alternate format question, the question will contain an audio clip that you must listen to in order to answer the question. Click on the Play button (a right-pointing arrow) to listen to the clip. A slider bar allows you to adjust the volume at which you hear the clip. If you want to listen to the audio clip more than once, you can click on the Play button again.

If the question is a graphics alternate format question, each of the four answer choices will be a graphic instead of text.

How Do I Use the Calculator?

Using the mouse, click on the Calculator button, and a drop-down calculator will appear on the computer screen. Use the mouse to click on the calculator keys. Remember, the diagonal or slash (/) key is used for division. When you are through with your calculations, click on the Calculator button again, and the calculator will disappear.

How Do I Select an Answer Choice for Traditional, Four-Option, Multiple Choice Questions?

You will use a two-step process to answer each question. Read the question and select an answer by using the mouse to click on the radio button preceding your answer choice. Your answer is now highlighted. When you are certain of your answer, click on the Next (N) button or the Enter key to confirm your answer. Your answer is now locked in and a new question will appear on the screen. *You are not able to change your answer after clicking on the Next (N) button or pressing the Enter key, so be certain of your answer before doing so.*

After your answer is entered into the computer, the computer selects a new question for you based on the accuracy of your previous answer and the components of the NCLEX-RN® exam test plan. If you answer a question correctly, the next question selected by the computer is more difficult. If you answer a question incorrectly, the next question selected by the computer is easier.

What If I Want to Change the Answer That I Have Highlighted?

If you want to change the highlighted answer, click on a different answer choice. Your answer is not locked in until you click on the Next (N) button or press the Enter key.

Even if you've never used a computer before, don't panic. You will be given instructions at the beginning of the test, and you will have to answer three tutorial questions before your test begins. These questions allow you to practice using the mouse to select an answer.

How Do I Select an Answer Choice for Select All That Apply Questions?

Read the question and click on the small box in front of the answer choice you want. A small check will appear in the box. Click on each answer choice that answers the question.

What If I Want to Change an Answer That I Have Checked?

If you change your mind and don't want an answer choice that you have selected, just click again on the small box in front of that answer choice and the check will disappear. When you are certain of your answer, click on the Next (N) button or press the Enter key to confirm your answer. Your answer is now locked in and a new question appears on the screen.

How Do I Select an Answer Choice for Hot Spot Questions?

To answer a hot spot alternate format question, just click on the area of the graphic or picture that answers the question.

What If I Want to Change the Area That I Have Selected?

If you change your mind and want to select another area of the graphic or picture, just use your mouse to click on the area that you want and the original selection disappears. When you are certain of your answer, click on the Next (N) button or press the Enter key to confirm your answer. Your answer is now locked in and a new question appears on the screen.

How Do I Enter an Answer Choice for Fill-in-the-Blank Questions?

To enter an answer for a fill-in-the-blank question, just use the keyboard to select the numbers or letters you want. If a unit of measurement already appears next to the answer box on the screen, be sure you enter *numbers* only into the answer box; adding a unit of measurement may cause your answer to be wrong.

What If I Want to Change What I Have Entered in the Text Box?

If you change your mind and want to enter another answer in the text box, just backspace over the answer you entered and then use the keyboard to enter another answer. When you are certain of your answer, click on the Next (N) button or press the Enter key to confirm your answer. Your answer is now locked in and a new question appears on the screen.

How Do I Select Options for Drag-and-Drop/Ordered Response Questions?

To put the responses in the correct order, click on the option you think should come first, hold down the button on the mouse, and drag the option over to the box on the right side of the screen. You may also highlight the option in the box on the left side and then click the arrow key that points to the box on the right side to move the option. Do the same with each response in the proper order.

What If I Want to Change the Order of My Responses?

If you change your mind about a response, click on it with the mouse and drag it back to the left side of the screen or use the arrow key as described above. To complete the question, you must move all options from the box on the left side of the screen to the box on the right side. When you are certain of your answer, click on the Next (N) button or press the Enter key to confirm your answer. Your answer is now locked in and a new question appears on the screen.

How Do I Enter or Change an Answer Choice for Chart/Exhibit, Audio, and Graphics Alternate Format Questions?

Chart/exhibit, audio, and graphics alternate format questions all use a four-option, multiple choice format, so you can enter or change your answer choices just as you would for traditional text-based, four-option, multiple choice questions.

Do I Get Any Breaks?

You will receive an optional break at the end of 2 hours of testing. There will be a pre-programmed prompt offering you a break. Leave the testing room, stretch your legs and eat your snack. Take some deep, cleansing breaths and get yourself ready to go back into the testing room. The computer will offer you another optional break after 3½ hours of testing. We recommend that you take it unless you feel you're on a roll.

You may take a break at any time during your test, but the time that you spend away from your computer is counted as a part of your five hours of total testing time. Kaplan recommends that you take a short (2 to 5 minute) break if you are having trouble concentrating. Take time to go to the restroom, eat your snack, or get a drink. This will enable you to maintain or regain your concentration for the test. Remember, every question counts! If you need to take a break, raise your hand to notify the test administrator. You must leave the testing room, and you will be required to take a palm vein scan before you are allowed to resume your test.

How Will I Know When My Test Ends?

A screen will appear on your computer that states, "Your test is concluded." You will then be required to answer several exit questions. These are a few multiple choice questions about your impression of the examination experience. They do not count toward your results.

How Long Will It Take to Receive My Results?

Your results are sent to you by your state board of nursing. Each state board determines when the NCLEX-RN® exam results are released. In the following jurisdictions, you may access your "unofficial" results 2 business days after taking your examination via the NCLEX® candidate website (for a $7.95 fee):

Alaska, Arizona, Arkansas, Colorado, Connecticut, District of Columbia, Florida, Georgia, Hawaii, Idaho, Illinois, Indiana, Iowa, Kansas, Kentucky, Louisiana, Maine, Maryland, Massachusetts, Michigan, Minnesota, Mississippi, Missouri, Montana, Nebraska, Nevada, New Jersey, New Mexico, New York, North Carolina, North Dakota, Northern Mariana Islands, Ohio, Oklahoma, Oregon, Pennsylvania, Rhode Island, South Carolina, South Dakota, Tennessee, Texas, U.S. Virgin Islands, Utah, Vermont, Virginia, Washington, Wisconsin, Wyoming

For most states, you will receive your official results approximately 6 weeks after your test date.

CHAPTER 13

TAKING THE TEST MORE THAN ONCE

Some people may never have to read this chapter, but it's a certainty that others will. The most important advice we can give to repeat test takers is: Don't despair. There is hope. We can get you through the NCLEX-RN® exam.

You Are Not Alone

Think about that awful day when the big brown envelope arrived. You just couldn't believe it. You had to tell family, friends, your supervisor, and coworkers that you didn't pass the NCLEX-RN® exam. When this happens, each unsuccessful candidate feels like the only person who has failed the exam.

How to Interpret Unsuccessful Test Results

Unsuccessful candidates on the NCLEX-RN® exam will usually say, "I almost passed." Some of you did almost pass, and some of you weren't very close. If you fail the exam, you will receive a Candidate Performance Report from NCSBN. In this profile, you will be told how many questions you answered on the exam. The more questions you answered, the closer you came to passing. The only way you will continue to get questions after you answer the first 85 is if you are answering questions close to the level of difficulty needed to pass the exam. If you are answering questions far above the level needed to pass or far below the level needed to pass, your exam will end at 85 questions.

Figure 13.1 on the next page shows a representation of what happens when a candidate fails in 85 questions. This student does not come close to passing. In 85 questions, this student demonstrates an inability to consistently answer questions correctly at or above the level of difficulty needed to pass the exam. This usually indicates a lack of nursing knowledge, considerable difficulties with taking a standardized test, or a deficiency in critical thinking skills.

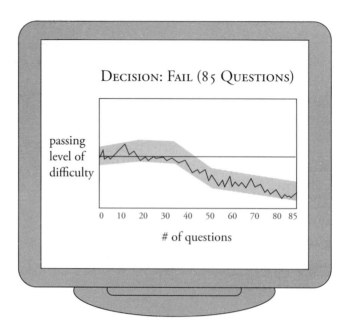

Figure 13.1

Figure 13.2 shows what happens when a candidate takes all 150 questions and fails. This candidate "almost passed." The candidate answers question 149, and the computer does not make a determination when it selects the last question. If the candidate's final ability estimate is at or above the passing standard after answering question 150, the candidate passes. If the final ability estimate is below the passing standard, the candidate fails.

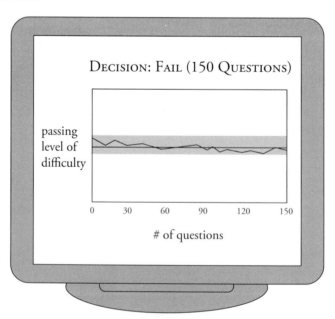

Figure 13.2

If you took a test longer than 85 questions and failed, you were probably familiar with most of the content you saw on the exam but you may have difficulty using critical thinking skills or taking standardized tests.

The information contained on the Candidate Performance Report helps you identify your strengths and weaknesses on this particular NCLEX-RN® exam. This knowledge will help you identify where to concentrate your study when you prepare to retake the NCLEX-RN® exam.

Should You Test Again?

Absolutely! You completed your nursing education to become an RN. The initial response of many unsuccessful candidates is to declare, "I'm never going back! That was the worst experience of my life! What do I do now?"

When you first received your results, you went through a period of grieving—the same stages that you learned about in nursing school. Three to four weeks later, you find that you want to begin preparing to retake the NCLEX-RN® exam.

How Should You Begin?

You should prepare in a different way this time. Whatever you did to prepare last time didn't work well enough. The most common mistake that candidates who failed make is to assume that they did not study hard enough or learn enough content. For some of you, that's true. But for the majority of you, memorizing more content does not mean more right answers. It could simply mean more frustration for you.

The first step in preparing for your next exam is to make a commitment that you will test again. Decide when you want to schedule your test and allow yourself enough time to prepare. Mark this test date on your calendar. You can do all of this before you send in your fees and receive your authorization to test. Remember, you cannot retake the NCLEX-RN® exam for 45 to 90 days, depending on your state board of nursing/regulatory body, so you may as well use this time wisely.

The next step is to figure out why you failed the NCLEX-RN® exam. Check off any reasons that pertain to you:

- ☐ I didn't know the nursing content.
- ☐ I memorized facts without understanding the principles of client care.
- ☐ I had unrealistic expectations about the NCLEX-RN® exam test questions.
- ☐ I had difficulty correctly identifying THE REWORDED QUESTION.
- ☐ I had difficulty staying focused on THE REWORDED QUESTION.
- ☐ I found myself predicting answer choices.
- ☐ I did not carefully consider each answer choice.
- ☐ I am not good at choosing answers that require me to establish priorities of care.
- ☐ I answered questions based on my real-world experiences.

☐ I did not cope well with the computer-adaptive test experience.

☐ I thought I would complete the exam in 85 questions.

☐ When I got to question 120, I totally lost my concentration and just answered questions to get through the rest of the exam.

After determining why you failed, the next step is to establish a plan of action for your next test. Remember, you should prepare differently this time. Consider the following when setting up your new plan of study.

You've seen the test.

You may wish that you didn't have to walk back into the testing center again, but if you want to be a registered professional nurse, you must go back. This time you have an advantage over the first-time test taker: you've seen the test! You know exactly what you are preparing for, and there are no unknowns. The computer will remember what questions you took before, and you will not be given any of the same questions. However, the content of the question, the style of the question, and the kinds of answer choices will not change. You will not be surprised this time.

Study both content and test questions.

By the time you retest, you will be out of nursing school for 6 months or longer. Remember that old saying, "What you are not learning, you are forgetting"? Because this is a content-based test about safe and effective nursing care, you must remember all you can about nursing theory in order to select correct answers. You must study content that is integrated and organized like the NCLEX-RN® exam.

You must also master exam-style test questions. It is essential that you be able to correctly identify what each question is asking. You will *not* predict answers. You will *think* about each and every answer choice to decide if it answers the reworded question. In order to master test questions, you must practice answering them. We recommend that you answer hundreds of exam-style test questions, especially at the application level of difficulty.

Know all of the words and their meanings.

Some students who have to learn a great deal of material in a short period of time have trouble learning the extensive vocabulary of the discipline. For example, difficulty with terminology is a problem for many good students who study history. They enjoy the concepts but find it hard to memorize all of the names and dates to allow them to do well on history tests. If you have trouble memorizing terms, you may find it useful to review a list of the terminology that you must know to pass the NCLEX-RN® exam. There is a list of those words at the end of this book.

Practice test taking strategies.

There is no substitute for mastering the nursing content. This knowledge, combined with test taking strategies, will help you to select a greater number of correct answers. For many students, the strategies mean the difference between a passing test and a failing test. Using strategies effectively can also determine whether you take a short test (85 questions) or a longer test (up to 150 questions).

Evaluate your testing experience.

Some students attribute their failure to the testing experience. Comments we have heard include:

"I didn't like answering questions on the computer."

"I found the background noise distracting. I should have taken the earplugs!"

"I looked up every time the door opened."

"I should have taken a snack. I got so hungry!"

"After 2½ hours I didn't care what I answered. I just wanted the computer to shut off!"

"I didn't expect to be there for 4 hours!"

"I should have rescheduled my test, but I just wanted to get it over with!"

"I wish I had taken aspirin with me. I had such a headache before it was over!"

Do any of these comments sound familiar? It is important for you to take charge of your testing experience. Here's how:

- Choose a familiar testing site.
- Select the time of day that you test your best. (Are you a morning person or an afternoon person?)
- Accept the earplugs when offered.
- Take a snack and a drink for your break.
- Take a break if you become distracted or fatigued during the test.
- Contact the proctors at the test site if something bothers you during the test.
- Plan on testing for 5 hours. Then, if you get out early, it's a pleasant surprise.
- Say to yourself every day, "I will pass the NCLEX-RN® exam."

CHAPTER 14

ESSENTIALS FOR INTERNATIONAL NURSES

Many of you have years of nursing experience in your home country. Now you are preparing for the NCLEX-RN® exam so you can be licensed to practice your profession in the United States. Because of Kaplan's extensive experience preparing nurses educated in other countries, we are very aware of the special issues that you face when trying to pass the NCLEX-RN® exam. Your special concerns will be discussed in this chapter.

Many nurses educated outside of the United States have not had the experience of taking a test that combines objective multiple choice questions with alternate format questions. Your testing experience may have been limited to oral exams or writing answers to essay and short answer questions. Multiple choice tests are used in the United States because they measure knowledge more objectively and are easier to administer to large groups of people. In order to pass the NCLEX-RN® exam, you must demonstrate that you are a safe and effective nurse by correctly answering predominantly multiple choice questions along with alternate format question.

NCLEX-RN® Exam Administration Abroad

NCSBN administers the NCLEX-RN® exam in selected international locations, including Australia, Canada, England, Hong Kong, India, Japan, Mexico, the Philippines, and Taiwan. (Testing is temporarily unavailable in Germany.) Please see **nclex.com** to locate a test center near you.

These sites provide greater convenience for international nurses to take the NCLEX-RN® exam. The international administration does not circumvent any regulations posed by the state boards of nursing, and the test sites are subject to the same security and procedures followed in U.S. test sites. If you choose to take the test at one of these sites, you must pay an additional $150 international scheduling fee plus a Value Added Tax (VAT) where applicable.

The CGFNS® Certificate

Before considering applications for licensure as a registered nurse in the United States, many U.S. state boards of nursing require internationally educated nurses to obtain a certificate from the Commission on Graduates of Foreign Nursing Schools (CGFNS®). Some states require applicants to complete this process before taking the NCLEX-RN® exam. The process of obtaining a CGFNS® certificate involves: (1) a review of your secondary and nursing education credentials and original nursing program, (2) passing the CGFNS® exam that tests nursing knowledge, and (3) obtaining a minimum score on a designated English language proficiency exam.

The CGFNS® exam is a two-part test of nursing knowledge. Nurses who pass this exam have been shown to be more likely to pass the NCLEX-RN® exam on the first try than nurses who have not. The CGFNS® exam can be taken overseas at a number of international testing sites run by CGFNS® or at selected sites in the United States.

Applications for the CGFNS® exam are free, and you may apply online at **cgfns.org**. Only online applications for the CGFNS® Certification Program are accepted. On the CGFNS® website, you will also find application deadlines and test dates. With an online application, you can submit your educational and professional documentation, choose a location and date for your exam, and pay fees by credit card. The online CGFNS Qualifying Exam® is administered in March, July, September, and November during a 5-day testing window in each of these months.

To find out about a particular state's requirements for international nurses, contact that state's board of nursing and request an application packet for initial licensure as an internationally educated nurse. You can also visit your chosen state or province's website using the key words "Board of Nursing" and the state or province name.

For detailed information regarding the CGFNS® English proficiency requirements, go to **cgfns.org**. The following information will help you register for the appropriate exams. Remember that these exam results are usually only valid for 2 years, so plan accordingly to avoid retakes. To learn more about preparing for these exams, see the Kaplan English Programs section at the end of this chapter.

> TOEFL®, TWE®, and TSE®
> Educational Testing Service
> P.O. Box 6151
> Princeton, NJ 08541-6151
> 1-800-468-6335 (United States, U.S. Territories, Canada)
> 1-609-771-7100 (all other locations)
> Fax: 1-610-290-8972
> Website: **www.ets.org/toefl**
>
> TOEIC® Testing Program
> Educational Testing Service
> Rosedale Road
> Princeton, NJ 08541
> Phone: 1-609-771-7170
> Fax: 1-610-628-3722
> Email: **toeic@ets.org**
> Website: **www.ets.org/toeic**
>
> IELTS® International
> Website: **www.ielts.org**

Work Visas

For the most current information on visa requirements, contact the nearest U.S. embassy or consulate in your home country or the nearest regional office of the U.S. Citizenship and Immigration Services if you already live in the United States. You can also contact the CGFNS® by telephone at 1-215-222-8454 or through its website at **cgfns.org**.

Nursing Practice in the United States

Some international nurses find nursing in the United States similar to nursing as they learned it in their country. For others, nursing in the United States is very different from what they learned or experienced in their country. The NCLEX-RN® exam may ask you questions about procedures that are unfamiliar to you. You may be asked questions about diets and foods that are new to you. In order to be successful on the NCLEX-RN® exam, you must be able to correctly answer questions about nursing as it is practiced in the United States.

Here is an overview of services and skills that U.S. nurses are expected to perform:

- Nurses are involved with prevention, early detection, and treatment of illness for people of all ages.
- Nurses care for the whole person, not just an illness. Their focus is on client needs; that is, how a client will respond to an illness.
- Nurses are professionals who are responsible for their actions.
- Nurses must communicate with clients and all the members of the health care team: other nurses, assistive personnel, physicians, dietitians, pharmacists, therapists, technicians, and social workers.
- Nurses serve as clients' advocates; that is, they counsel clients and make sure their rights are protected.
- Nurses help clients understand the health care system, and assist clients to make decisions about their health care.
- Nurses are assertive and ask questions of health care professionals when necessary, including physicians. Their style of communication is polite and professional but very direct.
- Nurses are responsible for meeting the needs of clients whose care involves high-tech equipment.
- Nurses are responsible for basing their actions on knowledge and acceptable nursing practice.
- Nurses, not families, are responsible for all the hands-on nursing care for clients in the hospital setting.
- Nurses are responsible for teaching clients and their families how to manage their health care needs.

U.S.-Style Nursing Communication

An issue of special concern for international nurses is therapeutic communication. Correctly answering the questions about communication can be difficult for some nurses educated in the United States. These questions become a special challenge to test takers for whom English is a second language, or for test takers who do not yet fully understand American-style communication.

Key features of U.S.-style communication in nursing:

- *Validate the client's experience and feelings by responding to the client verbally.* Ask questions that relate directly to what the client says.
- *Direct the client's behavior to promote comfort and well-being.* Do not patronize or reject the client by imposing a value judgment.
- *Maintain eye contact with the client, especially during conversation.* Lean forward to face the client. Nod, smile, or frown to demonstrate agreement or disagreement while listening.

Responses used in U.S. nursing are based on an assessment of the client's needs and are designed to foster growth and establish mutually formulated goals.

NCLEX-RN® exam questions concerning communication are best answered by:

- Conveying *respect* and *warmth*, making the client feel accepted and respected as an individual regardless of their words, actions, or behavior. This means that the nurse:
  - Assumes that all client behavior is purposeful and has meaning even though it may not make sense to others
  - Defines the social, physical, and emotional boundaries of the nurse-client relationship
  - Develops a contract with the client
  - Structures time to develop a nurse-client relationship
  - Creates a safe and secure environment
  - Accepts the dependency needs of the client while encouraging, assisting, and supporting movement toward health and independence
  - Intervenes when a client behaves inappropriately to directly reject the behavior but not the client
  - Intervenes directly to respond to the client, not to reinforce an inappropriate behavior

- Demonstrating *active listening* and *genuineness*. This means that the nurse:
  - Asks questions that relate directly to what the client says
  - Maintains good eye contact
  - Leans forward in the chair to face the client
  - Nods, smiles, or frowns to show agreement or disagreement
  - Understands that the personal feelings and past experiences of the nurse can negatively or positively affect relationships with clients

- Communicating *interest* and *empathy* by allowing the client to comfortably communicate concerns and behave in new ways. This means that the nurse:
  - Focuses conversation on the client's feelings
  - Understands that clients respond to the behavioral expectations of the nursing staff
  - Validates the client's feelings
  - Analyzes both verbal and nonverbal behavioral clues
  - Anticipates that there might be some difficulty as the client learns new behaviors

Nurses create barriers in the communication process when they demonstrate a poor understanding of the basics in therapeutic communication. They must convey respect, warmth, and genuineness through active listening and communicating interest and empathy about the concerns of clients, families, and/or staff.

Examples of barriers to communication:

- Minimizing concerns
- Giving false reassurance
- Giving approval
- Rejecting the person, not the behavior
- Choosing sides with the client, family member, or staff member in a conflict
- Blaming the external environment for the situation
- Disagreeing or arguing with the client or family member
- Offering advice about a situation
- Pressuring the client or family member for an explanation
- Defending one's own actions or behavior
- Belittling client, family member, or staff concerns
- Giving one-word responses to questions
- Using denial
- Interpreting or analyzing both verbal and nonverbal behavioral clues in the situation to the client
- Shifting the focus of the conversation away from the client, family member, or staff concerns
- Using jargon or medical terminology without explanation in conversation with the client and/or family
- Invalidating the client's, family member's, or staff's feelings
- Offering unrealistic hope for the future
- Ignoring client clues to help the client set appropriate limits on their behavior

The following are some questions that will allow you to practice the right approach.

Sample Questions

> *Directions:* Carefully read the question and all answer choices. Determine whether each option is an appropriate response. In the space at the right, record your decision ("Correct" or "Incorrect") along with the reason you believe that the nurse's response is correct or incorrect.

Questions	Reason the Option is Correct/Incorrect
1. A client has been hospitalized for 2 days for treatment of hepatitis A. When the nurse enters the room, the client says, "Leave me alone and stop bothering me." Which response by the nurse would be **most** appropriate? 1. "I understand and will leave you alone for now." 2. "Why are you angry with me?" 3. "Are you upset because you do not feel better?" 4. "You seem upset this morning."	
2. A client with a fractured arm tells the nurse, "I'm afraid to have the cast removed." Which response by the nurse would be the **most** appropriate? 1. "I know it is unpleasant. Try not to be afraid. I will help you." 2. "You seem very anxious. I will stay with you while the cast is removed." 3. "I don't blame you. I'd be afraid also." 4. "My aunt just had a cast removed and she's just fine."	

Questions	Reason the Option is Correct/Incorrect
3. A client comes to the clinic for a suspected pregnancy. The client tells the nurse, "I want to terminate this pregnancy because my spouse and I don't want to have children," and then begins to cry. Which statement by the nurse would be the **most** appropriate? 1. "Are you upset because you forgot to use birth control?" 2. "Why are you so upset? You're married. There's no reason not to have the baby." 3. "If you're so upset, why don't you have the baby and put it up for adoption?" 4. "You seem upset. Let's talk about how you're feeling."	
4. A client is in the terminal stages of carcinoma of the lung. A family member asks the nurse, "How much longer will it be?" Which response by the nurse would be **most** appropriate? 1. "I cannot say exactly. What are your concerns at this time?" 2. "I don't know. I'll call your family member's oncologist." 3. "This must be a terrible situation for you." 4. "Don't worry, it will be very soon."	

Questions	Reason the Option is Correct/Incorrect

5. A client is admitted to the hospital with a diagnosis of bipolar disorder. The client approaches the nurse and says, "Hi, baby," and opens the robe, under the client is naked. Which comment by the nurse would be **most** appropriate?

1. "This is inappropriate behavior. Please close your robe and return to your room."
2. "Please dress in your clothes and then join us for lunch in the dining room."
3. "I am offended by your behavior and will have to report you."
4. "Do you need some assistance dressing today?"

6. The nurse prepares to assist the client placed in Buck's traction with a bath. The client tells the nurse, "You're too young to know how to do this. Get me somebody who knows what they're doing." Which response by the nurse would be **most** appropriate?

1. "I am young, but I graduated from nursing school."
2. "If I don't bathe you now, you'll have to wait until I'm finished with my other clients."
3. "Can you be more specific about your concerns?"
4. "Your concerns are unnecessary. I know what I'm doing."

Questions	Reason the Option is Correct/Incorrect

7. A client with an abdominal mass is admitted to the hospital and scheduled for an exploratory laparotomy. The client asks the nurse, "Do you think I have cancer?" Which response by the nurse would be **most** appropriate?

1. "Would you like me to call your doctor so that you can discuss your specific concerns?"

2. "Your tests show a mass. It must be hard not knowing what is wrong."

3. "It sounds like you are afraid that you are going to die from cancer."

4. "Don't worry about it now; I'm sure you have many healthy years ahead of you."

8. A client is admitted to the postpartum unit following a miscarriage. The next day the nurse finds the client crying while looking at the babies in the newborn nursery. Which approach by the nurse would be **most** appropriate?

1. "There is a reason for everything. The miscarriage was for the best."

2. "Don't cry, it will be okay. You are young enough to have more children."

3. "Why are you looking at the babies in the nursery?"

4. "You seem to be grieving the loss of your baby. Please share what you're feeling."

Questions	Reason the Option is Correct/Incorrect
9. An older adult client is hospitalized with major neurocognitive disorder (NCD) due to Alzheimer disease. The client's adult daughter tells the nurse that caring for him is too hard, but that she feels guilty placing him in a nursing home. Which statement by the nurse would be **most** appropriate? 1. "It is hard to be caught between taking care of your needs and your father's needs." 2. "Would you like me to help you find a nursing home?" 3. "Don't feel guilty. The only solution is to place your father in a nursing home." 4. "I think I would feel guilty too if I had to place my father in a nursing home."	

Read the explanations to these questions and make sure that the American approach to these communications questions is understandable to you. It will help you to choose the right answer on the NCLEX-RN® exam.

Sample Questions Answers and Explanations

1. The answer is 4

(1) "I understand and will leave you alone for now." This is not the best approach because it does not promote further communication between the nurse and the client about how the client is feeling. In order to interpret this client's behavior, the nurse must first validate it with the client.

(2) "Why are you angry with me?" This response is incorrect. The nurse is drawing a conclusion about the client's behavior. This type of response is too confrontational. "Why" questions are considered nontherapeutic.

(3) "Are you upset because you do not feel better?" This answer is not the best choice. The nurse is drawing a conclusion about the client's behavior without validating it first. This question may also belittle the client's actual concerns.

(4) **"You seem upset this morning."** This is the correct answer choice because the nurse seeks to verbally validate the client's behavior rather than simply responding to the behavior. This promotes the nurse-client relationship by encouraging the client to share feelings with the nurse.

2. The answer is 2

(1) "I know it is unpleasant. Try not to be afraid. I will help you." It is not clear what concerns the client has about this procedure. The nurse should establish what they are before responding. The nurse falsely reassures the client by saying, "I will help you." Because you do not know the nature of the client's concerns, you cannot honestly offer help.

(2) **"You seem very anxious. I will stay with you while the cast is removed."** This is the best choice because the nurse responds to the client's feelings of fear. Doing so is consistent with therapeutic communication used in American nursing. This response also provides an additional opportunity for the nurse to remain with the client in a supportive capacity, enhancing the nurse-client relationship.

(3) "I don't blame you. I'd be afraid also." This answer is incorrect because it shifts the focus of the conversation from the client to the nurse. This sets up a barrier to further communication. The nurse concedes the issue too quickly, leaving the source of the client's fear unknown.

(4) "My aunt just had a cast removed and she's just fine." This choice shifts the focus of the conversation from the client to the nurse's aunt, who is of no concern to the client. It fails to explore the source of the client's anxiety and sets up a block to further communication.

3.   The answer is 4

(1) "Are you upset because you forgot to use birth control?" This response is inappropriate because it places blame on the client. The nurse should not assume that the client "forgot" to do something. It also fails to respond to the client's feelings and does not encourage the client to discuss concerns.

(2) "Why are you so upset? You're married. There's no reason not to have the baby." This response is inappropriate in terms of American therapeutic communication. It is harsh, presumptive, and assumes that the purpose of every marriage is to have children. This is not always the case in American culture. With this response, the nurse does not attempt to verify the reason for the client's tears, thereby discouraging further conversation about what the client is actually experiencing.

(3) "If you're so upset, why don't you have the baby and put it up for adoption?" This response is also inappropriate because it is a value-laden assumption placing positive value on adoption. Again, the nurse fails to explore with the client the reason for the client's tears, thereby discouraging further communication. The nurse is also offering advice.

(4) **"You seem upset. Let's talk about how you're feeling."** This is the best answer to this question. It promotes the nurse-client relationship and illustrates therapeutic communication used in American nursing. The nurse responds to the client's feelings in a nonjudgmental empathetic way.

4.   The answer is 1

(1) **"I cannot say exactly. What are your concerns at this time?"** This is the most appropriate response because it is unclear why the family member has approached the nurse at this point. Perhaps the client is in pain and the family member wants to discuss it with the nurse. It allows for that possibility. It is also direct and factually correct.

(2) "I don't know. I'll call your family member's oncologist." This is not the most appropriate response. It shifts the focus of responsibility from the nurse to the physician, which prevents a nurse–family member relationship from developing.

(3) "This must be a terrible situation for you." This is not the most appropriate response. It is a value-laden statement that fails to explore the family member's reason for approaching the nurse.

(4) "Don't worry, it will be very soon." This answer is inappropriate because it offers the family member false reassurance. It also offers advice by telling the family member not to worry. This statement is demeaning and may sound as if the nurse is too busy to discuss the family member's concerns.

5.   The answer is 1

(1)   **"This is inappropriate behavior. Please close your robe and return to your room."** This statement by the nurse is the correct answer choice. It responds to the client's behavior, sets limits on the behavior, and directs the client toward more appropriate social behavior in the milieu. This statement rejects the client's behavior, not the client as a person.

(2)   "Please dress in your clothes and then join us for lunch in the dining room." This answer is incorrect because ignores the behavior of the client improperly exposing the naked body. Instead it directs the client to dress and report to the dining room for lunch as though nothing has happened. This is inappropriate and nontherapeutic.

(3)   "I am offended by your behavior and will have to report you." This response is incorrect because it shifts the focus from the client to the nurse and the nurse's feelings. The nurse's personal feelings are irrelevant. Threatening to report the client is also punitive, which is nontherapeutic.

(4)   "Do you need some assistance dressing today?" This question fails to respond to the client's behavior. It is also a yes/no question, which is nontherapeutic.

6.   The answer is 3

(1)   "I am young, but I graduated from nursing school." This choice responds to only part of the message that the client sent to the nurse. It assumes that the nurse knows what the client's concerns are and agrees that there is some problem associated with being too young. Further clarification is necessary in this situation.

(2)   "If I don't bathe you now, you'll have to wait until I'm finished with my other clients." This response is nontherapeutic. It fails to explore the client's concerns about the nurse. It is an uncaring and punitive statement by the nurse that is inappropriate in a nurse-client relationship.

(3)   **"Can you be more specific about your concerns?"** This is the best answer choice because it seeks to validate the client's message. It is direct, not defensive, and allows the client to express their point of view.

(4)   "Your concerns are unnecessary. I know what I'm doing." This response dismisses the client's feelings by saying the client shouldn't be concerned. The nurse should not tell a client how the client should be feeling. While a response asserting the nurse's competence may sound like reassurance, the nurse has yet to validate the concerns that underlie the client's statement.

7. The answer is 2

(1) "Would you like me to call your doctor so that you can discuss your specific concerns?" This response is incorrect because it shifts the focus of responsibility from the nurse to the physician, thereby reducing the possibility of developing an ongoing nurse-client relationship.

(2) **"Your tests show a mass. It must be hard not knowing what is wrong."** This is the best answer choice because it responds to the client's feelings. It allows the client to continue to identify and express concerns regarding surgery, hospitalization, and the possibility of having a potentially life-threatening illness. The nurse validates that the client has valid concerns and invites the client to elaborate on them.

(3) "It sounds like you are afraid that you are going to die from cancer." This answer fails to validate with the client that "dying from cancer" is in fact the issue. The nurse reaches this conclusion on the basis of a brief question from the client without giving the client a chance to elaborate. This is inappropriate.

(4) "Don't worry about it now; I'm sure that you have many healthy years ahead of you." The nurse is telling the client how the client should feel, and then goes on to offer false reassurance. This response fails to address or explore the actual concerns of the client.

8. The answer is 4

(1) "There is a reason for everything. The miscarriage was for the best." This statement is insensitive to the client, offers false reassurance, and belittles the client's most immediate concerns.

(2) "Don't cry, it will be okay. You are young enough to have more children." This statement is insensitive to the grief that the client is experiencing. It also offers false reassurance by saying that the client can have other children.

(3) "Why are you looking at the babies in the nursery?" This is a "why" question, which may cause the client to become defensive. This response by the nurse also fails to respond to the client's immediate grief.

(4) **"You seem to be grieving the loss of your baby. Please share what you're feeling."** This is the best answer choice. This response promotes the nurse-client relationship, and allows for the identification of feelings and the expression of sadness. The client is in an acute stage of grief. Acknowledging the loss and offering support appropriately addresses this issue.

9. The answer is 1

(1) **"It is hard to be caught between taking care of your needs and your father's needs."** This is the most therapeutic response as it allows for continued development of a relationship with the family member of the client. This response allows the nurse to explore and validate the daughter's feelings about the nursing home placement.

(2) "Would you like me to help you find a nursing home?" This is not the best answer choice. It is a yes/no question and doesn't encourage discussion of the daughter's feelings.

(3) "Don't feel guilty. The only solution is to place your father in a nursing **home.**" Telling the adult daughter not to worry minimizes her concerns. Although it may be true that the daughter has done all that she can, this is not the best therapeutic response because it cuts off an opportunity for further conversation with the nurse.

(4) "I think I would feel guilty too if I had to place my father in a nursing home." This statement is value-laden and judgmental, and it blocks any further communication between the nurse and the client's daughter. It is not important what the nurse thinks about the daughter's decision, nor is it the nurse's role to make the daughter feel more guilty about her decision.

Language

English is the predominant language spoken and written in the United States, and the NCLEX-RN® exam is administered only in English. With the exception of the medical terminology, the reading level of the NCLEX-RN® exam is that of a junior in an American high school (11th grade). In order to be successful on the NCLEX-RN® exam, you must understand English—and the terminology—as it is used in the United States.

Vocabulary

Vocabulary can be a challenge for international nurses on the NCLEX-RN® exam. Not only must you know what each word means, but sometimes a word may have more than one meaning. You need to be able to correctly identify words as they are used in context. Refer to the NCLEX-RN® Exam Resources section in the back of this book for some of the commonly found words on the NCLEX-RN® exam. Some other ways to increase your vocabulary and learn how the words are used in everyday English include:

- Talking with Americans
- Watching American movies and television
- Reading American newspapers and magazines

Abbreviations

Many internationally educated nurses are unfamiliar with the abbreviations used in the United States. When studying, always look up unknown words in a medical dictionary. Consult the NCLEX-RN® Exam Resources section (Appendix C) in the back of this book for a list of abbreviations used by nurses in American health care settings.

As an internationally educated nurse, you face special challenges in preparing for the NCLEX-RN® exam. Following the tips and guidelines outlined in this book will increase your chances of passing the NCLEX-RN® exam and will allow you to reach your career goals.

Kaplan Programs for International Nurses

Knowing something about U.S. culture and how U.S. nurses fit into the overall health care industry is important for nurses trained outside the United States. If you are not from the United States, but are interested in learning more about U.S nursing, wish to practice in the United States, or are exploring the possibilities of attending a U.S. nursing school for graduate study, Kaplan is able to help you.

CGFNS® (Commission on Graduates of Foreign Nursing Schools) Preparation for International Nurses

Many U.S. state boards of nursing require internationally educated nurses to obtain a CGFNS® certificate before applying for initial licensure as a registered nurse. The certification process requires that a candidate pass a two-part test of nursing knowledge and demonstrate English language proficiency on the TOEFL® exam. Kaplan offers a comprehensive course of study to help you earn your CGFNS® certificate. To obtain information, please call 1-800-527-8378. Outside the United States, please call 1-212-997-5883 or log on to the website at **kaplannursing.com.**

Preparation for the NCLEX-RN® (National Council Licensure Examination) Examination for International Nurses

An internationally educated nurse must pass the NCLEX-RN® exam in order to obtain a license to practice as a registered nurse in the United States. Kaplan has a comprehensive course and review products to help international nurses pass this exam. To obtain information, please call 1-800-527-8378 (outside the United States: 1-212-997-5883) or log on to the website at **https://www.kaptest.com /ispn-cgfns/courses/ispn-cgfns-prep.**

Kaplan English Programs

In addition to Kaplan Nursing programs, Kaplan also offers English programs to help you improve your English skills and score on the TOEFL®. Kaplan's English Programs were designed to help students and professionals from outside the United States meet their educational and career goals. At locations throughout the United States, international students take advantage of Kaplan's programs to help them improve their academic and conversational English skills, raise their scores on the TOEFL® and other standardized exams, and gain admission to the schools of their choice. Our staff and instructors give international students the individualized instruction they need to succeed. The following sections provide brief descriptions of some of Kaplan's programs for non native English speakers.

English Language Programs

Kaplan offers a wide range of English language programs to help you improve your English quickly and effectively, regardless of your current level. Each of our programs has a special focus, allowing you to direct your study in a way that suits your particular language needs. All of the essential language skills are covered, and your fluency and confidence will increase rapidly thanks to Kaplan's communicative teaching method.

TOEFL® and Academic English

Kaplan's world-famous TOEFL® course prepares students for the TOEFL® iBT. Designed for high-intermediate to advanced-level English speakers, our course focuses on the academic English skills you will need to succeed on the test. The course includes TOEFL®-focused reading, writing, listening, and speaking instruction and hundreds of practice items similar to those on the exam. Kaplan's expert instructors help you prepare for the four sections of the TOEFL® iBT, including the Speaking section. Our simulated online TOEFL® tests help you monitor your progress and provide you with feedback on areas where you require improvement. We will teach you how to get a higher score!

Other Kaplan Programs

Since 1938, more than 3 million students have come to Kaplan to advance their studies, prepare for entry to American universities, and further their careers. In addition to the above programs, Kaplan offers courses to prepare for the SAT®, ACT®, GMAT®, GRE®, LSAT®, MCAT®, DAT®, USMLE®, and other standardized exams both online and at locations throughout the United States.

Applying to Kaplan English Programs*

To get more information, or to apply for admission to any of Kaplan's programs for non native English speakers, contact us at:

Kaplan English Programs
Phone: 1-800-818-9128 (within the United States)
Phone: +44 (0)20 7045 5000 (elsewhere)
Website: **kaplaninternational.com**

FREE Services for International Students

Kaplan now offers international students many services online—free of charge! Students may assess their TOEFL* skills and gain valuable feedback on their English language proficiency in just a few hours with Kaplan's TOEFL* Skills Assessment. Log on to **kaplaninternational.com** today.

---

*Kaplan is authorized under federal law to enroll nonimmigrant alien students.

Test names are registered trademarks of their respective owners.

PART FIVE

NCLEX-RN® EXAM RESOURCES

SUMMARY OF CRITICAL THINKING PATHS

The 10 charts in this appendix illustrate different paths you must choose from in order to correctly answer NCLEX-RN® exam questions. The stepping stones stand for steps that you must follow in order to find the correct answer for that question type. Use the chart to refresh your memory with respect to the various steps for each type of question. Tear out this page and refer to it to practice using this book's strategies when answering practice NCLEX-RN® exam-style questions.

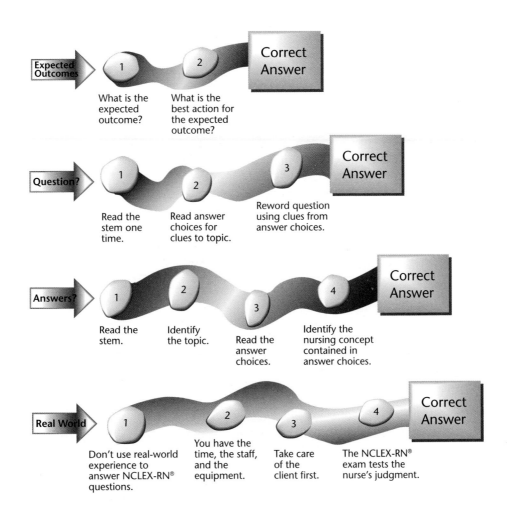

Expected Outcomes
1. What is the expected outcome?
2. What is the best action for the expected outcome?
→ Correct Answer

Question?
1. Read the stem one time.
2. Read answer choices for clues to topic.
3. Reword question using clues from answer choices.
→ Correct Answer

Answers?
1. Read the stem.
2. Identify the topic.
3. Read the answer choices.
4. Identify the nursing concept contained in answer choices.
→ Correct Answer

Real World
1. Don't use real-world experience to answer NCLEX-RN® questions.
2. You have the time, the staff, and the equipment.
3. Take care of the client first.
4. The NCLEX-RN® exam tests the nurse's judgment.
→ Correct Answer

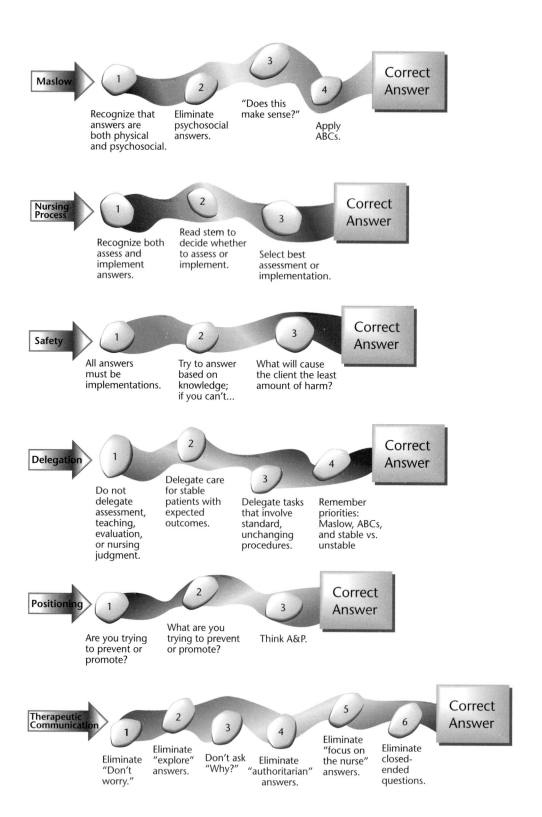

Maslow

1 — Recognize that answers are both physical and psychosocial.

2 — Eliminate psychosocial answers.

3 — "Does this make sense?"

4 — Apply ABCs.

Correct Answer

Nursing Process

1 — Recognize both assess and implement answers.

2 — Read stem to decide whether to assess or implement.

3 — Select best assessment or implementation.

Correct Answer

Safety

1 — All answers must be implementations.

2 — Try to answer based on knowledge; if you can't...

3 — What will cause the client the least amount of harm?

Correct Answer

Delegation

1 — Do not delegate assessment, teaching, evaluation, or nursing judgment.

2 — Delegate care for stable patients with expected outcomes.

3 — Delegate tasks that involve standard, unchanging procedures.

4 — Remember priorities: Maslow, ABCs, and stable vs. unstable

Correct Answer

Positioning

1 — Are you trying to prevent or promote?

2 — What are you trying to prevent or promote?

3 — Think A&P.

Correct Answer

Therapeutic Communication

1 — Eliminate "Don't worry."

2 — Eliminate "explore" answers.

3 — Don't ask "Why?"

4 — Eliminate "authoritarian" answers.

5 — Eliminate "focus on the nurse" answers.

6 — Eliminate closed-ended questions.

Correct Answer

NURSING TERMINOLOGY

abduction – movement away from the midline

abraded – scraped

acetonuria – acetone in the urine

adduction – movement toward the midline

afebrile – without fever

albuminuria – albumin in the urine

ambulatory – walking

amenorrhea – absence of menstruation

amnesia – loss of or defective memory

ankylosis – stiff joint

anorexia – lack of appetite

anuria – total suppression of urination

apnea – short periods when breathing has ceased

arthritis – inflammation of joint

asphyxia – suffocation

atrophy – wasting

auscultation, auscultate – to listen for sounds

bradycardia – heart rate lower than 60 beats per minute

Cheyne-Stokes respirations – alternating periods of apnea and hyperventilation

choluria – bile in the urine

client – individual, family, or group with whom the nurse interacts; includes significant others and populations

conjunctivitis – inflammation of the inner lining of the eyelid (conjunctiva)

copious – large in quantity, abundant

cyanotic – bluish in color due to poor oxygenation

defecation – bowel movement

dental caries – decay of the teeth

dentures – false teeth

diarrhea – excessive or frequent defecation and passage of liquid, unformed feces

diplopia – double vision

distended – appears swollen

diuresis – large amount of urine voided

dorsal recumbent – lying on back, knees flexed and apart

dysmenorrhea – painful menstruation

dyspnea – shortness of breath

dysrhythmia, arrhythmia – abnormal heartbeat

dysuria – painful urination

edematous – puffy, swollen

emaciated – thin, underweight

emetic – agent given to produce vomiting

enuresis – bed-wetting

epistaxis – nosebleed

eructation – belching

erythema – redness

eupnea – normal breathing

excoriation – raw surface

exhibit – an NCLEX question type that includes a client chart or medical record, which becomes visible when the exam candidate clicks an on-screen tab

exophthalmos – abnormal protrusion of eyeball

extension, extend – to straighten

fatigued – tired

feigned – pretended

fetid – foul smelling

fixed – motionless

flaccid – soft, limp, and flabby

flatus, flatulence – expulsion of gas from the digestive tract

flexion – bending

flushed – pink or hot

Fowler position – semierect, knees flexed, head of bed elevated 45–60 degrees

gavage – forced feeding through a tube passed into the stomach

glossy – shiny

glycosuria – glucose in the urine

gustatory – dealing with taste

heliotherapy – using sunlight as a therapeutic agent

hematemesis – blood in vomitus

hematuria – blood in the urine

hemiplegia – paralysis of one side of the body

hemoglobinuria – hemoglobin in the urine

hemoptysis – spitting of blood

horizontal – flat

hydrotherapy – using water as a therapeutic agent

hyperpnea – labored breathing characterized by deep and rapid respirations

hypertonic – concentration greater than body fluids

hypotonic – concentration less than body fluids

infrequent – not often

insomnia – inability to sleep

instillation – pouring into a body cavity

intermittent – starting and stopping, not continuous

intradermal – within or through the skin

intramuscular – within or through the muscle

intraspinal – within or through the spinal canal

intravenous – within or through the vein

involuntary – occurring without conscious control

incontinent – unable to control bladder or bowels

isotonic – having the same tonicity or concentration as body fluids

jackknife position – prone with hips over break in table and feet below level of head

jaundice – abnormal yellowness of the skin or whites of the eyes

knee-chest position – facedown, resting on knees and chest

kyphosis – humpback, concavity of spine

labored – difficult, requires an effort

lacerated – torn, ragged edged

lateral position – on the side, knees flexed

lithotomy position – on the back, buttocks near edge of table, knees well flexed and separated

lochia – drainage from the vagina after delivery

lordosis – swayback, convexity of spine

manipulation, manipulate – to handle

menopause – cessation of menstruation

menorrhagia – profuse menstruation

metrorrhagia – variable amount of uterine bleeding occurring at irregular intervals between expected menstrual periods

micturate – to pass urine, urinate

moist – wet

monoplegia – paralysis of one limb

mucopurulent – drainage containing mucus and pus

mydriasis – dilation of pupil

myopia – nearsightedness

myosis – contraction of pupil

nausea – desire to vomit

NCLEX integrated processes – themes fundamental to the practice of nursing that appear across the NCLEX Client Needs categories and subcategories; these include the nursing process, caring, communication, documentation, teaching, learning, and culture and spirituality

necrosis – death of tissue

nocturia – frequent voiding at night

obese – overweight

objective – involving verifiable information based on facts and evidence

oliguria – scant urination, less than 400 mL per 24 hours

orthopnea – inability to breathe or difficulty breathing while lying down

palliative – offering temporary relief

pallor – abnormal paleness of the skin

palpation, palpate – to feel with hands or fingers

paraplegia – paralysis of legs

paroxysm – a sudden or violent onset of symptoms (e.g., seizures, atrial fibrillation)

pediculi – lice

pediculosis – lice infestation

percussion, percuss – to strike

persistent – lasting over a long time

petechia – small rupture of blood vessels

photophobia – sensitity to light

photosensitivity – skin reaction caused by exposure to sunlight

pigmented – containing color

polyuria – excessive voiding of urine

prescription – an order, intervention, remedy, or treatment directed by an authorized health care provider

primary health care provider – a member of the health care team (usually a medical physician, nurse practitioner, etc.) who is licensed and authorized to prescribe for clients

profuse – large in amount

projectile – ejected or projected some distance

pronation – turning downward

prone – on abdomen, face turned to one side

prophylactic – preventative

protruding – extending outward

pruritus – itching

ptosis – drooping eyelid

purulent drainage – drainage containing pus

pyrexia – elevated temperature

pyuria – pus in the urine

radiating – spreading to distant areas

radiotherapy – using x-ray or radium as a therapeutic agent

rales, crackles – abnormal breath sounds

rapid – quick

rhinitis – inflammation of nasal mucosa causing swelling and clear watery discharge

rotation – movement in circular pattern

sanguineous drainage – bloody drainage

scanty – small in amount

semi-Fowler position – semi-erect, head of bed elevated 30–45 degrees

serous drainage – drainage of lymphatic fluid

Sims position – on left side, left arm behind back, left leg slightly flexed, right leg slightly flexed

sprain – wrenching of a joint

stertorous – characterized by snoring

stethoscope – instrument used for auscultation

strabismus – misalignment of visual focus

stuporous – partially unconscious

subcutaneous – under the skin

subjective – involving information that cannot be verified externally (e.g., sensations, opinions, emotions)

sudden onset – started all at once

superficial – on the surface only

supination – turning upward

suppurating – discharging pus

syncope – fainting

syndrome – group of symptoms

tachycardia – fast heartbeat, greater than 100 beats per minute

tenacious – tough and sticky

thready – barely perceptible

tonic tremor – continuous shaking

Trendelenburg position – flat on back with pelvis higher than head, foot of bed elevated 6 inches

urticaria – hives or wheals; eruptions on skin or mucous membranes

vertigo – dizziness

vesicle – fluid-filled blister

visual acuity – sharpness of vision

void – to urinate or pass urine

COMMON MEDICAL ABBREVIATIONS

ABC – airway, breathing, circulation

abd. – abdomen

ABG – arterial blood gas

ABO – system of classifying blood groups

AC – before meals

ACE – angiotensin-converting enzyme

ACS – acute compartment syndrome

ACTH – adrenocorticotrophic hormone

ad lib – freely, as desired

ADH – antidiuretic hormone

ADLs – activities of daily living

AFP – alpha fetoprotein

AIDS – acquired immunodeficiency syndrome

AKA – above-the-knee amputation

ALL – acute lymphocytic leukemia

ALP – alkaline phosphatase

ALS – amyotrophic lateral sclerosis

ALT – alanine aminotransferase

AMI – antibody-mediated immunity

AML – acute myelogenous leukemia

amt. – amount

ANA – antinuclear antibody

ANS – autonomic nervous system

AP – anteroposterior

A&P – anterior and posterior

APC – atrial premature complexes

aq. – water

ARDS – adult respiratory distress syndrome

ASD – atrial septal defect

ASHD – atherosclerotic heart disease

AST – aspartate aminotransferase

ATP – adenosine triphosphate

AV – atrioventricular

BCG – Bacille Calmette-Guerin

BID – two times a day

BKA – below-the-knee amputation

BLS – basic life support

BMR – basal metabolic rate

BP – blood pressure

BPH – benign prostatic hypertrophy

bpm – beats per minute

BRP – bathroom privileges

BSA – body surface area

BUN – blood urea nitrogen

C – centigrade, Celsius

c̄ – with

Ca – calcium

CA – cancer

CABG – coronary artery bypass graft

CAD – coronary artery disease

CAL – chronic airflow limitations

CAPD – continuous ambulatory peritoneal dialysis

caps – capsules

CBC – complete blood count

CC – chief complaint

CCU – coronary care unit, critical care unit

CDC – Centers for Disease Control and Prevention

CHF – congestive heart failure

CK – creatine kinase

Cl – chloride

CLL – chronic lymphocytic leukemia

cm – centimeter

CMV – cytomegalovirus

CNS – central nervous system

CO – carbon monoxide, cardiac output

CO_2 – carbon dioxide

comp – compound

cont – continuous

COPD – chronic obstructive pulmonary disease

CP – cerebral palsy

CPAP – continuous positive airway pressure

CPK – creatine phosphokinase

CPR – cardiopulmonary resuscitation

CRP – C-reactive protein

C&S – culture and sensitivity

CSF – cerebrospinal fluid

CT – computed tomography

CTD – connective tissue disease

CTS – carpal tunnel syndrome

cu – cubic

CVA – cerebrovascular accident or costovertebral angle

CVC – central venous catheter

CVP – central venous pressure

D&C – dilation and curettage

DCBE – double-contrast barium enema

DIC – disseminated intravascular coagulation

DIFF – differential blood count

dil. – dilute

DJD – degenerative joint disease

DKA – diabetic ketoacidosis

dL, dl – deciliter (100 mL)

DM – diabetes mellitus

DNA – deoxyribonucleic acid

DNR – do not resuscitate

DO – doctor of osteopathy

DOE – dyspnea on exertion

DPT – vaccine for diphtheria, pertussis, tetanus

Dr. – doctor

DRE – digital rectal exam

DVT – deep vein thrombosis

D/W – dextrose in water

Dx – diagnosis

ECF – extracellular fluid

ECG, EKG – electrocardiogram

ECT – electroconvulsive therapy

ED – emergency department

EEG – electroencephalogram

EHR – electronic health record

EMD – electromechanical dissociation

EMG – electromyography

ENT – ear, nose, and throat

ERCP – endoscopic retrograde cholangiopancreatography

ESR – erythrocyte sedimentation rate

ESRD – end-stage renal disease

ET – endotracheal tube

F – Fahrenheit

FBD – fibrocystic breast disease

FBS – fasting blood sugar

FDA – U.S. Food and Drug Administration

FFP – fresh frozen plasma

FHR – fetal heart rate

FHT – fetal heart tone

fl – fluid

FOBT – fecal occult blood test

4 × 4 – piece of gauze 4 inches by 4 inches; used for dressings

FSH – follicle-stimulating hormone

ft. – foot, feet (unit of measure)

FUO – fever of undetermined origin

g – gram

GB – gallbladder

GCS – Glasgow Coma Scale

GFR – glomerular filtration rate

GH – growth hormone

GI – gastrointestinal

gr – grain

gtt – drops

GU – genitourinary

GYN – gynecological

h, hrs – hour, hours

Hb, Hgb – hemoglobin

HCG – human chorionic gonadotropin

HCO$_3$ – bicarbonate

HCP – health care provider

Hct – hematocrit

HD – hemodialysis

HDL – high-density lipoprotein

HF – heart failure

Hg – mercury

HGH – human growth hormone

HHNK – hyperglycemia hyperosmolar nonketotic coma

HIPAA – Health Insurance Portability and Accountability Act

HIV – human immunodeficiency virus

HLA – human leukocyte antigen

H$_2$O – water

HR – heart rate

HSV – herpes simplex virus

HTN – hypertension

Hx – history

Hz – hertz (cycles/second)

IAPB – intra-aortic balloon pump

IBBP – intermittent positive pressure breathing

IBS – irritable bowel syndrome

ICF – intracellular fluid

ICP – intracranial pressure

ICS – intercostal space

ICU – intensive care unit

I&D – incision and drainage

IgA – immunoglobulin A

IM – intramuscular

I&O – intake and output

IOP – increased intraocular pressure

IPG – impedance plethysmography

IPPB – intermittent positive-pressure breathing

IUD – intrauterine device

IV – intravenous

IVC – intraventricular catheter

IVP – intravenous pyelogram or intravenous pyelography

JRA – juvenile rheumatoid arthritis

K$^+$ – potassium

kcal – kilocalorie (food calorie)

kg – kilogram

KO, KVO – keep vein open

KS – Kaposi's sarcoma

KUB – kidneys, ureters, bladder

L, l – liter

lab – laboratory

lb – pound

LBBB – left bundle branch block

LDH – lactate dehydrogenase

LDL – low-density lipoprotein

LE – lupus erythematosus

LH – luteinizing hormone

liq – liquid

LLQ – left lower quadrant

LOC – level of consciousness

LP – lumbar puncture

LPN – licensed practical nurse

Ⓛⓣ, Ⓛ – left

LTC – long-term care

LUQ – left upper quadrant

LV – left ventricle

LVN – licensed vocational nurse

m – minum, meter, micron

MAOI – monoamine oxidase inhibitor

MAST – military antishock trousers

mcg – microgram

MCH – mean corpuscular hemoglobin

MCV – mean corpuscular volume

MD – muscular dystrophy, medical doctor

MDI – metered dose inhaler

mEq – milliequivalent

mg – milligram

Mg – magnesium

MG – myasthenia gravis

MI – myocardial infarction

mL, ml – milliliter

mm – millimeter

MMR – vaccine for measles, mumps, rubella

MRI – magnetic resonance imaging

MS – multiple sclerosis

N – nitrogen, normal (strength of solution)

Na$^+$ – sodium

NaCl – sodium chloride

NANDA – North American Nursing Diagnosis Association

NG – nasogastric

NGT – nasogastric tube

NLN – National League for Nursing

NPO – nothing by mouth (nil per os)

NS – normal saline

NSAID – nonsteroidal anti-inflammatory drug

NSNA – National Student Nurses' Association

NST – non-stress test

O$_2$ – oxygen

OB-GYN – obstetrics and gynecology

OCT – oxytocin challenge test

OOB – out of bed

OPC – outpatient clinic

OR – operating room

OSHA – Occupational Safety and Health Administration

OTC – over-the-counter (drug that can be obtained without a prescription)

oz – ounce

$\bar{p}$ – with

P – pulse, pressure, phosphorus

PA chest – posterior-anterior chest x-ray

PAC – premature atrial complexes

PaCO$_2$ – partial pressure of carbon dioxide in arterial blood

PACU – postanesthesia care unit

PaO$_2$ – partial pressure of oxygen in arterial blood

PAD – peripheral artery disease

Pap – Papanicolaou smear

PC – after meals

PCA – patient-controlled analgesia

pCO$_2$ – partial pressure of carbon dioxide

PCP – *Pneumocystis jiroveci* pneumonia (formely *Pneumocystitis carinii* pneumonia)

PD – peritoneal dialysis

PE – pulmonary embolism

PEEP – positive end-expiratory pressure

PERRLA – pupils equal, round, react to light and accommodation

PET – postural emission tomography

PFT – pulmonary function test

pH – hydrogen ion concentration

PICC – peripherally inserted central catheter

PID – pelvic inflammatory disease

PIPEDA – Personal Information Protection and Electronic Documents Act

PKD – polycystic disease

PKU – phenylketonuria

PMS – premenstrual syndrome

PND – paroxysmal nocturnal dyspnea

PO, po – (per os) by mouth

pO$_2$ – partial pressure of oxygen

PPD – positive purified protein derivative (of tuberculin)

PPE – personal protective equipment

PPN – partial parenteral nutrition

PRN, prn – as needed, whenever necessary

pro time – prothrombin time

PSA – prostate-specific antigen

psi – pounds per square inch

PSP – phenolsulfonphthalein

PT – physical therapy, prothrombin time

PTCA – percutaneous transluminal coronary angioplasty

PTH – parathyroid hormone

PTSD – post-traumatic stress disorder

PTT – partial thromboplastin time

PUD – peptic ulcer disease

PVC – premature ventricular contraction

q – every

QA – quality assurance

QID – four times a day

qs – quantity sufficient

R – rectal temperature, respirations, roentgen

RA – rheumatoid arthritis

RAI – radioactive iodine

RAIU – radioactive iodine uptake

RAS – reticular activating system

RBBB – right bundle branch block

RBC – red blood cell or red blood count

RCA – right coronary artery

RDA – recommended dietary allowance

RF – rheumatic fever, rheumatoid factor

Rh – antigen on blood cell indicated by + or –

RIND – reversible ischemic neurologic deficit

RLQ – right lower quadrant

RN – registered nurse

RNA – ribonucleic acid

R/O, r/o – rule out, to exclude

ROM – range of motion (of joint)

RR – respiratory rate

Ⓡⓣ, Ⓡ – right

RUQ – right upper quadrant

Rx – prescription

s̄ – without

S., Sig. – (Signa) to write on label

SA – sinoatrial node

SaO$_2$ – systemic arterial oxygen saturation (%)

sat sol – saturated solution

SBE – subacute bacterial endocarditis

SDA – same-day admission

SDS – same-day surgery

S/E – side effects

sed rate – sedimentation rate

SI – International System of Units

SIADH – syndrome of inappropriate antidiuretic hormone

SIDS – sudden infant death syndrome

SL – sublingual

SLE – systemic lupus erythematosus

SMBG – self-monitoring blood glucose

SMR – submucous resection

SNF – skilled nursing facility

SOB – shortness of breath

sol – solution

sp gr – specific gravity

spec. – specimen

SpO$_2$ – oxygen saturation

SS – soapsuds

S/S, s/s – signs and symptoms

SSKI – saturated solution of potassium iodide

stat – immediately

STD – sexually transmitted disease

subcut – subcutaneous

sx – symptoms

Syr. – syrup

T – thoracic (followed by the number designating specific thoracic vertebra)

T, temp – temperature

T&A – tonsillectomy and adenoidectomy

tabs – tablets

TB – tuberculosis

T&C – type and crossmatch

TED – antiembolitic stockings

TENS – transcutaneous electrical nerve stimulation

TIA – transient ischemic attack

TIBC – total iron binding capacity

TID – three times a day

tinct, tr. – tincture

TLC – total lymphocyte count

TMJ – temporomandibular joint

TPA, t-pa – tissue plasminogen activator

TPN – total parenteral nutrition

TPR – temperature, pulse, respiration

TQM – total quality management

TSE – testicular self-examination

TSH – thyroid-stimulating hormone

tsp. – teaspoon

TSS – toxic shock syndrome

TURP – transurethral prostatectomy

UA – urinalysis

UAP – unlicensed assistive personnel

um – unit of measurement

ung – ointment

URI – upper respiratory tract infection

UTI – urinary tract infection

VAD – venous access device

VDRL – Venereal Disease Research Laboratory (test for syphilis)

VF, Vfib – ventricular fibrillation

VPC – ventricular premature complexes

VS, vs – vital signs

VSD – ventricular septal defect

VT – ventricular tachycardia

WBC – white blood cell or white blood count

WHO – World Health Organization

WNL – within normal limits

wt – weight

INDEX

C

Stem of multiple choice question, 36
  rewording the question, 60–62
Sterile techniques, 158
  burn cream application, 24
  catheter insertion, 47–48, 158, 253
Stethoscope, 193
  See also Auscultation
Stool impaction, 254
Strategies for taking exam
  about taking the exam, 5–6, 507–512
  answer choice elimination, 62–67
  bowtie questions, 57–58
  clues in answer choices, 70–74
  communication questions, 107–111,
    522–534
  critical thinking, 28–32, 59–60, 539–540
  drag-and-drop questions, 47–51
  dropdown questions, 51–54
  expected outcomes, 67–69, 78–80, 288
  fill-in-the-blank questions, 46, 509, 511
  highlight questions, 41–44
  hot spot questions, 44–45, 509, 510
  learning approach, 33–34
  Management of Care questions, 15–17,
    98–102
  matrix questions, 54–56
  multiple choice questions, 36–38, 510
  multiple response questions, 38–41
  nursing process, 21–24
  ordered response questions, 47–48, 509,
    512
  positioning questions, 102–107
  practicing the strategies of test taking,
    65–66, 112–114, 516
  preparation approach, 112–114
  priority question best answer, 84–98
  priority questions via Maslow, 85–89
  priority questions via nursing process,
    89–93
  priority questions via safety, 93–98
  real world *vs.* exam, 75–83
  retaking the exam, 513–517
  rewording the question, 60–62
  select all that apply questions, 510
  selecting best answer, 66–67
  study plan, 111–116
  successful test takers, 32–33, 62, 112–114
  trend questions, 58–59
  unsuccessful strategies, 33, 62, 111–112
Stress management, 191, 223
  caregivers, 216, 223
  coping mechanisms, 218–219, 223

crisis intervention, 219–220
  family dynamics, 221
Stroke
  dysphagia question strategy, 38–40
  prevention, 192
Study plan for exam, 111–116
Sublimation as coping mechanism, 219
Substance use disorders, 217–218
Successful test takers, 32–33, 62, 112–114
  See also Strategies for taking exam
  ineffective ways to prepare, 111–112
Suicide
  crisis intervention, 219–220
  implementing precautions, 320
Supervision of other health care workers,
    98–102, 120–121, 123
Supine position, 106
Support systems for clients, 223
  caregiver support, 216, 223
Suppression as coping mechanism, 219
Surgical asepsis, 158–159
Surgical procedure complications, 320
Susceptible hosts in chain of infection, 155

T

Taking the NCLEX-RN® exam, 5–6, 507–512
  retaking the exam, 513–517
  unable to take test on scheduled date, 507
TB education of client, 64
Teaching included on exam, 24
  See also Communication; Education of
    clients
Teamwork. *See* Collaboration
Technology
  automated drug dispensing systems, 290
  electronic health records, 125
  electronic medication administration
    records, 125
  ergonomics, 156
  fetal heart monitoring, 318
  use of, 125
Telehealth, 125
Terminal illness end-of-life care, 220
Terminology for exam. *See* Vocabulary
  for exam
Test Day, 115–116, 507–508
Testicular self-examination, 191
Textbook answer *vs.* real world, 75–83
Therapeutic communication,
    107–109, 223–224
  U.S. nursing communication, 522–523
    (*See also* Communication)

Therapeutic environment, 225
Therapeutic procedures, 321, 346
  unexpected response, 348
Time limit for exam, 5–6, 508
  breaks during exam, 5, 512, 517
  clock on computer screen, 508
Toddlers. *See* Preschool-age children
TOEFL®
  CGFNS® English language proficiency,
    519–520, 535
  contact information, 520
  Kaplan free online services, 535–536
  Kaplan programs for, 535–536
TOEIC® Testing Program, 520
Tonsillectomy postanesthesia, 93
Topical medications, 287
Total parenteral nutrition (TPN), 291
Total quality management (TQM), 127–128
Traction and fracture pain, 78
Transfusion of blood products
  procedure, 284–285
  transfusion reactions, 82–83, 285
Transmission-based infection
  precautions, 158
Trend questions, 58–59
Trendelenburg position, 106
Triage of clients, 124, 157
Tricuspid area, 45
Tube feedings, 256–257
Tuberculosis information, 64
Tunneled catheter, 285

U

Ultrasounds in prenatal care, 185
Umbilical prolapse, 17
Uniform Anatomical Gift Act (1968), 120
United States (U.S.)
  Kaplan programs for international nurses,
    534–536
  medical abbreviations, 545–550
  nursing communication, 522–523 (*See also*
    Communication)
  nursing practice, 521 (*See also* Nursing
    interventions)
  nursing vocabulary list, 541–543
Units of measure, 46
Unprotected sex, 192
Urethritis, 253
Urinary issues, 253
Urine specific gravity, 79
Urine specimen collection, 66–67